Medical Terminology
A Guide to Current Usage

PAUL M. DAVIES
TD MB BS DPH FRCR DMR

*Formerly Consultant Radiologist, Royal Surrey County Hospital
and St Luke's Hospital, Guildford*

Fourth Edition

HEINEMANN MEDICAL BOOKS

Heinemann Medical Books
An imprint of Heinemann Professional Publishing Ltd
Halley Court, Jordan Hill, Oxford OX2 8EJ

OXFORD LONDON SINGAPORE NAIROBI IBADAN KINGSTON

ISBN 0 433 07184 2

Formerly published as *Medical Terminology in Hospital Practice*
© Paul M. Davies, 1985

First published 1969
Second edition 1974
Reprinted 1976
Third edition 1978
Reprinted 1982
Fourth edition 1985
Reprinted 1987 (twice), 1989

Photoset by D. P. Media Limited, Hitchin, Hertfordshire
Printed and bound in Great Britain by
The Bath Press, Avon

Contents

Preface

The aim of this book is to help both students and members of professions allied to medicine to acquire a good working knowledge of medical terms in current use in medical practice. The designation 'professions allied to medicine' is used to indicate the nursing profession, physiotherapy, radiography and other paramedical professions.

The text also contains material designed to be of help to both trainee and established medical secretaries. It is arranged so that it may either be used as a source of ready reference or for more systematic study, and is supplemented in places by *special notes for diagnostic radiographers* given in smaller indented print.

In most cases, medical terms denoting the names of diseases are arranged to indicate how disease conditions affecting various systems of the body fit into a classification as being of congenital, traumatic, infective, neoplastic or other origin.

Short descriptions of various common or otherwise important disorders are also included in the text. It is, however, emphasised that these descriptions have the sole object of facilitating an understanding of medical terminology. They are not comprehensive accounts such as may be found in the many excellent textbooks available to the reader.

In preparing this, the 4th edition of this guide to *Medical Terminology*, a detailed revision of the text of the previous edition has been made and new material has been added in accordance with the ever-continuing advances in medical teatment and diagnosis. Particular attention has been paid in this revision to certain of the terms relating to imaging, biochemical investigations, immunity, the mononuclear phagocyte system (formerly called the reticuloendothelial system), shock, renal failure, lymphomas, myopathies and diseases of genetic origin.

Guildford   Paul M. Davies

Acknowledgements

I wish firstly to acknowledge my debt to Professor George J. Cunningham, Emeritus Professor of Pathology, Commonwealth University of Virginia, USA, and formerly Sir William Collins Professor of Pathology, Royal College of Surgeons of England. I am most grateful to him for writing forewords for the first and second editions of this work and for practical help and encouragement over many years.

With regard to this present edition, my sincere thanks are due to the following:

Miss Janet M. Smith, Top Grade Biochemist, Mayday Hospital, Croydon, for reading through the text and providing valuable suggestions and notes about present-day practice of clinical biochemistry;

Mr J. C. F. Peake, Principal Physicist, St Luke's Hospital, Guildford, for advice and notes about the technical and scientific aspects of medical imaging;

My many colleagues in the South West Surrey Hospitals who have patiently answered numerous queries about current usage of terms relating to the practice of medicine and its specialties, and to that of professions allied to medicine;

Mrs Caroline Sawers, Librarian, Guildford Postgraduate Medical Centre, for providing such excellent library facilities;

My wife Helen and my daughter Gwenda for their constant encouragement and valued help in the preparation of the work for publication;

Dr Richard Barling, Editorial Director, and other members of the staff of Heinemann Medical Books concerned with the publication of the book, for much appreciated guidance.

Paul M. Davies

PART I

Introduction

Some general aspects of medicine, medical terminology and the practice of medicine and allied professions

MEDICINE, DISEASE AND MEDICAL TERMINOLOGY

At the beginning of a study of medical terms it is most important to obtain a clear understanding of the meanings of the words medicine and disease.

Medicine is a term with three meanings, denoting:

(*a*) a drug—as in the expression taking medicine.

(*b*) the clinical specialty of medicine, as practised by physicians and concerned with the treatment of patients with drugs and other non-surgical measures.

(*c*) *all aspects of the science of the prevention, investigation and treatment of disease*—this latter being the principal sense in which the term is used.

Disease *is a condition in which some abnormality of structure or function, or of both structure and function, is present in some part or parts of the body.*

Thus a large part of medical science, being concerned with disease, consists of the study of abnormal conditions in the body.

However, the abnormal can be appreciated only in relation to a knowledge of normal conditions. Thus human **anatomy**—the study of normal body structures—and human **physiology**—the study of normal body functions—are integral branches of medicine and words relative to these subjects are regarded as medical terms.

Medical terminology is the study of words used to communicate facts and ideas particular to medicine, and is chiefly concerned with the present use and meaning of such words.

It may, however, be of interest to note in passing that a special characteristic of this subject is the great number of words encountered in medicine which are of direct, or indirect, Greek or Latin origin. This has resulted from the physicians of ancient Greece, notable among whom was Hippocrates (born circa 460 BC on the island of Cos), having been the first to introduce scientific methods into medicine and, later, after the decline of Greek civilisation, from the use of Latin as the international language for scholars throughout the Western world.

The Latin tongue obtained this dominant position through the rise of the power of Rome, but maintained it for many centuries after the fall of the Roman Empire (AD 476).

The meaning of a number of prefixes, suffixes and other word components of Greek or Latin origin are indicated in the Glossary.

The word **hospital** is derived from Latin, but authorities differ about whether it comes from the word in that language for a host or one meaning a guest.

Of necessity, the term disease occurs frequently in medical speech and writing, but an endeavour may be made to avoid undue repetition by employing other words which, when used in the right context, are its synonyms (i.e. words with similar meanings), e.g. disorder, illness, sickness, morbidity, malady, pathological condition, morbid condition, ailment.

Some general descriptive terms which may be applied when discussing different forms of illness are given below.

Description of disease	Meaning
Congenital	Present at birth.
Acquired	Acquired after birth.
Acute	Of rapid onset and progress.
Chronic	Of slow onset and progress.
Functional	Associated with abnormality of function but without demonstrable abnormality of structure.
Organic	Associated with structural abnormality.
Silent	Producing no symptoms or readily detectable signs.
Systemic	Involving the body (i.e. the system) as a whole.
Local	Involving only a part of the body (in contradistinction to systemic disease).

Causes and Classification of Disease

The causes of the abnormalities which constitute disease are many and varied. Some are known and others imperfectly understood or completely unknown. The study of the causation of diseases is called **aetiology** and closely related to this subject is **epidemiology**, concerned with the geographical distribution of various diseases, their frequency of occurrence, and their age, sex and racial incidence.

A useful classification which takes account of casual factors, in so far as these are known, is as follows:

Types of Diseases

Congenital—diseases which are present at birth as a result of the following.

(i) genetic factors, e.g. chromosomal disorders such as Down's syndrome; inherited disorders such as haemophilia and familial intestinal polyposis.

(ii) acquired *in utero* from environmental factors—e.g. congenital syphilis from maternal infection.

(iii) combined genetic and environmental factors—e.g. cleft palate, congenital pyloric stenosis, congenital heart disease.

[It should be noted that although the factors responsible for some congenital diseases are present at birth, signs and symptoms of these conditions may not develop until a varying period of time has elapsed. In some instances this may be many years.]

Traumatic (injuries)—due to:

(i) violence—e.g. fractures and dislocations;

(ii) mechanical irritation, e.g. bed sores;

(iii) external physical agents, e.g. thermal burns, frostbite, radiation injury;

(iv) external chemical agents, e.g. acid and alkali burns.

Infective—due to infection with pathogenic micro-organisms (disease-producing germs), e.g. influenza, measles, tuberculosis, malaria; and **Infestations**—due to worms, e.g. tape worm infestation.

Neoplastic—due to the pathological process called neoplasia (new growth) which results in formation of benign and malignant tumours.

Metabolic—due to:

(i) lack of essential food factors required for building and maintaining body tissues, e.g. rickets, due to lack of Vitamin D;

(ii) disorders of metabolism, i.e. the processes whereby absorbed foodstuffs are modified for tissue building and repair, and whereby waste products are broken down into the forms in which they can be excreted from the body—e.g. gout, which is a disorder of the metabolism of uric acid.

Chemical poisonings—due to entry of chemical poisons into the body, e.g. arsenic poisoning, poisoning from insecticides, lead poisoning.

Endocrine—due to disorders in endocrine (ductless) glands, e.g. goitre, pituitary dwarfism.

Allergic—due to various types of hypersensitivity, e.g. hay fever.

Psychiatric—due to abnormal conditions of the mind, e.g. anxiety states, depressive states, schizophrenia.

Iatrogenic—due to treatment given for other diseases, the term meaning produced by physicians, e.g. sensitivity reactions caused by penicillin.

Due to other causes and idiopathic—i.e. of unknown causation, e.g. idiopathic epilepsy, essential hypertension (high blood pressure of unknown cause).

Manifestations of Disease

The presence of disease may be revealed by the following.

Symptoms—abnormalities that are appreciable by the patient himself, e.g. pain, giddiness.

Signs—abnormalities appreciable to an observer, e.g. pallor, rise in body temperature.

Signs detectable by a medical practitioner during the course of an ordinary medical examination are often termed **clinical signs**, whereas those requiring specialised methods of detection may, according to their nature be designed as pathological signs, radiological signs, electro-cardiographic signs, etc.

It is desirable at this stage to consider the meaning of the term **clinical**. This word, although widely employed, is difficult to define. It is derived from the Greek word for a bed and originally meant at the bedside. It has now come to indicate the aspects of medical science most directly concerned with actual patients, e.g. a clinical demonstration is one in which patients are the main subject of the demonstration; a clinic is a building where patients attend for medical care or, alternatively, a session for medical diagnosis or treatment attended by patients, as in the expression 'the Monday morning surgical clinic'.

During the course of a disease, signs and symptoms may not be due to the original condition, but be manifestations of some disorder which has occurred as a direct consequence of the original disease. Such secondary disorder is referred to as a **complication**, e.g. pneumonia occurring as a complication of chronic bronchitis.

Practice of Medicine and Allied Professions and Technical Occupations

The practice of medicine is concerned with the prevention, investigation, diagnosis and treatment of disease; the care of the sick, the alleviation of suffering; and with the furtherance of medical knowledge and medical education.

Those who are qualified to practise medicine are, by established usage, commonly known as **doctors**, although their official designation is that of **medical practitioners**.

Medical practitioners in the United Kingdom as well as holding certain qualifications, recognised by law must be **registered** by the General Medical Council if they wish to practise. (*Note:* Newly qualified doctors are first conditionally registered and must spend a year in approved **preregistration posts** before full registration can be effected).

There are many careers within the medical profession but most medical men or women are engaged primarily in the following. **General medical practice—general medical practitioners**; usually referred to as **general practitioners** (GPs) or **family doctors**. **Specialist practice** (e.g. surgery, pathology, radiology) specialist medical practitioners, referred to as **specialists**. Senior specialists who hold established consultant post in hospitals, government departments, etc. are designated as **consultants**.

Note: The terms registrar and house officer often cause perplexity: a **registrar** is a doctor who is acquiring specialist experience and holds a registrar post in a hospital specialty (e.g. medical registrar, surgical registrar); a **house officer** is a junior doctor who is gaining experience within a hospital before embarking on a career as a specialist, family doctor, etc. He, or she, is frequently resident in the house, i.e. the hospital.

The practice of **community medicine** (public health)—concerned with the promotion of health and the prevention of disease. Doctors engaged in community health work have the professional assistance of **environmental health officers** (formerly called public health inspectors) and of **health visitors** (state registered nurses, with prescribed training in midwifery or obstetric nursing, who have passed a post-registration course in health visiting).

From time immemorial those engaged in the profession of medicine have required nursing assistance with their more serious cases of illness and the help of midwives in maternity work. It is interesting to note, therefore, that it was not until the latter half of the nineteenth century that the need was generally appreciated for establishing **nursing** and **midwifery** as fully recognised professions, with organised systems of practical and theoretical training. Indeed, but for the work of Florence Nightingale during and after the Crimean War (1854–56) the attainment of a recognised professional status by the nursing profession might have been delayed even longer.

During the earlier part of the twentieth century, the practice of these professions became regulated by law and their controlling bodies legally established. Thus, the Central Midwives Board was set up in 1902, and the General Nursing Council in 1919, by Acts of Parliament.

From requiring direct help, mainly in nursing and midwifery, and in pharmacy, progress has been such since the early years of this century that trained and skilled assistance is now an essential feature in many branches of medicine. This is particularly so in relation to many of the more complex techniques employed in hospital practice, where teamwork is vital for efficient diagnosis and treatment, and medical staff head teams which are often composed of members of a variety of other professions and technical occupations allied to medicine.

Hospital staff associated directly with the medical profession in the diagnosis and treatment of disease include:

Members of professions allied to medicine and other professions connected with medical diagnosis and treatment—nurses and midwives, *chiropodists, clinical biochemists, clinical psychologists, *hospital dietitians, hospital pharmacists, hospital physicists, *medical laboratory scientific officers, medical photographers, medical social workers (formerly called almoners), *occupational therapists, opticians (ophthalmic and dispensing), *orthoptists, psychiatric social workers, *physiotherapists, *radiographers (diagnostic and therapeutic), *remedial gymnasts, and speech therapists.

Staff in technical occupations connected with medical treatment and diagnosis—these include physiological measurement technicians in audiology, cardiology and neurophysiology; cardiographers, operating department assistants, pharmacy technicians, medical physics technicians, technicians in venereology, X-ray dark-room technicians, artificial kidney assistants, anatomical pathology technicians.

Note: with the exception of nurses and midwives, all those engaged in the professions and technical occupations listed above may be referred to as **paramedical staff**.

The roles of some of these hospital workers will be briefly indicated later, while discussing various methods of diagnosis and treatment. No account of medical practice can, however, be regarded as complete without emphasis on the importance therein of the work of **medical secretaries**.

Note: the medical and dental professions have always worked in close accord and many hospitals possess specialist departments of **oral surgery** in which, working under the direction of the dental surgeons, are dental therapists (formerly called dental auxiliaries), dental hygienists, dental surgery assistants and dental technicians. (The word **oral** means pertaining to the mouth.)

Linked with the oral surgery department, there may also be a department of **orthodontics**, a specialised branch of dentistry concerned with the prevention and treatment of irregularities of the teeth and of malocclusion (imperfect closure of the jaws).

The management of affairs relevant to the practice of medicine is termed **medical administration** and within an individual hospital the senior administrator is nowadays usually a lay official, designated as the **hospital administrator** (formerly known as the hospital secretary).

It will be appreciated that efficient medical administration, with good management and co-ordination of service departments, i.e. those concerned with accommodation, supplies, catering, finance, records, planning, laundry, engineering, building, maintenance and transport,

---

*Signifies a profession legally designated as 'Profession Supplementary to Medicine'.

Note: Occupational therapists, physiotherapists and remedial gymnasts are also designated as members of the 'Remedial Professions' and now have the assistance of staff who are graded as helpers in these three disciplines.

is an essential feature in the provision of hospital facilities for the diagnosis and treatment of disease.

It is also appropriate to refer here to the contribution to the care of the sick made by **hospital chaplains**, ordained ministers appointed to attend to the spiritual needs of hospital patients of various denominations.

Diagnosis of Disease

The term **diagnosis** denotes the measures taken to identify a particular disease and also the statement of the nature of a particular disease, once its presence has been established.

The making of a diagnosis in a patient with manifestations of disease is a logical prelude to the start of a rational form of treatment. It may also render possible the giving of a **prognosis**, i.e. a forecast as to the duration and outcome of the malady.

The first diagnostic procedure is to take a **clinical history** from the patient whenever practicable, but otherwise from parents, relatives or others with knowledge of the facts pertaining to the patient's illness.

Following history-taking, the next step is to carry out a **clinical examination** to determine the presence or absence of clinical signs of disease. The extent of this will vary considerably according to the nature of the condition suspected.

A full clinical examination may include simple physical methods such as inspection, palpation, percussion and auscultation (listening with a stethoscope, e.g. to heart or bowel sounds), and may also include inspection of the interior of the eyes with an instrument called an **ophthalmoscope**; inspection of the outer parts of the ears and ear drums with an **auriscope**, estimation of the systemic blood pressure with a **sphygmomanometer**, and simple testing of the urine for abnormal constituents such as sugar and the protein called albumen.

At the end of his clinical examination the medical practitioner will decide whether he can make a firm diagnosis or a provisional diagnosis, whether he wishes to subject the patient to some form of specialised investigation before making or finalising a diagnosis, or whether he wishes for a second opinion on the patient's condition from a specialist or other medical colleague. He will also determine whether to institute treatment himself, refer the patient elsewhere for treatment, or delay treatment pending the results of further investigation.

In most cases of illness, other than emergencies which may be sent direct to hospital, the practitioner first examining the patient will be a family doctor.

It is the role of the hospital services to provide both inpatient and outpatient facilities for patients who require investigations and treatments which are beyond the province of the family doctor, and also to provide facilities for dealing with various types of surgical and medical emergency (e.g. accidents, sudden illness, poisonings).

In referring a patient to hospital, the family doctor will decide, according to the nature or suspected nature of the patient's malady, to which department he should be referred in the first instance.

Hospital specialties are conventionally grouped into **clinical departments** which are concerned with both investigation and treatment and are responsible for the overall care of patients referred to them, and **special** departments which deal with some specialised aspects of either investigation or treatment.

Nomenclature and organisation of departments vary in different hospitals, but the following arrangement of principal departments is fairly representative of a large general hospital dealing with all types of illness and with maternity work.

Clinical Departments

Medicine	Surgery (including accident surgery)	Obstetrics and gynaecology
Ophthalmology (Eye diseases)		Otorhinolaryngology (Ear, nose and throat diseases)

Special Departments

Pathology	Diagnostic radiology and imaging (including ultrasound)
Rheumatology and rehabilitation	Radiotherapy and oncology
Occupational therapy	Nuclear medicine

A variety of investigations may be performed by the clinical departments and many of these will be indicated later (e.g. electrocardiography, electroencephalography, endoscopy, sight testing, audiometry).

The three major special departments concerned with diagnostic measures are as follows.

Department of pathology—wherein a wide range of laboratory investigations are performed. These include examination of specimens from the patient by macroscopic (naked eye), microscopic, chemical, physical, bacteriological, and virological methods. Such specimens may consist of secretions of the body (e.g. sputum), excretions (e.g. urine), body fluids (e.g. blood), smears containing body cells (e.g. as in cervical cytology), or portions of body tissue removed during the course of a surgical operation or at biopsy.

Biopsy is a diagnostic procedure in which a small fragment of tissue is removed from a living subject, specifically for microscopic examination. According to the site of the lesion it may be performed under local or general anaesthesia.

Pathology is the science of disease, and is that branch of medicine concerned with the investigation of disease processes in patients by methods such as those referred to above; it is also concerned with research into the basic nature of such processes and the study of their end results at **autopsy** or **necropsy** (post-mortem examination). Medical practitioners who specialise in this subject are termed **pathologists**, and working with them are **biochemists** and **medical laboratory scientific officers.**

The following are the main branches of pathology: **clinical biochemistry** (see below); **morbid anatomy**, dealing with structural changes produced by disease and including **histopathology**— the study of minute structural changes by microscopy; **medical microbiology**—the study of pathogenic micro-organisms which includes the studies of **bacteriology** (bacteria), **virology** (viruses) and **protozoology** (protozoa) (see p.34); and **haematology**—the study of the blood and its diseases, allied to which is **blood transfusion serology** concerned with all aspects (e.g. grouping, cross-matching, taking of blood) of providing blood suitable and safe for transfusion.

Marks defines **biochemistry** as 'the chemistry of living or once living things' and **clinical biochemistry** as 'the application of analytical chemical techniques to the prevention, investigation, treatment and understanding of disease' (Marks, V., 1984, personal communication). Referring to the organisational aspect of clinical biochemistry, Marks (1) states that this 'branch of the health industry . . . is a laboratory-based medical discipline. It employs the services of three historically, educationally professionally and financially distinct groups; namely medically qualified clinical biochemists—often known in the UK as chemical pathologists—hospital biochemists and medical laboratory technicians'.

An interesting development in biochemistry in the early 1960s was the simultaneous performance of multiple tests on specimens of blood by a system using a multichannel analyser and known as **automated analysis**.

It is also to be noted that an important function of clinical biochemists is the monitoring of the blood concentrations of certain drugs, e.g. digoxin and some cytotoxic and anticonvulsant drugs.

Department of diagnostic radiology and imaging—concerned originally, and still primarily, with the investigation of disease by X-rays, this department also carries out other forms of diagnostic imaging besides X-ray imaging, i.e. using radionuclides (in hospitals where there is no separate nuclear medicine department), ultrasound and thermographic methods. It is also, in the future, likely to be responsible for imaging using nuclear magnetic resonance (NMR), when this comes into general clinical use.

Radiology is the science of ionising radiations. The two main branches of medical radiology are called **diagnostic radiology** and

radiotherapy. Doctors who specialise in the former branch are known as **diagnostic radiologists**, or more shortly as **radiologists**; and working with them are professional staff called **radiographers** and also **dark room technicians**.

The term **imaging** denotes various scientific methods of producing, displaying and recording images of internal body structures and medical imaging consists of:

(i) **X-ray imaging**—involving basically the use of X-radiation to record images on X-ray films, referred to as radiographs and the display of images of internal structures on TV monitors. This last procedure is termed **X-ray screening**, the images initially being formed on a fluorescent screen and then intensified and converted into images on the monitor.

As an adjunct to both radiographic and screening examinations, substances called **contrast media** may be introduced into the body in order to delineate the interiors of hollow structures (e.g. gastrointestinal tract, urinary tract, blood vessels). Contrast media may absorb considerably more X-radiation (e.g. barium, iodine-containing media), or considerably less (e.g. air, oxygen) than do the body tissues, and thus be described as **radiopaque** or **radiotranslucent**.

Recent advances in X-ray imaging include the increasing use of **computerised tomography** (CT), sometimes called **computerised axial tomography** (CAT), employing head and body scanners; **digital subtraction radiography**, wherein unwanted backgound images are removed and of particular value in angiography, and **interventional radiology** in which a variety of percutaneous techniques are used in conjunction with X-ray imaging, or sometimes ultrasound imaging, for biopsy procedures or for treatment rather than diagnosis—e.g. control of haemorrhage by therapeutic embolisation and balloon angioplasty, treatment of arterial occlusion by transluminal angioplasty.

(ii) **radionuclide imaging**—see Department of nuclear medicine.

(iii) **ultrasound imaging**—involving the display on a TV monitor and recording of images produced by **echoes** (backward reflections) resulting from the passage of a beam of ultrasound waves into the body.

Such echoes are caused by the waves striking interfaces between organs and tissues, or certain structures within organs. The term **ultrasound** denotes high frequency vibrations beyond the range of audible sound.

Pulse–echo diagnostic methods of ultrasound use several different types of equipment:

● **A-scan equipment** giving data in one direction only as the traducer (the ultrasonic probe) is held stationary on the skin at the time of recording. It may be used to measure the distance of various structures from the surface of the body (e.g. midline structure of the brain), and also to measure the size of certain structures and organs (e.g. the biparietal diameter of the fetal skull). It can also be modified to show movement along the ultrasonic beam to produce a time-position, time-motion–TM mode, or motion–M-mode scan (e.g. to study motion of the heart valves).

• **B-scan equipment** gives an image of a two-dimensional body section which is built up by moving the traducer slowly over the skin. Such image may be of a horizontal, transverse of oblique plane according to the movement of the traducer.

• **Real Time scanners** which produce instantaneous views of body sections, enabling any movement within the section to be visualised.

Ultrasonic waves are also employed in **Doppler systems** which detect and measure movements within the body (e.g. fetal heart activity, blood flow in arteries and veins).

In **Duplex scanners**—Doppler and Real Time systems are combined.

(iv) **thermographic imaging**—an imaging method which records the emission of infra-red radiation from the body, producing a temperature pattern of the body surface. It is employed in the investigation of peripheral vascular disease (e.g. deep vein thrombosis) and in the study of superficial neoplasms.

(v) **nuclear magnetic resonance (NMR) imaging**—a method dependent on the magnetic properties of *protons* (nuclei of hydrogen atoms). NMR scanners use magnetic and radiofrequency fields to produce images of body sections very similar to those obtained with CT scanners.

This method which is sometimes more briefly referred to as **magnetic resonance** (MR) is at present undergoing clinical evaluation.

Department of nuclear medicine—concerned with both the investigation and treatment of disease by radioactive substances which are referred to as **radionuclides** or **radioisotopes** (or, when labelled with radioactive atoms for medicinal purposes, **radiopharmaceuticals**).

Investigations may be *in vivo* (in life, i.e. in the living body) or *in vitro* (in glass, i.e. in the laboratory). In *in vivo* investigations the distribution of a radionuclide within the body tissues may be demonstrated by moving detectors called **rectilinear scanners** or, more frequently, by stationary detectors called **gamma cameras**.

A few examples of the work of this department are: diagnostic use of radionuclides in renal disorders, suspected metastatic disease of bone and suspected pulmonary embolism; and the therapeutic use of these substances in primary polycythaemia and in metastatic and primary carcinoma of the thyroid gland.

Treatment of Disease

Treatment of disease may be by drugs (medicines)—medical treatment; by operation—surgical treatment; by physical methods—physiotherapy; by ionising radiation—radiotherapy; by psychological methods—psychotherapy; by other therapeutic methods; and by various combinations of these different forms of treatment.

The aspect of medicine dealing specifically with treatment is called **therapeutics**.

The term **therapy** means treatment of disease.

Some general aspects of therapy and of obstetric care will now be discussed:

Medical treatment—mainly treatment by medicines, i.e. by drugs, but includes other non-surgical measures such as dietetic therapy, rest, reassurance and often, of the highest importance, medical nursing care. The term medical is here used in its restricted sense as referring to the province of the physician, as opposed to that of the surgeon.

Drugs are used extensively in medical treatment and also as adjuvants in many other types of therapy. Some important types of drugs will be indicated later.

Surgical treatment—consists in most cases of treatment by **surgical operations** (i.e. procedures in which an instrument such as a scalpel or diathermy needle is used to cut into body tissues for therapeutic purposes), and any preoperative or postoperative measures necessary in conjunction with such operations. Certain non-operative techniques such as the closed reduction of fractures and dislocations and techniques using laser beams may also be regarded as forms of surgical treatment.

The term **surgery** means work by hand. Surgical operations, other than certain of those of a minor nature, fall within the province of the specialist **surgeons**, aided by other doctors who are specialist **anaesthetists**.

In the operating theatre, surgeons and anaesthetists are helped by both theatre nursing staff and trained assistants called **operating department assistants**.

In the surgical wards, skilled and efficient surgical nursing is of prime importance in postoperative management of most patients who are subjected to operation, while in many it is also a leading factor in preoperative treatment as well.

Intensive Care (Intensive Therapy)—this is provided in a special unit equipped for the concentrated medical attention and extra nursing facilities needed for gravely ill patients from any of the clinical departments—particularly immediately after serious major operations; in cases of severe shock following multiple injuries or other cause; cerebral compression; cardiac, respiratory, renal and liver failure; drug overdosage and near drowning.

Physiotherapy—this means treatment by physical (i.e. natural) methods, including measures such as the therapeutic use of exercise, light, heat, ultrasound, and water. A hospital physiotherapy department is staffed by **physiotherapists** usually under the general direction of a medical practitioner who is a specialist in **rheumatology and rehabilitation**. Physiotherapy has a wide application in both medical and surgical conditions, but finds its most extensive use in diseases and injuries of the locomotor system (i.e. the bones, joints and muscles).

Radiotherapy—consists of treatment by ionising radiation (see p.318) produced by, for example, superficial and deep X-ray apparatus, linear accelerators, betatrons, neutron generators, or ionising radiations emitted spontaneously by radium, radiocobalt, radiophosphorus, radioiodine, and other radionuclides (radioactive isotopes).

This form of therapy is chiefly employed for malignant new growths but is also used for some non-malignant conditions (e.g. certain types of skin disease).

A doctor who specialises in radiotherapy is called a **radiotherapist** and his technical assistants are called therapeutic **radiographers**. An essential adjunct to a radiotherapy department is a **department of medical physics** under the direction of a **hospital physicist** and staffed also with medical **physics technicians**. This department is concerned with the planning of treatments prescribed by radiotherapists, the care and the calibration of apparatus, the design and construction of specialised items of equipment, and so on; the care of radionuclides; and other tasks, among which are important duties relating to the protection of patients and staff against possible hazards arising from the diagnostic and therapeutic uses of ionising radiation.

The treatment of cancer by cytotoxic drugs and hormones also frequently falls within the province of radiotherapy departments. The increasing use of such methods either as adjuvants to, or substitutes for treatment with ionising radiation has led to many such departments now being called **departments of radiotherapy and oncology**, such a designation being more indicative of their role in modern hospital practice.

Psychiatric treatment—includes the use, in patients with disorders of the mind, of (*a*) medical measures (e.g. sedative drugs, stimulant drugs, antidepressant drugs, tranquillisers), (*b*) surgical measures—nowadays performed only to a very small extent, (*c*) physical measures (e.g. electroconvulsive therapy), and (*d*) **psychotherapy**, and **group therapy**—forms of treatment for mental illness which do not include medical, surgical or physical methods.

The study of the mind is called **psychology** and the branch of medicine which deals with diseases of the mind is termed **psychiatry** and is practised by doctors who are specialist **psychiatrists**. In the investigation of some aspects of mental illness, and also in the giving of some forms of treatment and rehabilitation work, psychiatrists are assisted by **clinical psychologists**, whose training includes the obtaining of a university honours degree in psychology. Also working within the field of mental illness and concerned with its social aspects are professional staff termed **psychiatric social workers**.

While psychiatric outpatient clinics are a common feature of general hospitals, facilities for the inpatient treatment of mental disorders are, to a large extent, mainly provided in special hospitals, termed **mental hospitals**, which aim at providing a therapeutic community where all staff of the hospital help with treatment. Modern thought, however, inclines to the view that such treatment would be better provided in special wards attached to general hospitals.

Terms relating to psychiatry will be further discussed in Part IV. **Other therapeutic methods**—these include:

- **chiropody**—the specialised treatment of foot disorders given by **chiropodists**, professional staff who have been trained in **podology**, i.e. the branch of medicine concerned with the study of human foot in health and in medical and surgical disease conditions;
- **diet therapy**—the word diet means a customary or prescribed form of feeding and the control of patient's feeding for therapeutic purposes is termed diet therapy. Therapeutic diets are planned and their provision is supervised by hospital dietetic departments in the charge of professionally trained **dietitians**. The hospital dietitian is also concerned with advising outpatients regarding their diets at home;
- **occupational therapy**—as defined by the Board of Education of the College of Occupational Therapy—is the treatment of physical and psychiatric conditions through specific selected activities in order to help people reach their maximum level of function and independence in all aspects of daily life (Gore, H. G. N., 1981, personal communication);
- **orthoptic treatment**—is a process of mental training, involving special eye exercises, employed in the treatment of squint and other disorders of normal binocular vision. Investigation and treatment of such conditions are carried out by **orthoptists**, working under the direction of ophthalmic surgeons or ophthalmic medical practitioners;
- **optical treatment**—is the correction of errors or refraction by spectacles or contact lenses. Sight testing and prescribing of spectacles and contact lenses may be performed by medical practitioners and also by qualified **ophthalmic opticians**, who may also supply visual appliances. **Dispensing opticians** supply visual appliances but do not test sight;
- **speech therapy**— is undertaken by **speech therapists** and, as described by Hatfield, is 'the scientific treatment of persons suffering from disorders of speech, language and voice. Suitable cases include defects of the peripheral speech organs (e.g. cleft

palate); articulatory and voice disorders of neuromuscular origin (e.g. cerebral palsy, Parkinson's disease); delayed or deviant speech in childhood; loss of spoken and written language due to cortical damage (aphasia, etc.); functional and organic voice disorders; and stammering'. (Hatfield, F. M., 1984, personal communication).

- **remedial gymnastics**—includes exercise therapy and recreational therapy. This form of treatment, which is of particular value of connection with rehabilitation of the sick and injured is administered by professionally trained **remedial gymnasts**, who, in a hospital, are members of a department of physical medicine.

In recent years the training programmes for physiotherapy and remedial gymnastics have moved closer together. As a result, the merging of these two professions is under consideration.

Assessment of the results of treatment may be made by clinical methods, and from the results of various forms of special investigations similar to those used in diagnosis, e.g. by pathology and radiology. In certain types of disease (e.g. diseases of the skin, tumours, lesions in certain internal structures capable of being photographed by what are termed endoscopic cameras) valuable records regarding progress under treatment may be obtained from **medical photography**. Records produced by qualified medical photographers are also of great value in various forms of research and in visual methods of instruction employed in medical education.

In many instances, social factors relating to a patient's home conditions, or his work, or provision for his dependants may be factors of considerable relevance to the treatment of his illness. It is the task of **medical social workers** (or in psychiatric departments, of **psychiatric social workers**), working in co-operation with the medical staff, to help patients with any personal problems that cause difficulties during illness.

Obstetric care—the specialty of **obstetrics** deals with the management of pregnancy, childbirth, and the **puerperium** (the period immediately following childbirth during which the uterus returns to its normal size and lactation commences).

In hospital, this specialty is usually linked in the same department with that of **gynaecology** which is concerned with diseases of the female reproductive system.

By obstetric care is meant the care of women during the different phases of the process of childbearing, given either by **obstetricians**, i.e. doctors practising **obstetrics**, or by **midwives** who also practise this specialty; and within certain legally defined limits, may carry out such practice independently of medical supervision.

The term **obstetrics** means literally 'to stand before' and the name of the specialty presumably derives from the position taken up by the doctor or midwife while assisting during childbirth. While medical or surgical treatment may be required for various types of obstetric disorder, the majority of so-called patients under the care of an obstetric department are normal healthy women and require supervision and assistance rather than therapy.

Note: in branches of medicine other than obstetrics, however, the word **patient** is generally understood to apply to a subject who requires investigation and treatment for some disease condition.

Some Drugs used in Medicine

A **drug**, as defined by Sears and Winwood (2) is 'any substance taken into the body, or applied to its surface, for the prevention or treatment of disease or symptoms'.

Thus, in medical terminology, the word has a much wider application than is usually appreciated by the general public, to whom it usually indicates a substance which is either a stimulant or a poison, or has dangerous habit-forming properties.

The prefix **pharm-** means pertaining to drugs. The study of drugs is called **pharmacology**, and the study of drugs used in medicine is referred to as **materia medica**.

In a hospital drugs are prepared, stored and dispensed in a department termed a **pharmacy** or **dispensary**. This is in the charge of a **hospital pharmacist**, under whom work **pharmacy technicians** (formerly known as dispensing assistants).

Important types of drugs used in medicine include the following.

Anaesthetics—used to produce loss of local sensibility, especially to touch and pain, i.e. **local anaesthetics** (e.g. cocaine and its derivatives); or **general anaesthetics** which cause a general loss of sensibility accompanied by unconsciousness (e.g. halothane, thiopentone—Pentothal). The word **anaesthesia** means without sensation.

Analgesics—pain-relieving drugs (e.g. morphine, aspirin).

Antibiotics—substances produced by living organisms which can destroy or prevent growth and multiplication of various pathogenic microbes (e.g. penicillin produced by a mould).

Anticoagulants—drugs which reduce the clotting power of the blood (e.g. heparin, phenindione—Dindevan).

Anticonvulsants—used in the treatment of epilepsy (e.g. phenobarbitone, phenytoin—Epanutin).

Antihistamines—drugs used to block the action of histamine. *Histamine* is a substance carried in the blood and tissues by cells known as *basophil leucocytes* in the former, and as *mast cells* when they migrate from the bloodstream into the tissues. When liberated from these cells it may cause allergic reactions of various types by stimulating nerve terminals, situated in blood vessels, skin and smooth muscle and called

H1 receptors. Antihistamine drugs may thus be described as H1 antagonists (e.g. promethazine—Phenergan; chlorpheniramine—Piriton).

Antihypertensives—drugs which lower the blood pressure and are also termed hypotensives (e.g. methyldopa—Aldomet; propranolol—Inderal).

Antimalarials—used in the prevention and treatment of malaria (e.g. chloroquinine, primaquine).

Antiseptics—chemical substances that render disease-producing microbes harmless by preventing their growth and multiplication (e.g. surgical spirit, chlorhexidine).

Aperients—substances which, when taken by mouth, promote bowel evacuation. Mild aperients are known as **laxatives** (e.g. liquid paraffin) and stronger aperients as **purgatives** (e.g. senna, castor oil).

Cytotoxic drugs—the name of these means cell-poisoning drugs. This class of drugs destroys cells and affects the cells of malignant tumours, and cells found in certain diseases of the blood, bone marrow, lymphatic and mononuclear phagocytic systems, more readily than normal cells. Two important types of cytotoxic drugs are the **antimetabolites**, which interfere with cell metabolism (e.g. cyclophosphamide) and **alkylating agents**, which produce a chemical reaction called alkylation (e.g. methotrexate). Certain vegetable extracts (e.g. vinblastine and vincristine, both extracts of periwinkle) and certain antibiotics (e.g. actinomycin D) also have cytotoxic properties.

Disinfectants (germicides)—chemical substances which destroy pathogenic microbes (e.g. lysol, phenol).

Diuretics—drugs that increase the secretion of urine by the kidneys (e.g. frusemide—Lasix).

Hormones—secretions of ductless glands and synthetic preparations identical with, or closely resembling these secretions (e.g. insulin, cortisone, oestrogens).

Hypnotics—drugs which induce sleep, and many of which also have analgesic (pain-relieving) properties (e.g. chloral, barbiturates).

Non-steroidal anti-inflammatory agents (NSAIs) used in rheumatic and other conditions for both anti-inflammatory action and pain relief (e.g. aspirin, phenylbutazone—Butazolidine), indomethacin—Indocid).

Oxygen—used to remedy deficient oxygenation of the blood, e.g. in cardiac or respiratory failure.

Radioactive isotopes—(see p 318).

Radiological contrast media—substances which when introduced into the body show up on radiographs or fluoroscopy in marked contrast against surrounding body tissue. They do this because they possess either a much higher atomic weight (barium sulphate and iodine preparations) or a much lower atomic weight (air, oxygen, carbon dioxide) than the substances composing the body tissue.

Steroids—a class of chemical substances which includes certain hormones produced in the cortex of the suprarenal glands and called **corticosteroids** (e.g. cortisol, corticosterone) and certain synthetic drugs (e.g. cortisone, prednisolone).

Sulphonamides—a particular class of chemical substance which can prevent the growth and multiplication within the human body of a wide range of bacteria (e.g. sulphadimidine, sulphathiazol).

Tranquillisers—substances which diminish anxiety and excitability by a sedative action on the nervous system (e.g. chlorpromazine and diazepam (Valium)).

Vaccines and sera—used in the prevention and treatment of various types of bacterial and viral infection.

Vitamin preparations—used for prevention and treatment of vitamin-deficiency disorders (e.g. vitamin C to prevent scurvy).

Drugs acting on the sympathetic nervous system—these are of two principal types: (i) **sympathetic stimulants**, acting on sites at nerve terminals, known as α- and β-adrenoreceptors, and found in effectors (muscles which contract and glands which secrete) innervated by the sympathetic nervous system (e.g. adrenaline, ephedrine); (ii) **β-receptor blocking agents** (β-blockers)—which inhibit stimulation of β-receptors (e.g. propranolol).

Drugs acting on the parasympathetic nervous system—these are, like the drugs acting on the sympathetic system, also of two main types: (i) **parasympathetic stimulants**—referred to as being cholinergic as they increase the action of acetylcholine, the chemical transmitter released at the endings of parasympathetic neurons supplying effector organs (e.g. physostigmine—Eserine); (ii) **Anticholinergic drugs**—which inhibit various parasympathetic activities (e.g. atropine, hyoscine, propantheline—Probanthine—and hyoscine-N-butylbromide—Buscopan).

(*Note:* the sympathetic and parasympathetic nervous systems together constitute the *autonomic (involuntary) nervous system*, see p 269).

Many of the types of drugs described above are used in diagnostic radiology as instanced by the use of:
  (i) general anaesthetics for certain special procedures (e.g. aortography, cerebral angiography) and local anaesthetics for others (e.g. bronchography, renal cyst puncture);
  (ii) analgesics (e.g. morphine, pethidine) tranquillisers (e.g. promethazine, diazepam) in premedication;
  (iii) antihistamines (e.g. Piriton), steroids (e.g. hydrocortisone), sympathetic stimulants (e.g. adrenaline) in the treatment of reactions to radiological contrast media;
  (iv) anticholinergic drugs to dry up bronchial secretions during general anaesthesia or bronchography (e.g. atropine) and to reduce muscle spasm during gastrointestinal examinations (e.g. Probanthine, Buscopan);
  (v) purgatives for bowel cleaning before abdominal X-ray examinations;

(vi) sulphonamides to prevent infection after catheterisation for cystography;

(vii) antiseptics for skin sterilisation (e.g. chlorhexidine).

Some other types of drugs used in the specialty include: bronchodilators used in treatment of reactions to contrast media (e.g. aminophylline, isoprenaline); octylnitrite, a vasodilator which also has an antispasmodic effect on the uterine tubes and the muscles at the lower end of the oesophagus, in cardiospasm; metochlorpramide (Maxolon) to promote gastric emptying during barium meal examinations; glucagon to secure temporary relaxation of the gastric musculature during double contrast barium meal examinations.

Many drugs, if taken into the body in amounts greater than those prescribed for medical treatment, will act as tissue poisons with resultant ill-effects which may, in many instances, be serious. The margin between the therapeutic dose and the amount which will cause drug poisoning is often small.

All medicinal products available in the UK are controlled by Part III of the **Medicines Act 1968** as either general sale list (GSL), pharmacy medicines (P), or prescription only medicine (POM).

Certain drugs possess habit-forming properties and are commonly referred to as **drugs of addiction**. These are subject to further legal controls under the **Misuse of Drugs Act 1971** and the **Misuse of Drugs Regulations 1973** and are designated as **controlled** (previously **dangerous**) **drugs**.

Treatment with chemical substances is called **chemotherapy**. The term was initially introduced in connection with the treatment of syphilis by arsenical compounds. In its modern usage it refers chiefly to the treatment of infections by sulphonamides, the use of cytotoxic drugs in malignant conditions and therapy with antituberculosis drugs.

Branches of Medicine and Surgery

A type of basic departmental hospital organisation was described on p 18.

Customarily there are several divisions within the major clinical specialties of medicine and surgery, the number and form of these varying according to the size of the hospital and the nature of its work.

Some of the principal divisions of medicine and surgery and the types of diseases or structures of the body with which they deal are:

Medicine	Surgery
General medicine	*General surgery*
	Accident surgery
Cardiology—heart diseases	*Cardiac surgery*—heart surgery
Dermatology—skin diseases	*Dental surgery*—surgery of the teeth
Endocrinology—endocrine diseases	*Ear, nose and throat surgery*

Genitourinary medicine (venereology)—sexually transmitted diseases

Geriatrics—diseases of old age

Neurology—diseases of the nervous system

Paediatrics—diseases of children

Psychiatry—mental diseases

Respiratory medicine—diseases of the chest

Rheumatology and rehabilitation—see p 23

Genitourinary surgery—urinary system of both sexes and male reproductive system

Ophthalmic surgery—eye surgery

Oral surgery—surgery of the mouth

Orthopaedic surgery—surgery of the bones and joints

Plastic surgery—surgical repair of damaged or defective tissues

Thoracic surgery—chest surgery

Note: Gynaecological surgery—surgery of the female reproductive system is within the province of the major specialty of gynaecology and obstetrics.

REFERENCES

(1) Marks, V. (1972). *Clinical Biochemistry: Trade or Profession*. Inaugural lecture. University of Surrey.
(2) Sears, W. G., Winwood, R. S. (1980). *Materia Medica for Nurses*. London: Edward Arnold.

PART II

Certain General Pathological Processes

The researches of pathologists have shown that certain series of changes from the normal may occur as common features in disorders which are otherwise of a different nature, and of widely different causation, e.g. changes due to inflammation are observed in disease due to such differing aetiology as infection, mechanical irritation, burns and over-exposure to ionising radiation.

Changes of this type, common to many different forms of disease are therefore known as **general pathological processes**. In contradistinction, abnormalities peculiar to individual diseases, or a group of related diseases, may be referred to as **specific pathological processes**. Where appropriate the latter will be mentioned when discussing terms referring to various types of diseases in Parts III, IV and V.

Some knowledge of the nature of the more important general pathological processes affords a valuable basis for the proper understanding of many medical terms.

This part of the book will accordingly give brief explanations of some of these processes—namely, certain manifestations of damage to tissue cells; infection, and processes concerned in immunity, inflammation and repair; some disorders of growth; cyst formation; some disorders of blood circulation; hypersensitivity, allergy and autoimmunity; and shock.

Manifestations of Damage to Tissue Cells

Necrosis

This term means death of tissue cells within a localised area.

If necrosis is accompanied or rapidly followed by putrefactive changes the condition then becomes one of **gangrene**.

Putrefaction is a type of tissue decomposition which results from infection with putrefactive bacteria. According to the type of putrefaction present, gangrene may be either **moist** or **dry** in type.

Degeneration

This is a condition in which structural changes are produced in tissue cells as a result of damage initially insufficient to cause necrosis. The changes may, however, progress to necrosis or, alternatively, if the causal factors cease to operate they may sometimes regress with a return to normality of the affected cells.

Degeneration is of various types. One form is called **fatty degeneration** (fatty change) and is characterised by the accumulation of fat in specialised cells of organs such as the heart and liver. It may result from a variety of causes, among which are lack of adequate oxygen supply, dietetic deficiencies, excess consumption of alcohol and severe infections.

Other forms of degeneration include the conditions called **cloudy swelling** and **hyaline**, **fibrinoid**, **mucoid** and **amyloid degeneration**.

In the last named, an abnormal protein substance called **amyloid** appears in the walls of blood vessels and in the connective tissues of muscles and various internal organs. Its presence is associated with the clinical conditions known as **primary amyloidosis** and **secondary amyloidosis**. In the former, which is very rare, the disorder develops without apparent cause, whereas in the latter it is secondary to some other condition, such as severe chronic infection, Hodgkin's disease or rheumatoid arthritis.

Pathological Calcification

This term describes the abnormal deposition of calcium salts in the soft tissues of the body.

In the form of pathological calcification called **dystrophic calcification**, calcium salts are deposited in tissues that have been killed or injured by disease. This process is a common feature in sites of healed tuberculous infection and may also be seen as a result of certain other inflammatory conditions, in some types of neoplasm, in some forms of arterial disease (e.g. atheroma) and in old blood clots.

Calcium deposits may also occur in previously healthy tissue as a result of another form of pathological calcification called **metastatic calcification**. This process occurs in certain disorders associated with high concentrations of calcium in the blood, e.g. hyperparathyroidism, overdosage with vitamin D.

Both types of pathological calcification may, if the deposits are of sufficient size, be demonstrated by X-rays. Dystrophic calcification, showing the sites of healed primary tuberculous infection in cervical, mesenteric and hilar lymph nodes, and in the lungs, is a frequent chance finding on radiographs of the neck, abdomen and chest. It may also be seen in the lesions of postprimary pulmonary tuberculosis; renal tuberculosis; a variety of benign and malignant neoplasms; certain benign breast disorders; as a result of injuries or inflammatory conditions of ligaments and tendons; in the aorta and peripheral and other arteries in a disease called atheroma; and also frequently in clots which form in small veins in the pelvic cavity and when calcified are termed **phleboliths**.

Infection, Immunity, Inflammation and Repair

Infection

Infection is said to be present when pathogenic micro-organisms (disease-producing germs) have established themselves in the tissues of some part or parts of the body and are able to survive and reproduce themselves therein.

Micro-organisms (also known as microbes) are minute living organisms of such a size that they can either be observed only under a microscope (by light or electron microscopy), or are so small that they are ultramicroscopic, i.e. beyond the range of visibility of any known microscopic methods.

It will be appreciated that the presence of bacteria, known as **commensals**, living normally on the external and certain of the internal surface of the body (e.g. within the mouth or bowel) without causing harmful effects, does not constitute infection. Certain commensals can, however, develop pathogenic properties if they are carried to organs or tissues in sites different from those in which they noramlly exist, e.g. the *Escherichia coli* is normally a commensal in the bowel, but if it gains access to the urinary tract it may cause severe bladder and kidney infections.

Infection results in tissue damage and, in the vast majority of cases in the production of clinical signs and symptoms of infective disease.

In some types of infection, however, it is possible for an individual to acquire the infection without developing any signs or symptoms of its presence. This is known as **subclinical infection** and the affected subject is called a **healthy carrier** of the disease in question, because he carries its causative micro-organisms. These he may transmit to others, who may then develop clinical signs and symptoms. Cases with subclinical infection are not uncommon in epidemics of poliomyelitis (infantile paralysis), and various epidemics of typhoid fever have been traced to infection of water or food supplies by healthy carriers.

A person may also become a healthy carrier as a result of survival of pathogenic micro-organisms within his body after otherwise apparently complete recovery from an infective illness and disappearance of all clinical signs and symptoms.

Germs that are harmful are termed medically **pathogenic** (disease-producing) **micro-organisms** (microbes) or, more shortly, **pathogens**. They are of four main varieties—namely **bacteria**,

viruses, fungi and **protozoa**. Minute organisms known as **rickett-siae** are of intermediate type between bacteria and viruses; others known as **chlamydiae** possess properties which relate them to bacteria.

Bacteria are of different types, among which are **cocci, bacilli**, and **spirochaetes**. Bacteria liberate poisonous substances called **toxins**. There are two varieties, **exotoxins**, which diffuse out from living bacteria, and **endotoxins**, which are only liberated when bacteria die.

Viruses are only able to reproduce in living cells. Like bacteria, they are also of different types, e.g. pox viruses and herpes viruses.

Bacteria, fungi and protozoa are all visible by ordinary microscopic methods. Many viruses are visible by electron microscopy and a few types may be identified by light microscopy—but others are ultramicroscopic.

Some examples of infective diseases caused by micro-organisms are the following.

Bacteria—pneumococcal pneumonia (*pneumococcus*), tuberculosis (*tubercle bacillus*); syphilis (*Treponema pallidum*).

Viruses—common cold, measles, poliomyelitis.

Fungi—ringworm, athlete's foot.

Protozoa—malaria.

Micro-organisms may gain access to the body by **inhalation** (being inspired into the respiratory tract), **ingestion** (being swallowed in food or drink), by **inoculation** through wounds in the skin and sometimes by penetration of undamaged skin. They may also enter the body through the external ear, anal canal, vagina and urethra.

Clinical signs and symptoms of infective disease may present in the form of (*a*) local manifestations due to inflammatory reaction (see p 37) at sites of infection e.g. swelling, redness, heat and pain; and (*b*) general manifestations, e.g. **pyrexia** (fever, i.e. rise in body temperature above normal), **headache**, **anorexia** (loss of appetite) and **malaise** (a feeling of being generally out-of-sorts).

The body possesses the following defence mechanisms against infection.

Surface defence mechanisms which seek to prevent entry of pathogens into its tissues. Thus the skin and, to a lesser extent, the mucous membranes lining its interior structures provide barriers to such entry. Among other such mechanisms are also the destruction of bacteria by the acidity of the gastric juices and removal of particulate matter by coughing.

Internal defence mechanisms—some of which are inherited and others acquired.

Inherited mechanisms include: (i) the presence in the bloodstream of naturally occurring non-specific antibodies; (ii) the inflammatory reaction and the property of **phagocytosis** (the ability of certain cells to take up invading micro-organisms and foreign particles into their cytoplasm) possessed by the polymorphonuclear leucocytes (neutrophils) of the blood, and the macrophages of the mononuclear phagocyte system (formerly known as the reticuloendothelial system); (iii) the presence of **complement** (a chemical agent which destroys bacteria by dissolving their cell membranes) in the circulation and its participation in certain immunity reactions.

Acquired mechanisms comprise the ability of the body to react to invasion of its tissues, by pathogens, by producing a specific immune response (see later).

It should be emphasised that these various inherited and acquired mechanisms act in concert, e.g. the inflammatory reaction enables a concentration of phagocytes, antibodies and immune cells at a site of infection.

Immunity

The acquired internal defence mechanisms against infection referred to above, require the ability of the body, when invading pathogens gain entry to its tissues, to recognise the 'foreignness' of the proteins contained within them, and then to react by producing either **specific antibodies** or **specific immune cells** with actions antagonistic to the invaders. This is referred to as producing a **specific immune response**.

Substances capable of producing an immune response are known as **antigens**, and are mainly proteins but include a small number of carbohydrates. The immune response is specific for any given antigen or related group of antigens and involves, firstly, recognition of the antigen (often referred to as the ability to differentiate between self and non-self) and then a reaction to it. In the case of infection this reaction is beneficial, helping to overcome a first attack of infection and, by secondary responses, preventing or modifying further attacks of infection for a variable time, i.e. providing an immunity of variable degree and duration. The word **immunity** means exemption.

Not all immune responses however, are beneficial. In some cases they may be responsible for various disorders, some of which are serious—e.g. tissue rejection after transplant operations, reactions to the transfusion of incompatible blood, certain hypersensitivity reactions and autoimmune diseases.

Antibodies produced by an antigenic stimulus are proteins of the type called **gammaglobulins** (immunoglobulins). They are manufactured by B-lymphocytes which are mature plasma cells. As antibodies operate in a fluid medium, they are said to be responsible for **humoral immunity** (humour in this context meaning fluid).

Specific immune cells are lymphocytes of a type called T-lymphocytes, which in some incompletely understood manner are modified or influenced by the thymus gland, and are said to be responsible for **cell-mediated immunity**.

Immunity, of varying duration, against a number of infective diseases may be artifically induced by active or passive immunisation procedures.

Active immunisation is obtained by giving a vaccine by injection, by mouth, by scarification of the skin, or by multiple pressure technique (e.g. vaccination against smallpox) and often confers a long-lasting protection. The vaccine may consist of (i) living but attenuated (weakened) pathogens (e.g. BCG vaccination against tuberculosis); (ii) dead pathogens (TABC vaccination); (iii) modified bacterial toxins called toxoids (e.g. tetanus toxoid).

Passive immunisation is used to confer short-lived protection, e.g. during an epidemic of an infective disease. It may include the injection of antibody (e.g. gammaglobulin to prevent measles) or injection of blood serum from immunised animals (e.g. antitetanus serum obtained from horses).

Defective immune responses occur in some conditions termed **immunodeficiency disorders**. These include the conditions called **agammaglobulinaemia** and **hypogammaglobulinaemia** in which there is a deficiency of humoral immunity and the more recently described **acquired immune deficiency syndrome** (**AIDS**), a viral infection in which cellular immunity is defective. Among the features of this latter condition, which occurs principally in male homosexuals and drug addicts, may be the development of Kaposi's sarcoma, a rare neoplasm usually occurring in the skin.

Immunodeficiency may also be created deliberately when **immunosuppressive therapy** using drugs (e.g. azothioprine) is administered to prevent **tissue rejection**, consequent on transplant operations, in which tissues and organs (e.g. kidney, heart, liver) are obtained from other individuals.

Antigenic properties are sometimes also acquired by substances which are integral constituents of the body (see **autoimmunity**).

Inflammation

This process is the local reaction of the body to any form of damage to its cells.

The most common cause of inflammation is infection, but it also occurs in response to cellular damage from many other types of injury, e.g. by mechanical trauma, external physical and chemical agents.

Several different types of inflammation are described. These are, however, all essentially variants of the same basic pathological process, which is defensive in nature and tends to localise the effects of the damage and where possible prevent their extension to other organs and tissues.

The inflammatory reaction results in the production of an **inflammatory exudate** in the tissue spaces in the affected area. This consists of blood cells and plasma, together with antibodies, which leak blood through openings in the walls of capillaries.

In acute inflammation, the exudate is rich in both cells and fluid, whereas in chronic inflammation it is predominantly cellular in type consisting mainly of white blood cells, of the types called lymphocytes and plasma cells, and of macrophages (see p 200).

White cells of the variety called polymorphonuclear leucocytes, or polymorphs, are found in great numbers in the exudate of acute inflammation and, as the reaction subsides, increasing numbers of macrophages appear at the site of the reaction. Both polymorphs and macrophages possess the ability to take up foreign matter, such as the bodies of infecting micro-organisms, into their cytoplasm. This is called **phagocytosis** and the plasma in the inflammatory exudate possesses naturally occurring antibodies which render bacteria more readily susceptible to phagocytic action.

The property of phagocytosis is also possessed by static cells of the mononuclear phagocyte system which are found in sites as lymph glands, liver, bone marrow and spleen and are also called macrophages. These cells, which form an important secondary line of defence against infection, are designed to clear the lymphatic circulation and bloodstream of invading microbes.

The course of an inflammatory reaction varies greatly according to the nature of the tissue damage by which it is evoked, and when such damage is slight it may subside at an early stage. This is spoken of as **resolution**, a term indicating a return to normal after a disease process.

When tissue damage is pronounced and results from bacterial infection, the reaction may proceed to **suppuration**, i.e. the formation of pus. **Pus** is a yellowish fluid composed of fluid from the blood, dead and living bacteria, white blood cells and dead tissue cells. It lies initially within a cavity in the tissue which is formed as a result of tissue destruction. A cavity which contains pus is known as an **abscess**.

In many sites, abscess cavities, unless relieved by surgical incision, tend to enlarge and ultimately rupture, either on the surface of the body or into some hollow cavity or hollow organ. An infective **sinus** is a track produced by pus when discharging itself from an abscess cavity. A sinus is open at one end only. An abscess may sometimes burst in two directions and then a track with two open ends called a **fistula** is formed. A fistula may lead from skin to mucous membrane or from one cavity of the body to another.

An **ulcer** is an open sore caused by an inflammatory process breaking through the skin or a mucous membrane.

An area that is the subject of an acute inflammatory reaction appears red and hot owing to its having a temporarily increased blood supply, an essential feature of the reaction. It is also swollen because of the presence of an exudate in its tissue spaces and is painful and tender to the touch, as a result of increased tension within these spaces and pressure on sensory nerve endings in the vicinity. Presumably the heat and redness caused by acute inflammation were responsible for the name inflammation which means literally a setting on fire.

When an inflammatory reaction caused by bacterial infection fails to localise and to destroy the invading micro-organisms, one or more of the following may ensue:

- spread of infection into the draining lymphatics causing **lymphangitis** (inflammation of lymph vessels) and **lymphadenitis** (inflammation of lymph glands);
- spread of the infecting micro-organisms by the blood to distant tissues where they may cause **metastatic infections** (secondary infections).

When pyogenic micro-organisms are carried in large numbers in the blood and cause multiple secondary abscesses in various structures, the condition is described as **pyaemia**; (**pyogenic** means pus-producing.)

The presence of multiplying pyogenic micro-organisms in the bloodstream is termed **septicaemia** (blood poisoning).

Repair

Injuries (e.g. fractures and wounds) and also disease processes (e.g. infections and resultant inflammatory reactions) which cause death of body cells in localised areas produce a loss of continuity in tissues of affected regions.

When any such loss of continuity occurs, natural processes are quickly set in motion in an effort to restore tissue continuity. Such processes constitute **repair**.

Note: cells and tissues killed by disease are subjected to the action of phagocytes. Phagocytic action by macrophages is generally efficacious in removing small areas of necrotic material and in separating off larger areas from surrounding living tissue, e.g. as in the separation of a slough from a boil.

In some tissues the specialised cells retain their powers of multiplication through life (e.g. bone, surface epithelium of skin, fibrous tissue, liver) and repair is thus achieved by multiplication of undamaged specialised cells. This is known as **regeneration**.

In other tissues (e.g. muscle, cartilage) the specialised cells lose their powers of multiplication. Regeneration is thus not possible and deficiencies are restored by a process termed **repair by fibrosis** (repair by organisation), usually referred to more shortly as **fibrosis**.

This includes, first, the ingrowth of **granulation tissue** consisting of loops of new capillaries, macrophages, and young fibroblasts (connective tissue cells) forming a loose vascular connective tissue. This is then slowly converted first into **fibrous connective tissue** and then, in time, into dense, avascular **scar tissue**.

Scar tissue has a tendency to contract and thus may, as in the case of contractures after severe burns, cause marked deformities.

Tissue damage in chronic inflammatory disorders often results in marked fibrosis and subsequent scarring. In some such disorders the reparative processes are accompanied by abundant formation of granulation tissue. This is often so in conditions such as tuberculosis, syphilis, actinomycosis and leprosy which consequently may be described as **chronic granulomas**.

A process analogous to repair by fibrosis is seen in the central nervous system where damage to the specialised cells is repaired by ingrowth of the neuroglia, the specialised supporting connective tissue of the central nervous system. This type of repair is called **gliosis**.

Reparative fibrosis and subsequent contraction of scar tissue within the wall of a hollow structure (e.g. oesophagus, bowel, common bile duct, urethra) may produce an area of permanent narrowing of the structure referred to as a **stricture** or **stenosis**.

Fibrosis in sites such as the pleural, pericardial and peritoneal cavities frequently results in bands of fibrous scar tissue joining opposing surfaces of these cavities. Such bands are called **adhesions** and may sometimes cause serious ill-effects (e.g. intestinal obstruction due to peritoneal adhesions).

The process of repair may be slowed or, in some instances, prevented entirely by several factors, among which are chronic infection, deficient blood supply, vitamin C deficiency, presence of foreign bodies, and the necessity to attempt to bridge large defects by newly formed tissue.

Conversely, repair may be hastened by effecting close apposition of the sides of the gap in the tissues (e.g. as in the suture of an uninfected incised wound or surgical incision) and obtaining what is termed **healing by first intention** (primary union).

In contradistinction to healing by first intention is **healing by second intention** (healing by granulation, secondary union), in which the tissue defect is gradually filled by ingrowth of granulation tissue which is converted first into fibrous connective tissue and ultimately into scar tissue.

In some individuals overgrowth of fibrous tissue during healing may result in the production of tumour-like masses in scars, known as **keloids**.

Plain radiographs may, in many infective or other inflammatory disorders, show evidence of soft-tissue swelling (e.g. around inflamed joints); inflammatory exudate (e.g. in the lung alveoli in pneumonia); or abscess formation (e.g. in bone infections, lung abscess, infection of the subphrenic space).

Contrast radiology is widely used to demonstrate certain types of ulceration (e.g. barium meals to demonstrate peptic ulceration); to demonstrate stricture formation; and to investigate infective sinuses (sinography) and fistulae (fistulography).

Fibrosis, resulting from damage to lung tissue, may be evidenced in chest radiographs by abnormal dense linear shadows, together with displacements of structures such as the heart, trachea and pulmonary blood vessels which appear to be pulled towards the fibrotic areas.

By reason of their increased blood supply, areas of acute or subacute inflammation may be demonstrated as 'hot spots' on thermograms.

Both ultrasound and CT are widely employed in both the demonstration and the percutaneous drainage of internal abscesses.

Disorders of Growth

Growth in excess of normal caused by an increase in the size of individual cells, **hypertrophy**, or to increased cell-division, **hyperplasia**, may develop as a manifestation of disease.

A complete failure of development called **agenesis** or **aplasia**, a failure of development of organs or tissues to normal size called **hypoplasia**, and a shrinkage in size of organs and tissues, termed **atrophy**, may also occur as a result of various morbid conditions.

Disordered growth of cells resulting in developmental abnormality is called **dysplasia**, and a change in tissue cells from one type to another, **metaplasia** (e.g. change in type of epithelial cells due to chronic irritation).

Some forms of hypertrophy (e.g. enlarged muscles in athletes) and hyperplasia (e.g. increased numbers of red blood cells in people living at high altitudes) are physiological, however, and not pathological. A generalised tissue atrophy is, moreover, frequently seen as a physiological process in old people.

Another form of growth disorder is called **neoplasia**.

Neoplasia

This term means new growth and refers to the formation of **neoplasms** or **tumours**. Neoplasms consist of masses of abnormal cells which grow at the expense of surrounding normal body tissues and carry out no useful function in the body. In pathology the term tumour is used as being synonymous with the term neoplasm. In the widest sense, however, a tumour is any form of swelling. The study of neoplasms is called **oncology**.

Neoplasms fall into two major divisions, the **benign** (innocent) and the **malignant**.

Benign neoplasms—are usually of slow growth. They tend to displace normal tissues and seldom cause serious effects unless they grow in, or press on, important organs. A capsule of fibrous tissue is often formed around them. They do not spread to distant organs and tissues.

Malignant neoplasms—are often of rapid growth. They tend to infiltrate widely into surrounding tissues and often cause ulceration. They cause serious general effects in the body, and, unless successfully treated, will eventually prove fatal. Fortunately with modern methods of therapy many types of malignancy are curable, particularly if diagnosed at an early stage of their development. They have a marked tendency to spread to distant organs and tissues, forming **metastases** (secondary growths) there. In the type of malignant neoplasms called **carcinomas** such metastatic spread occurs both via the lymphatics and bloodstream. In the type called **sarcomas**, distant spread is usually only via the bloodstream. **Carcinomas** are malignant tumours of epithelia, whereas **sarcomas** are derived from various types of connective tissue (including bone and cartilage).

Neoplasms whose cells show a similarity to those of their tissue of origin are described as being **differentiated**. Those, on the other hand, in which such similarity is absent are said to be **undifferentiated** or **anaplastic** in type.

The word **cancer** may be used either in a restricted sense as a synonym for carcinoma or, in a wider sense, to indicate all forms of malignant disease (e.g. cancer research and cancer prevention). Both terms derive from the Latin for a crab.

Carcinogenesis means production of cancer and cancer-producing agents are called **carcinogens**.

The term **carcinoma-in-situ** indicates a localised carcinomatous growth, which does not show any evidence of invasion of its surrounding tissues or of distant spread.

All forms of diagnostic imaging may be employed in the diagnosis of neoplastic disease, as may various pathological investigations including biochemical tests and the microscopic investigation of material obtained by biopsy or operation.

Benign neoplasms frequently require surgical treatment. Surgery, radiotherapy and chemotherapy (with cytotoxic drugs or hormones) are used either singly or in differing combinations in the treatment of malignant disorders.

The cells of many malignant neoplasms are more sensitive to damage from ionising radiation than those of surrounding normal tissues. It is on this fact that the use of radiotherapy in malignant disease is based, and neoplasms which respond well to this form of treatment are said to be **radiosensitive**.

Some malignant cells are known to have antigenic properties and the nature of resultant immune reactions, together with the possibilities of utilising such reactions in cancer prevention and treatment, is the subject of much current research. A considerable amount of research is also being conducted into the roles of both genetic and environmental factors in various types of neoplastic disorders.

Cyst Formation

Cysts are abnormal cavities which may form in the body as a result of widely differing pathological processes (e.g. developmental error, trauma, infection, obstruction of glandular ducts and neoplastic disease). They contain either fluid or semifluid material, or air, and possess a lining membrane.

Disorders in Blood Circulation

Haemorrhage

Means bleeding and may occur as a result of trauma or disease affecting the walls of blood vessels. A number of diseases of widely different causation may cause bleeding into the skin or internal organs. **Epistaxis** is bleeding from the nose; **haematemesis**, vomiting of blood; **haemoptysis**, coughing up of blood from the respiratory tract, **haematuria**, blood in the urine. **Melaena** is the passage of stools which are coloured black because of the presence of altered blood from some portion of the alimentary tract. Haemorrhage from the pregnant uterus, during the later weeks of pregnancy but before delivery, is called **antepartum haemorrhage**.

Hyperaemia

This term describes a condition in which there is an excessive amount of blood present in a part or parts of the body. **Congestion** is a synonymous term. **Local hyperaemia** may result from inflammation or obstruction of veins. **General venous congestion** is seen in right-sided heart failure, when the right ventricle of the heart can no longer adequately pump blood, returned from the veins, out into the pulmonary circulation.

Anaemia

Means that blood is lacking in either or both normal haemoglobin content or numbers of red cells, or that there is a deficiency in the total amount of blood in the body.

Ischaemia (Local Anaemia)

Means a localised deficiency of blood in a part of the body, e.g. **ischaemic heart disease**—due to disease of coronary arteries resulting in a diminution of the blood supply to the heart muscle.

Thrombosis

Means the formation of a **thrombus** (clot) in the interior of a blood vessel or the heart. The main cause of thrombosis is damage to the walls of blood vessels or the endocardial lining of the heart. Infection is a common cause of thrombosis, as is the arterial disease called **atheroma**.

Thrombi which block the interior of large vessels may be demonstrated radiographically by arteriography or phlebography, as appropriate.

Pathological calcification may occur in old thrombi. Calcified thrombi in veins are called **phleboliths**. Small phleboliths are frequently seen in the pelvic cavity. While they are of no pathological significance, they may be of importance radiologically as intravenous urography may sometimes be required to distinguish between a phlebolith and a calculus (stone) in the lower end of a ureter.

The important condition of deep vein thrombosis will be referred to in Part IV when discussing diseases of veins and also in connection with its causal role in pulmonary embolism (see p 105).

Embolism and Infarction

A portion or the whole of a thrombus may become detached and be carried in the bloodstream to another part of the body. This process is called **thromboembolism**, or more shortly **embolism** and the detached fragment of blood clot is called an **embolus**.

This fragment will ultimately be transported into a blood vessel which is too small for it to pass through. It will then be arrested in its progress and be said to be **impacted**.

An embolus can originate in a vein or an artery, or in the interior of the heart. When arising in a systemic vein, or in the right side of the heart, it will ultimately impact in the arterial side of the pulmonary circulation. When arising in an artery or in the left side of the heart, however, it will impact in an artery in some site such as the brain, spleen, kidney, lower end of the aorta, or in a limb artery.

Impaction of an embolus in an artery will deprive an area of tissue of its blood supply. Unless such a supply can be provided from other arterial vessels in the immediate vicinity this will result in the death of an area of tissue. An area of dead tissue produced as a result of embolism or of thrombosis is called an **infarct**.

It should be noted that embolism may also occur as a result of entry into the circulation of air, tumour cells or fat globules.

Note: In a technique used in interventional radiology, an artery may be deliberately blocked by the introduction into its lumen of a balloon, blood clot from the patient's own blood, plastic sponge material such as gelfoam, or muscle. This technique is called **therapeutic angiographic embolisation** and may be employed for uncontrollable bleeding or as a preoperative measure to secure a bloodless field at certain operations. These and other indications for its use are discussed in detail by Dick (1).

Oedema (Dropsy)

Is a condition of swelling of soft tissues, resulting from the presence of excessive fluid in their tissue spaces. The fluid consists of plasma from the bloodstream and may accumulate in the tissues as a result of obstruction to veins, inflammatory conditions, certain types of heart and kidney disease, protein deficiency, or allergic disorders. Oedema may also be caused by obstruction of lymphatic vessels. The swollen arm that may follow radical amputation of the breast is an example of lymphatic oedema. It is thought that this condition may well result from the extensive removal of lymphatic tissue in this operation.

In patients with oedema, concomitant exudation of plasma in the peritoneal cavity or pleural cavities may occur, resulting in **ascites**, in the former instance, and **pleural effusion** in the latter.

Oedema fluid has a scattering effect on X-rays, when present in any large quantity, necessitating the use of increased kilovoltage when taking radiographs or carrying out fluoroscopy. This applies particularly to abdominal examinations in patients with ascites and chest examinations in those with pleural effusions.

Acute Circulatory Failure (Shock)

This condition is of several different types and has various causes. It results in deficient oxygenation of tissue cells and the clinical condition known as **shock**.

Four principal varieties of shock are: (a) **hypovolaemic shock**—due to diminished volume of blood in the circulation e.g. caused by haemorrhage or burns; (b) **cardiogenic shock**—due to diminished output of blood by the heart e.g. as a result of myocardial infarction; (c) **neurogenic shock**—due to circulatory disturbance from nervous causes e.g. severe pain or fright; (d) **septicaemic shock**—occurring in certain severe infections.

Common clinical features of shock are giddiness, pallor, coldness, anxiety, fainting, rapid pulse and lowered blood pressure.

A patient with hypovolaemic shock, and resultant lowered venous pressure, may need to be examined by chest X-ray to show the position of a **CVP line**, a fine intravenous catheter the tip of which is inserted into the right atrium to monitor the central venous pressure (CVP). This is an important measure in prevention of overloading of the circulation during fluid-replacement therapy.

Hypersensitivity and Allergy

Hypersensitivity is a condition in which the body reacts abnormally to the entry, or contact with its surface, of certain foreign materials. The term **allergy** is sometimes used as a synonym for hypersensitivity, but is perhaps better reserved for the type of hypersensitivity resulting from abnormal specific immune responses.

It was noted on p 35 that pathogenic bacteria and viruses have antigenic properties—i.e. the production of antigen-antibody reactions of a defensive nature designed to benefit an infected individual.

In contradistinction, allergic reactions are thought to be caused by the occurrence of abnormal antigen-antibody reactions which cause damage to tissue cells, and result in undesirable and sometimes dangerous clinical manifestations.

A variety of agents, protein or carbohydrate may act as antigens and provoke allergic reactions in susceptible individuals.

Among the clinical disorders in which allergy is a basic factor or is thought to play some role are bronchial asthma, hay fever (due to hypersensitivity to grass pollens), eczema, food allergy (e.g. allergic disorder after eating shellfish), certain types of reaction to various drugs (e.g. drug rashes caused by penicillin or sulphonamides), serum sickness caused by injection of therapeutic sera, allergic reactions to iodine-containing contrast media.

It is also to be noted that many authorities regard acute rheumatism and acute glomerulonephritis as being primarily due to allergic reactions resulting from streptococcal infection.

One type of severe and sometimes fatal acute allergic reaction is seen in the conditions called **anaphylactic shock**, in which the outstanding feature is a sudden general circulatory collapse.

Certain important effects seen in allergic disorders are due to the liberation within the tissues of a substance called **histamine** (see p 26). In the treatment of allergic disorders such effects may be controlled by giving **antihistamine drugs**.

The suprarenal hormone hydrocortisone is frequently effective in suppressing allergic reactions.

The injection or less commonly the oral administration of iodine-containing radiological contrast media may, in some individuals cause reactions which are allergic in type, e.g. urticaria (nettlerash), swelling of eyelids and other soft tissues of face and neck, spasm of bronchial muscles causing dyspnoea (difficulty in breathing).

Antihistamine drugs, and hydrocortisone are widely used in the prevention and treatment of such reactions.

Autoimmunity

Allied to allergy (see above) is the phenomenon of **autoimmunity** wherein certain substances within the tissues of an individual develop antigenic properties and cause the formation of so-called **auto-antibodies**. These may then result in various types of antigen-antibody reaction in the body of such an individual.

Such reactions are widely considered as being the basis of a number of diseases which are termed **autoimmune diseases**, and are therefore said to arise from a failure by the body to differentiate self from non-self (see p 35).

Some authorities consider that auto-immunity may play some part in the causation of rheumatoid arthritis and there is general agreement in classifying the uncommon conditions called Hashimoto's thyroiditis and disseminated lupus erythematosus as autoimmune diseases.

The presence of different kinds of autoantibodies in blood serum may be demonstrated by a series of tests the results of which produce what is termed an **autoimmune profile**.

REFERENCES

(1) Dick, R. (1977). Radiology now. Therapeutic angiographic embol-isation. *British Journal of Radiology*; **50**: 241–2.

PART III

Certain Infective Diseases

Diseases caused by invasion of the tissues by pathogenic micro-organisms, i.e. bacteria, viruses, rickettsiae, fungi and protozoa, are called **infective diseases**. As they can be transmitted from one individual to another, either by direct contact or by some intermediate agent (e.g. infected water or food, insect carriers), they are sometimes referred to as **communicable diseases**.

The term **contagious diseases** is of rather ill-defined usage, but is generally employed in respect of those infective disorders which are transmissible by direct contact.

Any system of classification of infective diseases is likely to lead to some overlapping of various groups. In this explanation of medical terms, the conditions referred to will be described under the following headings: infectious fevers, pyogenic infections, tuberculosis, sexually transmitted (venereal) diseases; some other infective diseases.

Tropical infections will be referred to in Part V of the book, and some other types of infective diseases will be referred to in Part IV, when discussing terms referring to diseases of the various systems of the body.

It is important in the consideration of infective disease to make special note of the following:

- the meanings of the terms infection, inflammation, and immunisation (see Part II).
- the use of the suffix **–itis** to indicate inflammatory conditions, e.g. parotitis, inflammation of the parotid salivary glands.
- the terms **pyrexia**, **tachycardia**, **headache**, **anorexia** and **malaise** (see p 34).
- **septicaemia** (see p 38).
- **toxaemia**—the word **toxin** means a poison, and toxaemia is a condition wherein bacteria toxins, or other poisonous substances are present in the general circulation causing effects such as malaise, weakness, furring of the tongue and pyrexia.
- **lesion**, a word meaning injury and conveniently applied to any form of structural damage caused to body tissues by disease.

- **focus** (plural: foci)—a term used in one of its senses to indicate an area of disease, e.g. as in 'primary tuberculous focus'.
- **complications**—additional pathological conditions developing during the course of a disease.
- **sequelae** (singular: sequel)—pathological conditions which follow a disease and which are considered to have developed as a result of such disease.

INFECTIOUS FEVERS

By common usage, those of the infective diseases which are termed infectious consist of several acute infective disorders which, being readily transmissible, show a tendency to appear periodically in **epidemics**, i.e. outbreaks which affect fairly large numbers of individuals and which sometimes have a wide geographical distribution.

Fever and **pyrexia** are synonymous terms indicating a rise in body temperature above its normal level of 36.9°C. The adjective febrile means pertaining to a fever and any febrile illness may, until the course of the fever is established, be referred to as **pyrexia of unknown origin (PUO)**.

Included among disorders which may be classified as infectious fevers are what are sometimes called common childhood ailments, i.e. measles, German measles, whooping cough, mumps and chickenpox. Also included are conditions such as smallpox, diphtheria, scarlet fever, typhoid fever and cerebrospinal fever.

All these fevers possess what is called an **incubation period**, i.e. the time between acquiring the infection and the appearance of the first clinical signs and symptoms. These latter, which are often of a non-specific type, herald the approach of the main clinical features of the illness and are known as **prodromal symptoms** and **signs** (e.g. headache, dizziness, general malaise, pyrexia, tachycardia).

Another feature common to most of these diseases is the development, at some stage, of multiple inflammatory skin lesions, referred to in lay parlance as spots, which form a **rash** (synonyms: **eruption**, **exanthem**).

A rash may consist of **macules**—spots or blotches which are not raised above the surrounding skin; **papules**—spots which are raised above the skin (sometimes referred to as pimples); **vesicles**—small blisters containing clear fluid and **pustules**, small blisters containing pus; or mixed forms of these lesions. A rash may also be described as **petechial**, when it is composed of small purplish spots called **petechiae**, which are due to blood effused beneath the epidermis; or as **purpuric** when haemorrhages beneath the skin produce large purple spots or patches.

The infectious fevers discussed in this section are caused by either bacterial or viral infection, and in many of them active and passive methods of immunisation (see p 36) are employed in their prophylaxis (prevention). Immune sera may also be used to treat some of these illnesses.

Measles (Morbilli)

This virus infection has an incubation period of about 10–14 days. Its name probably originally meant spots and a prominent feature is the appearance of a widespread rash, usually on the fourth day of the illness.

Characteristic early features are conjuctivitis and the development of white spots in the mouth, the so-called **Koplik's spots**.

Bronchopneumonia and otitis media are the most frequent complications, and the former may be of serious import in infants.

Active immunisation may now be undertaken with measles vaccine. Those exposed to infection may be given temporary protection by human gammoglobulin (immunoglobulin), an extract of blood serum containing antibodies against the causal virus.

German Measles (Rubella)

The alternative name of rubella derives from the redness of the rash which develops in this virus disease. Another characteristic is glandular enlargement, which may be widespread. The incubation period is about 14–21 days.

The infection is generally mild but unfortunately if contracted during the first three months of pregnancy may lead to subsequent birth of a child with serious disabilities such as congenital heart disease, congenital cataract (opacity of the lens of the eye) or congenital deafness.

The presence or absence of immunity may be established by a blood test for rubella antibodies.

Temporary protection may be given during early pregnancy by administration of human immunoglobulin, but it is desirable that girls, who have not contracted the disease before they attain child-bearing age, should be actively immunised with rubella vaccine.

Whooping Cough (Pertussis)

This is a bacterial infection due to an organism called *Bordetella pertussis*, and has an incubation period of about 8–14 days.

The infection causes a catarrhal inflammation of the upper respiratory tract and a dry cough which becomes paroxysmal in type. The fits of coughing often end with an inspiratory noise described as a 'whoop'.

Among the serious complications which may occur are bronchopneumonia, atelectasis (collapse) of segments of lung tissue, and **convulsions**, i.e. fits in which abnormal movements occur owing to involuntary muscular contractions, and in which there may often be an accompanying loss of consciousness.

Antibiotics may be used in treatment.

Prophylactic vaccination may be carried out when considered desirable.

Mumps (Epidemic Parotitis)

This virus infection causes acute inflammatory changes in the parotid salivary glands (i.e. parotitis) and occasionally in the submandibular salivary glands as well.

The incubation period is about 14–21 days.

The disease is not itself serious but may, if contracted after puberty produce serious complications among which are **orchitis** (inflammation of the testes), **oophoritis** (inflammation of the ovaries) and **pancreatitis** (inflammation of pancreas). Orchitis may result in sterility.

There is no specific treatment for mumps.

The name of the condition appears to derive from the abnormal appearance of the face, produced by the parotid swellings, the word mumps originally indicating an abnormal facial expression.

Chickenpox (Varicella)

This is a mild virus infection unconnected with chickens, but owing the second part of its name to the fact that at one time a disease with a rash exhibiting the formation of pocks, i.e. spots of vesicular or pustular type, was referred to as a pox.

Chickenpox has an incubation period of about 14–21 days and its causal virus is indistinguishable from that of herpes zoster (shingles).

The disease is characterised by a vesicular rash. In the earlier stages of the disease, it is sometimes difficult to differentiate between the rashes of chickenpox and the much more serious condition of smallpox.

There is no specific treatment.

> Pneumonia is an uncommon complication of chickenpox and may cause disseminate small nodular areas of consolidation which may subsequently undergo pathological calcification and thus be demonstrable on chest radiographs.

Smallpox (Variola)

This virus disease, thought to be non-existent at the time of writing, can occur in the form of **classical smallpox (variola major)** which is serious and not infrequently fatal; and in a much milder form called **alastrim (variola minor)**.

The incubation period is 12 days. The rash is at first macular and then goes through papular, vesicular and pustular stages (see p 48), the latter being due to secondary bacterial infection of the vesicles. The difficulty which can occasionally occur in differentiating smallpox from chickenpox has been referred to when discussing the latter condition.

In its severer forms the infection is accompanied by marked pyrexia and considerable toxaemia. **Myocarditis** (inflammation of the heart muscle), and virus **pneumonia** (inflammation of the lung) are among the complications.

There is no specific therapy but penicillin or other antibiotics are of value in diminishing the effects of secondary infection and preventing complications.

A high degree of protection against smallpox may be obtained by active immunisation with a vaccine of calf lymph, containing the live related virus which causes **cowpox (vaccinia)**.

Vaccination against smallpox with vaccinia virus was first carried out in England in 1796 by Edward Jenner, a Gloucestershire physician.

Diphtheria

The word diphtheria means a membrane and the name of this disease derives from the fact that the inflammatory exudate, formed at the site of infection, coagulates to form a characteristic false membrane.

The causal pathogen is a bacterium known variously as the *Corynebacterium diphtheriae*, the *Klebs-Loeffler bacillus*, or the *diphtheria bacillus*.

Infection occurs most commonly in the throat, producing faucial diphtheria (i.e. so named from the pillars of the fauces, between which lie the tonsils), but can also develop in the nose or larynx and, rarely, in the skin (cutaneous diphtheria).

In addition to local effects, damage in distant tissues may be caused by reason of the fact that the causal bacteria secrete a highly poisonous exotoxin, which is absorbed into the bloodstream and is transported around the body.

Diphtheria exotoxin is particularly likely to affect the heart muscle, causing a toxic **myocarditis** (inflammation of the heart muscle); and the nervous system leading to disorders such as **palatal paralysis** (paralysis of the muscles of the soft palate); **ciliary paralysis** (paralysis of ciliary muscles, the muscles of the eye responsible for visual accommodation); **respiratory paralysis** (paralysis of the respiratory muscles) and **peripheral neuritis** (a condition in which nerve damage causes various forms of sensory disturbance and weakness of motor muscles in the limbs). Peripheral neuritis is also referred to as **polyneuritis** or **peripheral neuropathy**.

The incubation period of diphtheria is 2–8 days. Treatment is with diphtheria antitoxin and penicillin.

Active immunisation consists of vaccination with some form of diphtheria toxoid (i.e. toxin modified so as to render it harmless but retaining its antigenic properties), e.g. APT, TAF.

As a result of widespread active immunisation, diphtheria is now very uncommon in the UK. A skin test, called the **Schick test**, is employed to investigate the presence or absence of immunity to the disease.

Scarlet Fever (Scarlatina)

This is due to a variety of *streptococcus*, which differs from other types of streptococci in that it secretes an exotoxin which produces the scarlet rash that gives this fever its name.

The incubation period is about 1–8 days. Treatment is with penicillin and complications during the course of the disease are uncommon. Acute **nephritis** (inflammation of the kidney) or rheumatic fever may occur after an attack of scarlet fever and it is thought they may be due to a state of hypersensitivity resulting from the streptococcal infection.

Scarlet fever may also be classified as a pyogenic infection (see later).

Typhoid and Paratyphoid Fevers (Enteric Fevers)

Typhoid means resembling typhus. Typhus means a stupor and both typhus fever (see p 60) and typhoid fever are severe infections which may result in a stuporous or comatose condition in the patient.

The paratyphoid fevers A, B and C run a similar but generally milder course than typhoid fever. Together with typhoid, they constitute the **enteric fevers**, enteritis (i.e. inflammatory changes in the bowel) being a prominent feature in all these conditions which are due to bacteria belonging to a group of intestinal pathogens known as salmonellae.

These fevers are spread by water or food containing the causal bacteria as a result of contamination by the excreta of either patients suffering from the disease, or of **healthy carriers**. The latter are individuals who have apparently recovered from an attack of the disease but continue thereafter, often for many years, to excrete typhoid or paratyphoid bacilli in their urine or faeces.

The main features of typhoid fever are initially **septicaemia** (a condition in which the causal pathogens are present and multiplying in the bloodstream); a fever producing a characteristic step-ladder temperature chart; a scanty rash consisting of rose-spots; diarrhoea with so-called pea-soup stools, starting during the second week of the disease; and the development of a stuporous state.

Blood culture (i.e. the growing of any pathogens present in the blood on suitable bacteriological media) during the earliest stages of the infection, and, subsequently, performance of a test on the blood called the **Widal test** are important diagnostic investigations in enteric fevers.

The incubation period of this group of fevers is about 7–14 days. Complications due to enteritis are haemorrhage from ulcers in the small intestine and perforation of this part of the bowel. Other complications include **cholecystitis** (inflammation of the gall bladder).

Either chloramphenicol or ampicillin, which are both antibiotics, are often of great value in treatment. Cases must be nursed with barrier precautions.

Active immunisation with **TABC vaccine** is employed with the object of reducing the incidence of the disease. These initials indicate the vaccine is constituted so as to produce antibodies against typhoid and paratyphoid fevers A, B and C.

Meningococcal Meningitis (Cerebrospinal Fever)

This is a bacterial disease due to an organism called the *meningococcus*. The infection begins in the nasopharynx and from here the pathogens enter the bloodstream causing a septicaemia. In most instances the infection later becomes localised in the meninges, thus accounting for the descriptive name of meningococcal meningitis. The disease used to be called **spotted fever**, as a purpuric rash not infrequently develops at an early stage of the disease.

Neck rigidity is an important sign of meningeal irritation due to inflammatory changes in the meninges.

The causative micro-organisms can be demonstrated by microscopy of stained films made from a sample of cerebrospinal fluid obtained by lumbar puncture.

Complications include various paralyses of cranial nerves, bronchopneumonia and hydrocephalus.

Treatment is by penicillin, sometimes supplemented by sulphonomides.

Besides the meningococcus a number of other bacteria can cause acute meningitis e.g. *pneumococcus*, *haemophilus influenzae*, etc.

PYOGENIC INFECTIONS

When certain bacteria, such as the *staphylococcus*, *streptococcus*, *meningococcus*, *gonococcus*, *Escherichia coli* and *bacillus proteus* cause infection, they provoke an inflammatory reaction which often results in **suppuration**, i.e. the formation of pus. The word **pyogenic** means producing pus and infections characterised by purulent inflammatory exudates are therefore frequently termed **pyogenic infections** (**purulent** means consisting of pus).

The pathogens most commonly responsible for such infections are the staphylococcus and the streptococcus.

Two pyogenic infections, scarlet fever and meningococcal meningitis, have already been referred to as they may also be classified as infectious fevers. Gonococcal infection will be considered later when discussing terms relating to venereal diseases.

Staphylococcal Infections

These tend usually to take the form of localised abscesses. They may sometimes progress to **staphylococcal septicaemia** or **pyaemia**, but these latter conditions are not common.

Some important conditions caused by staphylococcal infection are as follows.

Skin and subcutaneous tissues: **furuncle** (a small abscess due to infection in a hair follicle or sweat gland known more widely as a **boil**); **carbuncle** (a condition akin to a boil but larger, consisting of several adjacent abscess cavities within a localised area of inflammation); **paronychia** (infection of the tissues around a fingernail, known also as a **whitlow**); **pulp infection of a finger**; **wound infections**, including also wounds involving other tissues besides the skin and subcutaneous tissues (a **wound** is a gap in an external or internal body surface caused by injury).

Bone—**staphylococcal osteomyelitis** (inflammation of bone).

Lung—**staphylococcal pneumonia** (inflammation of lung tissue).

Treatment of staphylococcal infections is by antibiotic drugs. Surgical treatment may also be required to drain abscesses.

Streptococcal Infections

In contradistinction to staphylococci, streptococci tend to produce diffuse spreading inflammatory lesions.

Involvement of draining lymph vessels and glands, causing respectively **lymphangitis** and **lymphadenitis**, is not uncommon and spread to the blood causing **streptococcal septicaemia** occasionally occurs.

Some important conditions caused by streptococci are as follows.

Skin and subcutaneous tissues—a spreading inflammation of connective tissue called **cellulitis**. A severe form of cellulitis is seen in the streptococcal infection called **erysipelas**, a term meaning redness of the skin. (In olden days erysipelas was known as St Anthony's fire.)

Pharynx—**streptococcal tonsillitis**. Infection of the throat with a certain type of streptococcus causes **scarlet fever** (see p 52).

Ear—**otitis media** (inflammation of the middle ear).

Bone—**streptococcal osteomyelitis** (inflammation of bone).

Heart—**subacute bacterial endocarditis** (see p 72).

Many authorities also consider that the disease called **rheumatic fever**, and certain types of the kidney disorder called **nephritis**, are manifestations of a state of hypersensitivity produced as a direct result of streptococcal infection in the tonsils or elsewhere in the pharynx.

Female genital tract—**puerperal sepsis** (see p 193).

Streptococcal infections are treated by antibiotics and in some instances also by adjuvant surgery.

TUBERCULOSIS

The basic lesions in this disease are small nodules of chronic inflammatory tissue, which develop at sites where the invading pathogens establish themselves. These nodules are termed **tubercles** and the causative micro-organisms, which belong to a class of bacteria termed acid-fast bacilli, are called *tubercle bacilli* or, alternatively, *mycobacteria tuberculosis* or *Koch's bacilli* after Robert Koch, the famous German bacteriologist.

Tuberculosis means a condition in which tubercles are present.

A first infection with the disease constitutes **primary tuberculosis**, and most individuals who live in civilised communities contract such an infection but, in most instances, in so mild a form that no recognisable ill-effects ensue. Common sites of primary tuberculosis are in the respiratory and alimentary tracts and their draining lymph glands. In subsequent years, sites of former lesions may be rendered apparent by small areas of pathological calcification in the lung and hilar lymph glands, or in lymph glands in the neck or mesentery.

Infection may be (i) with *human type tubercle bacilli* derived from inhalation of air or ingestion of food contaminated by the sputum of another human being with active tuberculosis, or (ii) with *bovine type tubercle bacilli* found in milk and milk products obtained from infected cattle. This type of infection is now uncommon in the UK as a result of tuberculin-testing of dairy herds and pasteurisation of milk.

Once it has subsided, the initial infective process gives the affected individual a varying degree of immunity against further tuberculous infection. Sometimes, however, primary tuberculosis may cause clinical signs and symptoms of some severity and may also produce **metastatic tuberculous infections**. These latter result from tubercle bacilli entering the bloodstream or lymphatic channels, and thus being carried to distant organs and tissues where they produce secondary (metastatic) infective lesions.

Note: The word **metastasis** (plural: metastases) indicates a secondary lesion of a disease, occurring in a site at a distance from the first or primary centre of disease. While it is used with reference to various infective disorders, this term finds its widest use in relation to malignant disorders.

Metastatic tuberculosis may supervene during the active stage of primary tuberculosis but occurs much more frequently as a result of reactivation of *tubercle bacilli* which have been lying dormant in an apparently healed primary focus of infection. It is found in sites such as the lungs, bones and joints, kidneys, uterine tubes, peritoneum and meninges; and, when tubercle bacilli are able to enter the bloodstream in large numbers, it may occur in a generalised form called **miliary tuberculosis**, with disseminate lesions in many different organs.

In addition to reactivation of an old tuberculous focus, infection occurring subsequent to primary tuberculosis may result from reinfection, with *tubercle bacilli* from a source outside the body. It is believed that reinfection may be a cause of the condition termed **postprimary pulmonary tuberculosis**, particularly in older subjects (see p 99), but that this type of infection is more commonly due to reactivation of a former tuberculous lesion.

Metastatic tuberculosis infection and tuberculosis due to reinfection may both be described as forms of **secondary tuberculosis**.

Postprimary pulmonary tuberculosis can also produce metastatic tuberculous lesions through spread of bacilli by the blood and lymphatics. Extension of this type of disease, however, occurs more commonly through direct spread in the sputum of the *tubercle bacilli* to other sites in the respiratory system and also the digestive system. This type of spread may cause complications such as tuberculous bronchopneumonia, tracheobronchial tuberculosis, tuberculous laryngitis, intestinal tuberculosis, and tuberculous infection in the region of the anus. This latter is very rarely associated with fistula formation resulting in a condition known as **fistula-in-ano**.

Note: tuberculosis is only one of a number of causes of fistula-in-ano.

Susceptibility to tuberculosis infection may be investigated by **tuberculin testing**. In this procedure a substance obtained from tubercle bacilli, and called tuberculin, is injected into the skin by intradermal injection as in the **Mantoux test**, or by a mechanical device making multiple minute punctures as in the **Heaf test**.

Negative reactors to tuberculin tests may be actively immunised by injection of an attenuated (weakened) strain of tubercle bacillus called the *Bacillus–Calmette–Guérin*. This procedure is generally termed **BCG vaccination**.

Measures to raise the general resistance to infection such as adequate rest, adequate diet and fresh air, are important in the treatment of tuberculosis. Chemotherapy with **antituberculous drugs** such as ethambutol and rifampicin is extensively employed and surgery is required in some types of lesion.

Calcification in cervical, hilar, or mesenteric lymph glands, and in lung tissues showing sites of former primary tuberculous infection is a common incidental finding in radiographs of the neck, chest and abdomen.

Radiological investigation plays an important part in the detection and assessment of the progress under treatment of postprimary pulmonary tuberculosis; and also in those cases of primary tuberculosis in which the infection is severe enough to produce clinical signs and symptoms of disease. It is also of great value in the diagnosis of tuberculous infection in the urinary system, locomotor system and female reproductive system.

SEXUALLY TRANSMITTED (VENEREAL) DISEASES

As indicated by their modern designation 'sexually transmitted' and their older designation 'venereal' (derived from the Latin word meaning love) infections of this type are usually, but not invariably, transmitted by sexual intercourse.

Syphilis

This infection may be congenital (due to infection of a fetus in-utero from the maternal bloodstream) or acquired and is due to a spirochaete (a type of bacterium) called *Treponema pallidum*.

Acquired Syphilis

This disease is first manifested in the form of a primary stage. Subsequently other stages of infection may develop if it is untreated or inadequately treated. The various stages of acquired syphilis are described as follows.

Primary syphilis—characterised by the development of a **primary sore**, or **chancre**, which is usually on the genital organs. It appears about a month after the infection is contracted.

Secondary syphilis—appears about six weeks after the development of the primary sore. At this stage, dissemination of spirochaetes, by the bloodstream, has resulted in generalised infection of the body tissues. Common manifestations are skin rashes, sore throat, pain in bones, etc. Sometimes localised nodular thickening develop on bony surfaces. These are called **periosteal nodes**.

Latent syphilis—a stage after healing of the secondary lesions, in which there are no clinical signs and symptoms of active disease. This stage may last many years.

Tertiary syphilis—in this stage, lesions confined to a particular organ or tissue are often seen. The lesions are of many types: among them are swellings called **gummas**, syphilitic **osteitis** (inflammation of bone), syphilitic disease of the heart and aorta, and manifestations of **neurosyphilis** (i.e. syphilitic infection of the nervous system) of the type called **meningovascular syphilis**.

Quaternary syphilis—two types of neurosyphilis may occur at this stage, namely, **tabes dorsalis** (locomotor ataxia) and **general paralysis of the insane** (dementia paralytica).

Congenital Syphilis

A pregnant woman who has syphilis in either active or latent form can transmit the infection to her unborn child. This may result in either abortion, stillbirth, or the birth of a living child whose tissues are widely infected with spirochaetes.

Thus, in congenital syphilis there is no primary stage and the manifestations of the disease are usually referred to as early and late.

Signs of **early congenital syphilis** usually begin to appear during the early weeks of life, e.g. loss of weight, inflammation of bone and cartilage around the nasal cavities causing a condition known by the descriptive name of **snuffles**, inflammatory lesions in bone, fissures around the mouth, skin rashes.

In **late congenital syphilis** infection of bone is also common, as are inflammatory changes in the cornea of the eye, known as **interstitial keratitis**, and other eye lesions. Neurosyphilitic lesions may also occur. The permanent teeth may be deformed and the incisors may be of a type called **Hutchinson's teeth**.

> The periosteal nodes of secondary syphilis, and the bone lesions which may develop in the tertiary and congenital forms of the disease, produce changes demonstrable by radiography. Syphilitic disease of the aorta and heart may also produce radiographic evidence of their presence.

Investigation of a suspected case of syphilis may consist of demonstration of the causal spirochaetes in material obtained from the primary sore by dark ground microscopy and various tests on samples of blood and cerebrospinal fluid. These latter include the **Wassermann reaction** and now more widely used **VDRL** (VD Research Laboratory), **FTA** (fluorescent treponemal antibody) and **TPHA** (*Treponema pallidum* haemagglutination) tests.

The treatment of syphilitic infection is principally by penicillin.

Gonorrhoea

In males, the initial result of this infection is an acute inflammation of the urethra with consequent production of a purulent urethral discharge. It is from this discharge that the name of the disease derives, gonorrhoea meaning a flowing of seminal fluid although, in reality, the flow is of pus formed in the urethra.

Infection is due to a bacterium called the *gonococcus* or, alternatively, the *Neisseria gonorrhoeae*, and gonorrhoea is thus sometimes referred to as **neisserian infection**.

In females the disease usually begins as a **urethritis** (inflammation of the urethra) or **cervicitis** (inflammation of the cervix of the uterus).

Direct spread of pathogens along the genital tract to the prostate gland in the male, or the uterine tubes in the female, may cause respectively **prostatitis** (inflammation of the prostate gland) or **salpingitis** (inflammation of the uterine tubes).

Gonococci rarely spread by the bloodstream but if they do so may cause metastatic inflammatory lesions in other structures such as **iritis** (inflammation of the iris diaphragm of the eye), **arthritis** (inflammation of joints), **bursitis** (inflammation of bursae), and **fasciitis** (inflammation of fasciae).

In males the urethritis may sometimes result in a localised area of narrowing in the urethra, called a **urethral stricture**.

Infants born to infected mothers may show evidence of an eye infection, called **ophthalmia neonatorum** (eye inflammation of the newly born) about three days after birth. This condition may be due to organisms other than the gonococcus, e.g. staphylococcus. It can lead to blindness in the more severe types of case.

The treatment of gonorrhoea is primarily by penicillin, but other drugs may be necessary when the causative organisms belong to strains which do not exhibit a normal susceptibility to the action of this antibiotic, and are thus termed penicillin-resistant.

Other Sexually Transmitted Diseases

The other principal diseases:

Non-specific urethritis—a disease predominantly of males which nowadays has a greater incidence in Britain than gonorrhoea but is not always of venereal origin. It occasionally occurs together with symptoms of conjunctivitis and arthritis in so-called **Reiter's syndrome**.

Note: a **syndrome** is a combination of symptoms which occur together.

Chancroid (soft sore)—due to *Haemophilus ducreyi*.

Lymphogranuloma venereum (LGV), also known as **lymphogranuloma inguinale**—a tropical infection due to a species of *chlamydia*.

Granuloma inguinale—a bacterial infection due to *Donovania granulomatis*.

Genital herpes—an infection due to the herpes simplex viruses (the virus also responsible for labial herpes see p 229). It is transmitted by sexual intercourse, and sometimes by other forms of direct physical contact, and produces small vesicles (blisters) on and around the genital organs. These lesions subsequently develop into painful ulcers, which are slow to heal and may recur. Enlarged inguinal glands and general systemic upset may be features of the disease.

Acquired immune deficiency syndrome (AIDS) and **viral hepatitis**—both these diseases can be transmitted sexually as well as by other means (see pp 36 and 135).

SOME OTHER INFECTIVE DISEASES

Tetanus, typhus fever, actinomycosis, glandular fever, Weil's disease and undulant fever will be discussed briefly in this section. Coryza and influenza and certain other virus infections will be referred to when discussing infections of the respiratory tract. Infections which occur chiefly in tropical climates will be discussed in Part V.

Tetanus (Lockjaw)

This disease is due to a bacterium, called the *Clostridium tetani*, which lives normally in the intestines of horses and sheep. Infection is caused by soil contaminated by the excreta of such animals entering wounds. Such contamination is common in cultivated ground and in road dust. Active immunisation with tetanus toxoid is a highly efficient method of prophylaxis.

While tetanus produces a localised type of infection in a wound, the causal pathogens secrete a powerful exotoxin which spreads both locally and to the central nervous system, producing muscle spasms and rigidity. The former usually begin in the muscles of mastication (eating). Spasm of these muscles is called **trismus** and results in inability to open the mouth, thus explaining the term **lockjaw**, which is also used to describe the disease. The word tetanus is derived from a Greek word meaning to stretch.

The onset of trismus is followed, after a varying interval, by the appearance of generalised muscle spasms which not infrequently result in death from exhaustion or cardiac failure or complicating pneumonia.

Antitoxin and sedatives and muscle relaxants are employed in treatment and highly skilled nursing is of prime importance.

Typhus Fever

The word typhus means a stupor. There are various forms of typhus fever, such as **epidemic typhus** (transmitted by lice), **endemic typhus** (transmitted by rat fleas) and **scrub typhus** (transmitted by small parasitic insects of the variety called mites).

The most important of these is epidemic typhus, an acute and sometimes fatal fever which tends to appear in epidemic form during wars and times of famine.

An **endemic disease** is one which characteristically occurs more or less constantly in a particular region or locality. Endemic typhus tends to be confined to certain regions in the tropics and subtropics and does not show the widespread incidence which can develop in epidemic typhus, when conditions are suitable for the spread of this latter disease.

The above-mentioned forms of typhus are all caused by various types of rickettsiae (see p 34). Some other febrile rickettsial infections are often described as being members of the so-called typhus group of fevers, e.g. **Q (Query) fever, Rocky Mountain spotted fever, trench fever**.

In epidemic, endemic and scrub typhus, the diagnosis may be confirmed by a blood test for anti-rickettsial antibodies called the **Weil-Felix reaction**.

Actinomycosis

Actinomycosis, thought formerly to be a fungus disease, is caused by a bacterium called *Actinomyces israeli*.

Infection with this organism leads to chronic inflammatory lesions in the tissues. The common sites for primary infection are the face and jaws, the intestine and the lung. Metastatic spread of the disease is not uncommon.

Pulmonary actinomycosis may be either primary or metastatic. Extension of disease to the chest wall and erosion of ribs are sometimes seen as complications of the lung lesions.

The ileocaecal region is a common site for intestinal actinomycosis, and the early signs and symptoms of this condition may be confused with those of appendicitis.

The formation of small abscess cavities and multiple sinuses is a frequent feature of actinomycotic lesions. Actinomycotic pus contains characteristic small granules known as **sulphur granules** on account of their yellow colour.

Weil's Disease

A disease due to a spirochaete called the *Leptospira icterohaemorrhagiae*. As indicated by the name of this pathogen, jaundice (icterus) and haemorrhages into mucous membranes are prominent clinical features in most cases. Kidney damage also frequently occurs and may lead to renal failure.

Infection is derived from food or water, contaminated with rat's urine, or less commonly from a rat bite. The causal spirochaete is a natural parasite of rats and is of world wide distribution.

Weil's disease is uncommon in Britain. It was named after Adolf Weil, a German physician.

Undulant Fever (Abortus Fever)

This infection, worldwide in distribution, is caused by *Brucella abortus*, a species of the Brucella genus of bacteria named after Sir David Bruce, a British Army surgeon.

The disease is contracted through contact with infected cattle or by drinking unpasteurised milk from infected cows. It is characterised by a swinging type of fever, hence the name undulant fever. Headache, arthritis, splenic enlargement, and, rarely, infective lesions in spinal vertebrae demonstrable by radiography, are among the other features of the disease.

Treatment is by antibiotics.

The related condition, **Malta fever** (Mediterranean fever) is classified as a tropical disease and is caused by drinking milk from goats infected with another species of Brucella called *Brucella melitensis*.

PART IV

Diseases of the Various Systems of the Body and Obstetric Terms

---

The various terms indicated on p 47 as meriting special notice with reference to infective disease are also highly relevant to descriptions in this part of the book. Also of considerable importance are the following:

prefixes:	**dys-**	difficult, e.g. dysphagia—difficulty in swallowing.
	haem-	blood, e.g. haemorrhage—a flow of blood.
	hydro-	fluid, e.g. hydrothorax—fluid in the pleural cavity.
	pneumo-	air (or gas), e.g. pneumothorax—air in the pleural cavity.
	py-	pus, e.g. pyogenic—pus-producing.
suffixes:	**-ectomy**	removal, e.g. gastrectomy—removal of stomach.
	-itis	inflammation, e.g. gastritis—inflammation of stomach.
	-oma	tumour, e.g. epithelioma—epithelial tumour.
	-oscopy	visual examination, e.g. gastroscopy—visual examination of the interior of the stomach by a gastroscope.
	-osis	a condition of, or indicating a degenerative condition, e.g. diverticulosis, a condition of diverticula and spondylosis, a degenerative disorder of the vertebrae.
	-ostomy	making an opening into, e.g. gastrostomy—making an opening into the stomach.
	-otomy	making an incision into or through a structure, e.g. laparotomy—making an incision into the abdominal cavity.

In addition to the prefixes and suffixes are: the word **lesion**, meaning an injury and widely used to indicate any form of structural damage to the body tissue, caused by disease; and the word **lumen** describing the space in the interior of any hollow structure, e.g. the lumen of the intestine, indicating the space enclosed by the intestinal wall.

CARDIOVASCULAR SYSTEM

Some Anatomical and Physiological Considerations

The **cardiovascular system** is concerned with the circulation of blood throughout the body and consists of the heart and the blood vessels.

The circulation is maintained by the pumping action of the heart muscle which pumps blood into (*a*) the *pulmonary circulation*, wherein deoxygenated blood is reoxygenated while passing through the capillaries in the lungs; and (*b*) the *systemic circulation*, wherein oxygenated blood is carried to the various organs and tissues of the body. The main arterial trunk in this circulation is the *aorta* which arises from the left ventricle. All the blood passing through the systemic circulation returns to the right side of the heart, via the *superior vena cava* or *inferior cava*, and then passes through the pulmonary circulation and is re-oxygenated.

During its course some of the blood in the systemic circulation passes through (*c*) the *portal circulation* on its return journey to the heart. The main vessel of the portal circulation is the *portal vein*, which is formed by the union of the *superior mesenteric* and *splenic veins* and carries venous blood, from the small and large intestine and the spleen, to the liver. Having passed through the liver capillaries, this blood is carried by the *hepatic veins* to the inferior vena cava.

The heart muscle is termed the *myocardium* and is lined by a membrane, the *endocardium*, which also covers the cusps of the heart valves. On its outer aspect the myocardium is covered by the inner and outer layers of a membrane called the *pericardium*.

In early fetal life the heart consists of a single tube which subsequently becomes folded and divided into the *right atrium* and *left atrium*, separated by the *interatrial septum*, and the *right ventricle* and *left ventricle*, separated by the *interventricular septum*.

The period during which the heart muscle contracts is called *systole*, and that during which it relaxes, *diastole*. The pressure maintained in the circulation by the pumping action of the heart is called the *blood pressure* and is normally about 40–60 millimetres of mercury (mm Hg) higher in systole than in diastole.

The pumping action of the heart results in each period of systole causing an expansile impulse throughout the arteries. This impulse may be felt in superficial arteries (e.g. the radial, femoral and carotid arteries) and is known as the *pulse*.

The output of the heart at each beat and the number of beats per minute may both be increased by the action of the sympathetic nervous system. Such action occurs as a result of the liberation of adrenaline at certain nerve terminals and the resultant stimulation of sites termed β-receptors, and found in the heart and other effector organs and tissues.

The prefix **card-** and the adjective **cardiac** mean pertaining to the heart but are sometimes also used with reference to the cardiac orifice of the stomach.

Blood vessels consist of *arteries*, *veins* and *capillaries*. Small arteries may be termed *arterioles* and small veins described as *venules*.

Arteries and arterioles possess three coats (*a*) the *adventitia*—an outer coat composed of fibrous and elastic tissue, (*b*) the *media*—composed of smooth muscle and elastic tissue, (*c*) the *intima*—composed of endothelium lining the *lumen* (interior) of the vessel.

The prefix **angio-** means pertaining to a blood vessel, **arterio-** pertaining to an artery, **phlebo-** and **veno-** pertaining to a vein.

Some General Aspects of Cardiovascular Diseases

Diseases of the cardiovascular system may be congenital or acquired. Traumatic, infective and, rarely, neoplastic diseases may affect this system, but of much greater incidence among the acquired disorders are many of unknown or incompletely understood causation, e.g. hypertension (high blood pressure), coronary artery disease, and other forms of atheromatous disease, rheumatic heart disease, deep vein thrombosis. Heart disease occurring as secondary effect of chronic lung disease and known as **pulmonary heart disease**, is also common.

Among the clinical symptoms and signs which may be associated with heart disease are: **dyspnoea** (difficult breathing, shortness of breath) on exertion or at rest; pain in the chest on exertion; **oedema** (swelling) around the ankles and elsewhere in the soft tissues; **cyanosis** (blueness of the skin and mucous membrane); abnormalities in the rate and rhythm of the heart; cardiac enlargement and the presence of abnormal cardiac murmurs (heart sounds).

Various signs and symptoms caused by disordered blood circulation may occur in regions affected by diseases of blood vessels, sometimes with accompanying pain.

The branch of medicine concerned with diseases of the heart is called **cardiology**, and working within this speciality are two grades of technicians, known respectively as physiological measurement technicians in cardiology, and as cardiographers.

Special Methods of Investigation

In ordinary clinical examination, **auscultation** (listening) with a stethoscope and **estimation of the systolic** and **diastolic blood pressure** with a **sphygmomanometer** are important procedures in many types of cardiovascular disease, as may also be various forms of plain radiography and certain pathological investigations. In addition, certain specialised examination methods may be used and among these are the following.

Electrocardiography—the suffix **-graphy** is derived from the Greek word for writing and in this context denotes the making of a record. This procedure records minute electrical currents produced by contractions of various parts of the heart muscle. The recording may be effected so as to produce an image that can be recorded as a tracing on a screen or on photographic paper. This procedure is of great value in the investigation of many heart disorders, e.g. coronary thrombosis, disorders of cardiac rate and rhythm, heart block.

Ultrasound cardiography (UCG)—also referred to as **echocardiography**—a method of special value in investigating disorders of the mitral and aortic valves, and of pericardial effusions, and the group of disorders of the heart muscle termed the cardiomyopathies.

Cardiac catheterisation—an investigation where a long, thin, flexible catheter (tube) is inserted into the lumen of a fairly large superficial artery or vein (e.g. femoral or brachial artery; an antecubital vein, femoral vein) and manipulated under X-ray control to enter either the left or right side of the heart.

Valuable information may be obtained by recording pressures in various heart chambers and great vessels, and also by withdrawing samples of blood from such sites and analysing their oxygen content.

Abnormal openings between various chambers of the heart (called **septal defects**) may also be shown by cardiac catheterisation and it is frequently convenient to combine this procedure with certain forms of contrast radiography (e.g. angiocardiography, coronary arteriography), the contrast medium being injected through the catheter at the conclusion of the other investigations.

Angiography—this term describes various forms of X-ray investigation whereby blood vessels are filled with radiographic contrast media and demonstrated by fluoroscopy or by taking radiographs. Cinéradiography is used in several instances.

Among such investigations are angiocardiography (demonstrating the interiors of the chambers of the heart), coronary arteriography, pulmonary arteriography, aortography, cerebral arteriography, peripheral arteriography and various forms of phlebography (contrast radiography of veins, also known as venography).

Nuclear cardiology—investigation of cardiac function, circulation time, presence of myocardial infarcts, etc., by radionuclide imaging techniques.

Performance of various tests, which determine the response of the heart to exercise, and are called **exercise tolerance tests**.

Biochemical investigations, e.g. estimating certain serum enzymes in the diagnosis of myocardial infarction.

Congenital Diseases of the Heart (Congenital Morbus Cordis)

Congenital diseases of the heart are a group of conditions resulting from errors of development of the heart and the great vessels arising from it. They vary greatly in severity, ranging from small isolated defects of little clinical importance to severe multiple abnormalities, resulting in early death of the patient. Their cause is unknown, although an association has in some cases been shown between infection with **rubella** (German measles) in early pregnancy and the subsequent birth of an infant with congenital cardiac disease.

Congenital cardiac lesions are frequently associated with congenital defects in structures elsewhere in the body.

In some types of congenital heart disease a communication exists between the two sides of the heart permitting the passage of blood from one side of this organ to the other. This is known as a **shunt**. When a patient has a **right-to-left shunt**, deoxygenated blood is passed to the left side of the heart and thus into the systemic circulation. This results in **cyanosis**, i.e. blueness of the skin and mucous membranes, and accounts for infants with a certain type of heart disease being described as blue-babies.

Valuable information about the presence and nature of a shunt may be derived from cardiac catheterisation and angiocardiography.

Some of the principal types of congenital heart disease will now be indicated. It should, however, be remembered that in many cases congenital defects may be multiple and a combination of different lesions may be found in the same patient.

Fallot's tetralogy—Fallot was a French physician and the term **tetralogy** indicates that a combination of four anomalies are found: (i) stenosis (narrowing) of the pulmonary artery; (ii) a defect in the inter-ventricular septum; (iii) an aorta which, instead of arising solely from the left ventricle, 'overrides' the interventricular septum and thus receives blood from the right and left ventricle, i.e. there is a right-to left shunt; (iv) an enlarged right ventricle.

The principal clinical features are cyanosis and shortness of breath.

Radiographs may show that the heart shape resembles a boot and that there is a deficiency of vascular markings in the lungs resulting from the narrowing of the pulmonary artery.

Suitable cases are treated by surgery.

Isolated pulmonary stenosis—a condition in which narrowing occurs at the pulmonary valve or just below the root of the pulmonary artery in the portion of the right ventricle called the *pulmonary conus*. There is no shunt in this condition, and no cyanosis:

This defect varies considerably in severity. It may cause little disability or, alternatively, it may result in severe breathlessness and progress to cardiac failure. Selected cases are treated by an operation called **pulmonary valvotomy**.

Patent ductus arteriosus—the *ductus arteriosus* is a vessel which during fetal life, when the lungs need very little blood, carries most of the blood from the pulmonary artery into the aorta. When respiration starts, immediately after birth, the lungs need all the blood in the pulmonary artery so the ductus normally closes shortly after birth.

Failure of closure constitutes the condition of patent ductus arteriosus. After birth the pressure of blood is higher in the aorta than the pulmonary artery; thus the direction of blood flow through the ductus is reversed and the anomaly results in excess blood in the lungs. It is to be noted that, although there is a shunt present, in this instance it is from left to right so there is no cyanosis.

Breathlessness on exertion is the cardinal symptom, which may be delayed until adult life is reached. Patients with a patent ductus show a special liability to develop an infective cardiac disease called **subacute bacterial endocarditis**. On this account surgery in childhood is often advised for mild cases as well as for those who suffer from disability due to the disease.

Coarctation of the aorta—the term **coarctation** means a narrowing, and in this condition there is congenital stenosis in the distal part of the arch of the aorta.

As a result of this stenosis, there is high blood pressure in the head, neck and arms and low blood pressure in the lower part of the trunk and legs. To remedy this deficient circulation in the lower part of the body, a **collateral circulation** is developed by enlarging the **anastomoses** (communicating channels) between arteries arising above and below the narrow segment of the aorta. As a result of this, one of the clinical signs of the condition is the presence of dilated arteries over the chest and back.

On X-ray films a characteristic notching of the ribs may be seen, resulting from enlargement of the intercostal arteries produced by collateral circulation through these vessels. The actual coarctation can be demonstrated by arch aortography.

The degree of aortic narrowing varies considerably and in some cases there may be no symptoms until late in life. In young patients operation may be advised, the narrow area of the aorta being resected.

Some patients with coarctation of the aorta may develop haemorrhage from small **congenital aneurysms** at the base of the brain, which frequently occur in association with this disease. An **aneurysm** is a localised dilatation of a blood vessel.

Atrial septal defect (auricular septal defect)—in this disease there is a defect in the interatrial (interauricular) septum between the two atria of the heart. Consequently there is a left-to-right shunt which increases the amount of blood in the right side of the heart and in the pulmonary artery. Breathlessness is the cardinal symptom of the disease. The shunt being from left-to-right there is normally no cyanosis, but in severe cases reversal of the shunt may sometimes occur.

The onset of symptoms are often delayed until adulthood. Treatment is surgical in suitable cases.

Atrial septal defect may be found in combination with **congenital mitral stenosis** (narrowing of the orifice of the mitral valve, which lies between the left atrium and left ventricle). The combination of these two anomalies is known as **Lutembacher's syndrome**, after the French physician R. Lutembacher. A **syndrome** is a combination of symptoms.

Ventricular septal defect—there are two types of ventricular septal defect: (i) a small defect, which may cause an abnormal cardiac murmur but which generally gives rise to no disability. This type is known as **Maladie de Roger**; (ii) a large defect in the interventricular septum, with a large left-to-right shunt. Like an interatrial septal defect this leads to excess blood entering the right side of the heart and pulmonary circulation. Certain types of interventricular septal defects may be closed surgically.

Dextrocardia—a condition in which the apex of the heart is found on the right side (**dextro-** means right). In uncomplicated cases the heart is a complete mirror image of the normal heart and the aortic knuckle is also found on the right side.

Dextrocardia is often found to be associated with a similar reverse position of the abdominal viscera, i.e. the liver lying in the left side of the abdomen, and the stomach in the right side. This is termed **transposition of the viscera**.

Some other types of congenital heart disease. There are a great variety of different types of congenital disease. Some of the rarer forms are described by the following names:

Bicuspid aortic valve, **congenital aortic stenosis** (narrowing of aortic valve), **double aortic arch**, **Eisenmenger's syndrome**, **persistent truncus arteriosus** (the aorta and pulmonary artery possess a communication of varying size owing to failure in the development of the septum between them), **pulmonary atresia** (failure of development of the orifice of the pulmonary valve), **right-sided aortic arch**, **transposition of the great vessels** (the aorta arises from the right ventricle and the pulmonary artery from the left ventricle in this condition which is associated with septal defect), **tricuspid atresia** (failure of development of the tricuspid valve orifice between the right atrium and right ventricle), **anomalous pulmonary venous drainage** (some, or all, of the blood from the lungs drains into the right atrium; either directly or indirectly, e.g. via the superior or inferior vena cava, or other vessel. There is an associated intracardiac shunt.

Inflammatory Diseases of the Heart

The most important of these are **rheumatic heart disease**, an inflammatory condition whose exact cause has not been determined, and **bacterial endocarditis**, in which the inflammatory lesions develop as a result of infection.

Syphilitic aortic regurgitation is secondary to syphilitic inflammation of the aorta and will be referred to later when discussing diseases of arteries.

Inflammatory changes in the heart muscle may also develop as a complication of certain other infections (e.g. diphtheria, pyogenic infections, pneumonia, typhus) causing **myocarditis**, or in some instances a disorder referred to as **cardiomyopathy**; this latter term meaning disease of the heart muscle. (*Note*: cardiomyopathy may be due to causes other than infection, e.g. chronic alcoholism, vitamin deficiency—see later).

Inflammatory changes in the pericardium cause **pericarditis** and may result in the formation of a thick scanty inflammatory exudate— **dry pericarditis**, or the formation of an abundant fluid exudate— **pericardial effusion**. Among the causes of pericarditis are acute rheumatism, pyogenic infections, tuberculous infection and involvement of the pericardium by neoplastic (malignant) disease.

Pericarditis, especially tuberculous pericarditis, may result in fibrosis, contraction and pathological calcification in the pericardium, changes which impede the pumping action of the heart and constitute the disorder referred to as **chronic constrictive pericarditis**. This disorder is frequently amenable to surgical treatment.

Rheumatic Heart Disease

As has been stated by Duthie (1) the term **rheumatism** has been loosely applied to all conditions causing pain and stiffness in the muscles and joints.

Rheumatic heart disease, however, results from a specific type of rheumatic disorder termed **acute rheumatism** or a similar but less acute disorder called **subacute rheumatism**.

As indicated by Brimblecombe and Barltrop (2) the term **acute rheumatism** includes rheumatic fever, carditis, rheumatic nodules, erythema marginatum and chorea occurring singly, or in combination. **Rheumatic fever** is characterised by acute inflammatory changes in joints, often of a fleeting nature. **Erythema marginatum** is a skin disorder. **Chorea** may be referred to as rheumatism of the nervous system (p 286).

The principal pathological features of acute and subacute rheumatism are the occurrence of foci of inflammation in the connective tissues of affected structures. These foci produce **arthritis** in the joints, **carditis** in the heart and **chorea** when they occur in the nervous system. In the majority of sites the inflammatory changes resolve without causing permanent damage. This, however, does not always occur in the heart, where serious damage often results from fibrosis. This develops during healing of the lesions and causes chronic heart disease. Moreover, as recurrent attacks of acute rheumatism are common, each new attack may cause further cardiac damage.

The cause of acute rheumatism has not been established, but many authorities regard it as a manifestation of allergy to streptococcal infection in the throat. Its chief incidence is seen in childhood.

Rest and the administration of salicylate drugs and penicillin are important treatment measures during the acute stages of the condition. Subsequently, small doses of penicillin may be given as a prophylactic against further streptococcal infection because this latter carries a high risk of causing recurrence of acute rheumatism.

Any type of cardiac involvement in acute and subacute rheumatism is referred to as **rheumatic carditis**. Different types of this condition may be described as **rheumatic endocarditis**, **myocarditis** or **pericarditis** according to the part of the heart principally involved. Sometimes in cases with marked involvement of the pericardium an effusion may form between the two layers of pericardium. This is known as a **rheumatic pericardial effusion** and produces an appearance of gross cardiac enlargement on radiographs.

In the frequent instances when permanent cardiac damage follows rheumatic carditis, several different sequelae may develop, according to the extent and distribution of the lesions in the heart. The principal types of these are as follows.

Chronic rheumatic valvular disease of the heart—this is produced by fibrosis of the endocardial covering of the cusps of the cardiac valves. It may result in a valvular orifice becoming narrowed, i.e. in **valvular stenosis**, or in thickened valve cusps becoming unable to close a valvular orifice properly, i.e. in **valvular incompetence**. Alternatively, there may be a combination of stenosis and incompetence. One or more valves may be affected.

The chief types of chronic valvular disease caused by acute and subacute rheumatism are, first, **mitral stenosis** (narrowing of the orifice of the mitral valve) and, second, **aortic incompetence**, also known as **aortic regurgitation** (a condition in which the aortic valve cannot close properly). Much less common are **mitral incompetence, aortic stenosis** and **tricuspid valvular disease**.

Radiologically, cases with chronic valvular disease frequently show alterations in the shape of the heart which differ according to the valve or valves involved. There is often demonstrable cardiac enlargement, which, in advanced cases, may be very great. Pathological calcification in the mitral or aortic valves may sometimes be observed on fluoroscopy.

In mitral stenosis, enlargement of the left atrium may be demonstrable by plain radiography. Such enlargement may also be shown, by barium swallow, to cause displacement of the oesophagus.

A pericardial effusion may produce on X-ray films a characteristically shaped enlargement of the heart shadow with an absence of pulsation along its borders on fluoroscopy. This type of effusion may also be detected by ultrasound.

Many cases of mitral stenosis are now amenable to surgical treatment; the stenosis being relieved by an operation called **mitral valvotomy**; or, alternatively, the diseased valve may be replaced by an artificial valve.

Aortic stenosis may also be treated by either valvotomy or valve replacement, and aortic imcompetence by valve replacement.

Chronic myocarditis (myocardial fibrosis)—a sequel of myocardial involvement leading to fibrosis of varying extent in the heart muscle. When the fibrosis is extensive the pumping action of the heart may be seriously impeded.

Adherent pericardium—this condition is uncommon, but may be a sequel to marked involvement of the pericardium (whether resulting in an effusion, or not) in rheumatic carditis. The two layers of the pericardium become bound together in places by fibrous adhesions and this may seriously impede the heart's action and lead to cardiac enlargement. Pathological calcification may occur in the diseased pericardium.

Cardiac failure—heart failure may occur during the active phase of rheumatic carditis or as a result of any one of its sequelae.

Bacterial Endocarditis (Infective Endocarditis)

Bacterial endocarditis is a condition in which inflammatory changes occur in the endothelial coverings of the cardiac valves as a result of direct invasion by pathogenic bacteria. It is of two types, acute and subacute.

Acute bacterial endocarditis—a rare condition in which acute endocarditis usually occurs in the course of a general septicaemia caused by infection with organisms such as staphylococci, streptococci or pneumococci.

Subacute bacterial endocarditis—this disease is most frequently caused by infection with a type of streptococcus called *streptococcus viridans*. This organism is found as a normal inhabitant of the upper respiratory tract. If, however, it gains access to the bloodstream and invades the endocardium of the cardiac valves, it is capable of causing serious damage to these latter structures. Such damage is usually seen only in those whose hearts are already abnormal as a result of, either previous rheumatic endocarditis, or congenital heart disease. The inflammatory changes result in deposits of fibrin and blood platelets on the surface of the valve cusps. Such deposits are called **vegetations** and they can also form on artificial heart valves, which may therefore also be the site of infective endocarditis (**prosthetic endocarditis**). Fragments of vegetations may become detached forming emboli in the bloodstream and these may lodge in sites such as the skin, kidneys, spleen and brain.

Among the clinical features are fever, wasting, anaemia, enlargement of the heart and spleen, abnormal cardiac murmurs and signs and symptoms due to embolism.

The diagnosis is initially made on clinical grounds but can often be confirmed bacteriologically by growing the causal streptococci from a sample of blood. The test employed is called a **blood culture**.

Standard treatment is by prolonged therapy with appropriate antibiotic drugs.

Coronary Heart Disease (Coronary Insufficiency, Coronary Artery Disease)

This disease, which appears to be of increasing prevalence, is a common cause of disability and death in the UK especially in men.

A notable report of a joint working party of the Royal College of Physicians of London and the British Cardiac Society (3) refers to evidence that the causes of coronary heart disease are largely 'environmental and rooted in the modern affluent way of life'. Cigarette smoking, physical inactivity and high lipid concentrations in the blood plasma are indicated as risk factors.

Note: **lipids** are fatty substances, absorbed in the diet, transported in the blood and stored in the tissues as a source of energy. They include *triglycerides* (neutral fats); *compound lipids*, (classified into phospholipids, sphingomyelins, galactolipids); *sterols* (e.g. cholesterol and ergosterol); *fat soluble vitamins A, D, E* and *K*; and *prostaglandins*. Lipids are transported in the bloodstream in combined lipid and protein complexes called *lipoproteins*. These lipoproteins are of four main types: chylomicrons, and very low density, low density and high density lipoproteins referred to respectively by the letters VLDL, LDL and HDL. Abnormalities in the metabolism or transport of cholesterol, resulting in high plasma concentrations of this lipid substance (hypercholesterolaemia), are thought to be important factors in the causation of atheroma (see below). Animal fats, e.g., meat fat, butter and eggs, are rich sources of lipids. Substitution in the food of polyunsaturated fats of vegetable origin for animal fats can lower the amount of lipids in the blood. The term **hyperlipidaemia** indicates an increase of blood lipids above the normal.

The basic pathological process in coronary heart disease is the development of atheroma (degenerative arterial disease) in the coronary arteries, which arise from the ascending aorta and carry the blood supply of the heart muscle. The atheromatous changes produce areas of narrowing in the interiors of the arterial vessels in the coronary circulation, thus diminishing the supply of blood available to areas of the myocardium.

The term **ischaemia** has already been noted as indicating a localised deficiency of blood supply and coronary atheroma is the commonest cause of what is termed **ischaemic heart disease**, some authorities use this term and coronary artery disease as synonyms.

Clinically, coronary heart disease is manifested by angina pectoris and by coronary thrombosis.

Angina Pectoris (Angina of Effort)

Angina is cardiac pain which occurs when the blood supply to the myocardium is inadequate to meet increased demands arising from some physical exertion. It usually starts in the chest but may radiate to other regions. It is characteristically relieved by rest, and an attack may be cut short by taking a tablet of drug called glyceryl trinitrate (trinitrin). The long-term treatment includes the avoidance of undue exertion, and sedatives and beta-blocking drugs may be prescribed e.g. propranolol (Inderal).

In selected cases of angina, coronary bypass graft surgery may improve the myocardial blood supply and relieve the pain.

Demonstration of the extent of the atheromatous changes by coronary arteriography is an important measure in the assessment of patients for whom coronary surgery or transluminal angioplasty is contemplated.

True angina is sometimes mimicked by pain known as **pseudo-angina**. This may be caused by chronic inflammation of the oesophagus or by **Tietze's disease**, a condition in which there is a painful swelling of one or more rib cartilages.

Coronary Thrombosis (Coronary Occlusion, Myocardial Infarction, Cardiac Infarction)

The pathology of this form of coronary artery disease is largely explained by its several alternative names, given above. Sudden occlusion (blockage) of a coronary artery by the formation of a thrombus (clot) in an area of narrowing produced by atheromatous change in the arterial wall, deprives an area of myocardium of its blood supply. Arterial anastomoses (communicating channels) being poorly developed in the coronary circulation, the occlusion results in the death of an area of myocardium, the dead tissue being termed a **myocardial** or **cardiac infarct**.

The severity of the condition varies considerably according to the size of the vessel which is occluded. In most instances the onset is heralded by severe chest pain of sudden onset.

The dead muscular tissue of a cardiac infarct is, in the course of time, removed and converted into fibrous tissue, leaving an area of permanent weakness in the wall of the heart.

Coronary thrombosis usually presents a fairly characteristic clinical picture. Electrocardiography is a valuable procedure in this condition. Evidence of damage to the heart muscle may be shown by demonstrating raised blood levels of the enzymes *aspartate aminotransferase* (AST), *creatine kinase* (CK) and *lactic dehydrogenase* (LD). (*Note: enzymes* are substances found in living organisms which promote, or speed up chemical reactions, without themselves undergoing any change. They are nearly all protein in nature.)

A chest X-ray may be requested as a matter of some urgency when it is suspected that the disorder is complicated by heart failure. The radiograph is then of particular value in showing the presence or absence of pulmonary oedema (see p 79), as this influences the decision whether the treatment should include the giving of diuretics, i.e. drugs which increase the secretion of urine by the kidneys and therby decrease the amount of fluid in the lung alveoli.

The initial treatment of coronary thrombosis is rest and measures to relieve the pain associated with this condition. The heart is monitored, in order to detect any abnormalities of rhythm of the heart beat, and anticoagulant drugs may be given to prevent venous thrombosis and resultant pulmonary embolism. Later treatment may involve coronary by-pass surgery, or a procedure termed transluminal angioplasty, particularly in patients with angina.

Hypertensive Heart Disease

The term **hypertension** used with reference to the cardiovascular system, and without qualification, refers to **systemic arterial hypertension** and indicates an arterial blood pressure greater than normal in the systemic circulation (cf pulmonary hypertension and portal hypertension).

Hypertensive heart disease is a disease of the heart resulting from the increased load on the heart arising from the presence of sustained high blood pressure.

Hypertension is, in the vast majority of cases, of unknown origin and usually of the type termed **essential hypertension**, the word essential indicating that it is a primary condition and not secondary to any known cause (cf primary essential emphysema).

Some cases of essential hypertension, in which the disease is especially severe and rapidly progressive, fall into a subgroup called **malignant hypertension**.

Hypertension, in some cases, is secondary to renal (kidney) disease and is then called **hypertension of renal origin** (see p 163). In other cases it may be secondary to endocrine disorder, toxaemia of pregnancy, or certain types of drug treatment.

In most types of chronic hypertension there is widespread narrowing of small arterial vessels which causes increased resistance in the peripheral part of the circulation. The left ventricle, therefore, has to work harder to maintain its output against this resistance. As a result, it hypertrophies and eventually areas of fibrosis may develop in the myocardium. Ultimately, the condition may progress to one of heart failure.

Left ventricular enlargement in hypertensive heart disease may be demonstrated on plain chest radiographs and by fluoroscopy. Suspected hypertension of renal origin is investigated by isotope renography, intravenous urography, and sometimes also by renal arteriography.

In the treatment of the more severe types of hypertension, drugs which lower the blood pressure and are thus known as **hypotensive drugs** (e.g. methyldopa, clonidine, propranolol) are widely used.

It is to be noted that hypertension and coronary heart disease quite often coexist in the same patient.

Chronic Valvular Disease of the Heart

This term is usually used for acquired disorders of the heart valves. Acute rheumatism has already been noted as a common cause of valvular disease, particularly of mitral stenosis and aortic regurgitation. Syphillitic aortis has been indicated as causing syphilitic aortic regurgitation. The arterial disease atheroma which affects the coronary circulation in coronary heart disease can also affect the cusps of the aortic valve and is an important cause of aortic stenosis (narrowing of the orifice of the aortic valve).

Disturbances of Cardiac Rate and Rhythm (Cardiac Arrhythmias)

In health the average normal heart rate is, in a subject at rest, taken as 72 beats a minute. The beats are regularly spaced and of equal volume.

An abnormally rapid heart rate is called **tachycardia**, and an abnormally slow rate **bradycardia**.

Terms used to describe abnormalities of rhythm include the following.

Extrasystoles—premature contractions, which in the absence of organic heart disease are not of significance.

Paroxysmal tachycardia—intermittent attacks of tachycardia which may occur without apparent cause in some instances, but in others may be associated with coronary artery disease and other serious types of organic heart disease.

Atrial fibrillation (auricular fibrillation)—an abnormality of cardiac rhythm resulting from very rapid irregular and intermittent contractions of muscle fibres in the atrial walls. The ventricles, as a result, also contract irregularly and often at an increased rate.

Atrial fibrillation is a common complication of rheumatic mitral stenosis and of heart disease associated with overactivity of the thyroid gland. It is frequently a precursor of heart failure.

Digitalis is extensively used in the treatment of fibrillation, but in some cases periodic measurement of blood plasma concentrations of this drug are important to obviate toxic effects from too high a dosage. Another drug called quinidine may be employed in selected cases.

Heart block—contractile impulses in the heart begin in a structure called the *sino-atrial node* (the pacemaker of the heart), pass through the atrial walls to the *atrioventricular node* and are conducted to the walls of the ventricles via the *atrioventricular bundle of His*. Involvement of this last structure, by various forms of disease processes (e.g. coronary artery disease, rheumatic heart disease) may cause partial or complete, temporary or permanent, interruption of the conduction of contractile impulses producing various degrees of the condition described as heart block. In **complete heart block** the contraction of the ventricles is quite independent of that of the atria.

Heart block is frequently complicated by periodic attacks of loss of consciousness called **Stokes–Adams attacks**. One method of treating patients with such attacks is by some form of battery-operated **cardiac pacemaker**, which has one of its electrodes either passed into the cavity of the right ventricle or attached to the outer surface of the heart. The heart beat is thus artificially paced by electrical stimulation.

Chronic Pulmonary Heart Disease

This type of heart disease is also referred to as **cor pulmonale**, and is discussed by Turner (4) as a sequel to certain disorders of the lungs and pulmonary circulation.

It occurs when the right ventricle has to work against an increased resistance in the pulmonary circulation, such as may develop in a common lung disorder called emphysema, in various types of pulmonary fibrosis, and as a result of severe chronic bronchitis.

Cor pulmonale is a common cause of right ventricular failure.

Pulmonary Hypertension

This is a condition of raised blood pressure in the pulmonary circulation. It may result from lung disorders that cause chronic pulmonary heart disease or from other heart diseases in which there is either increased flow of blood through the lungs (e.g. some congenital septal defects, patent ductus arteriosus) or increased back pressure within the pulmonary circulation (e.g. mitral stenosis), or it may be of unknown origin.

Typical changes in the pulmonary arteries may be demonstrable on radiographs.

Thyrotoxic Heart Disease

This term describes heart disease secondary to hyperthyroidism (thyrotoxicosis), i.e. overactivity of the thyroid gland. The disorder of cardiac rhythm called atrial fibrillation is common in this type of heart condition.

Cardiomyopathies

These are an ill-defined group of disorders, in which the chief feature is disease of the myocardium, developing from causes other than ischaemic heart disease, hypertension or acute rheumatism. They may occur in association with, or as a result of, a large variety of different conditions, e.g. alcoholism, nutritional deficiencies, connective tissue diseases, or endocrine diseases, or be of unknown cause.

Heart Failure (Cardiac Failure)

Heart failure is a condition that occurs when, as a result of disease, the heart can no longer pump out blood in amounts adequate to maintain the circulation. It may be of sudden or slow onset. According to its cause and severity it may prove rapidly or eventually fatal; or, alternatively, it may slowly improve. It should not be confused with **cardiac**

arrest, a condition of complete cessation of the contractions of the heart muscle, which is fatal unless the heart beat can be restarted within a short period.

Heart failure usually develops in the first instance in one ventricle and then, unless relieved, eventually involves the opposite ventricle too.

Left Ventricular Failure

In this type, as a result of diseases which impose an undue strain on the left ventricle (e.g. hypertensive heart disease, a proportion of cases of coronary heart disease, aortic incompetence, coarctation of the aorta), the left ventricle dilates and blood accumulates in the pulmonary circulation causing overfilling of lung vessels—a condition referred to as **congestion**. When severe this may result in fluid leaking out of the pulmonary capillaries into the lungs causing **pulmonary oedema**. The patient is short of breath and often suffers from paroxysms of difficulty in breathing. These paroxysms are called **cardiac asthma** on account of a superficial resemblance to attacks of bronchial asthma.

Fluid in the pleural cavity may also be found. This is termed a **hydrothorax**, and can be a feature of either left or right-sided ventricular failure.

In left ventricular failure the right ventricle has to work against an increased pressure of blood in the pulmonary circulation. If left ventricular failure is not relieved, it will therefore eventually result in superadded right ventricular failure.

Right Ventricular Failure

This type of failure is encountered in conditions which impose undue strain on the right ventricle, e.g. diseases of the lungs which lead to pulmonary heart disease and heart diseases that are associated with pulmonary hypertension. It may also occur as a sequel to left ventricular failure, as discussed above.

When the right ventricle fails, blood accumulates in the veins and capillaries of the systemic circulation. This results in cyanosis, oedema and enlargement of the liver. Effusion of fluid into the pleural and peritoneal cavities occurs in some cases. Pulmonary congestion is seen in certain types of right ventricular failure, e.g. when due to mitral stenosis. This causes shortness of breath and may be associated with haemoptysis.

The abnormality of the rhythm of the heart beat called **atrial fibrillation** frequently occurs in right ventricular failure.

X-ray films are of value in cases of cardiac failure as a means of demonstrating the size and shape of the heart, overfilling of lung vessels, pleural effusions, and pulmonary oedema.

Rest, a low salt diet, sedation and the administration of digitalis, are basic forms of treatment in heart failure. Drugs that increase the flow of urine and therefore called **diuretics** are employed to reduce oedema. Oxygen is given to patients with cyanosis and dyspnoea.

Cardiac Arrest

This term describes the cessation of the pumping action of the heart and consequent halting of the circulation of blood through the blood vessels. It is accompanied by cessation of respiration and is therefore frequently referred to as **cardiorespiratory arrest**.

The condition may be due to various causes, among which are diseases of the cardiovascular and respiratory systems (e.g. coronary thrombosis, pulmonary embolism, etc.), head injuries and chest injuries.

Clinically, cardiac arrest is evidenced by unconsciousness, absent pulses, absence of respiration and dilated pupils.

Persistence of the condition for more than about three minutes may lead to serious and permanent brain damage, the brain tissues being particularly sensitive to deprivation of a normal supply of oxygenated blood.

To be effective, resuscitation measures must therefore be instituted without any delay. Immediate measures comprise external cardiac compression (external cardiac massage) and artificial ventilation (artificial respiration) by the mouth-to-mouth or mouth-to-nose method. If these are not rapidly successful more complex procedures are required. These may include internal cardiac compression (internal cardiac massage), intubation of the trachea and ventilation of the lungs, and intravenous or intracardiac injection of various drugs.

In patients who are shown by electrocardiography to exhibit abnormal contractions of the ventricles of the heart of a type called **ventricular fibrillation**, a procedure called **defibrillation** is required to restore normal cardiac rhythm. This involves the momentary passage through the heart of a high voltage electric current.

Some Terms used with Reference to Cardiac Surgery

Hypothermia—the use of this term in connection with cardiac surgery indicates methods used in association with general anaesthesia to obtain an appreciable lowering of body temperature. By such means the oxygen needs of the body are reduced, making it possible for the circulation to be arrested for a short time, during which cardiac surgery of short duration may be carried out. The word hypothermia means low temperature.

Cardiopulmonary bypass (heart-lung machine)—a machine whereby the blood is drawn off the venous side of the systemic circulation, oxygenated and pumped back into the arterial side; the heart and lungs being bypassed. It is used for cardiac operations of long duration.

Blalock's operation—one type of operation employed in treating Fallor's tetralogy.

Valvotomy—an operation designed to enlarge a narrowed cardiac valve orifice.

Valve replacement—the replacement of a diseased heart valve by an artificial valve such as a Starr-Edwards prosthetic heart valve of ball and cage type, or by a homograft valve (a **homograft** or **allograft** is a structure grafted from an individual of the same species).

Open and closed cardiac surgery—open cardiac surgery consists of surgical operations on the interior of the heart performed under direct vision. Other forms of heart operation, including those on the interior of the heart by indirect methods, are closed cardiac surgery.

Cardiac pacing—surgical measures concerned with the introduction into the body of cardiac pacemakers (see p 77).

Coronary bypass surgery—undertaken to relieve angina; it involves bypassing a diseased segment, or segments of coronary arteries by venous grafts, which are then connected to the aorta or the proximal part of the coronary system.

Cardiac transplantation—replacement of a diseased heart by a heart taken from a donor shortly after death. The first man-to-man cardiac transplant operation was performed in the Union of South Africa in 1967.

Diseases of Arteries

Arterial disease may be congenital, traumatic, inflammatory or due to other and unknown causes.

Some important arterial disorders are as follows.

Atheroma (atherosclerosis)—the name of this disease derives from the Greek word for gruel, a substance to which the atheromatous lesions in affected arteries were thought to bear some resemblance. Its alternative name **atherosclerosis** should not be confused with **arteriosclerosis** which means hardening of the arteries, and is a term which is applied to any form of disorder in which arterial walls become thickened and hard in texture as a result of degenerative changes in the muscle and elastic tissues of their media.

Atheroma is a degenerative condition of unknown origin, which is extremely common in middle-aged and elderly people. It may also occur in young people suffering from diabetes mellitus.

The basic features of the disease are the patchy deposition of lipids (fatty substances) and the occurrence of areas of thickening, which may develop into dense raised plaques in the intima of affected arteries. These latter accordingly develop areas of narrowing within their interiors and this diminishes their blood-carrying capacity. Moreover, the presence of atheroma predisposes to occlusion of arteries as a result of thrombosis, and may also lead to a complication called **aneurysm formation**. An **aneurysm** is a localised dilation of a vessel wall, usually formed as a result of undue stretching of a diseased area under the pressure of the circulating blood.

Clinical manifestations resulting from diminution or deprivation of blood supply may occur in tissues supplied by atheromatous arteries. Among the clinical disorders due to atheroma are:

(i) **angina** and **coronary thrombosis**, both resulting from atheroma of the coronary arteries (see p 75).

(ii) **mental changes**, **cerebral thrombosis** and **cerebral haemorrhage** due to atheroma of the arteries supplying the brain;

(iii) **peripheral vascular disease** resulting from atheroma of the limb arteries (usually those of the leg) and often also from atheroma of the lower part of the abdominal aorta and external iliac arteries. The chief symptoms are coldness of the limb and a type of pain in the legs called **intermittent claudication**. This resembles angina, in that it appears with exertion and is relieved by rest. Thrombosis is a not uncommon occurrence in peripheral vascular disease. In lower limb arteries it may sometimes lead to gangrene, especially in diabetic subjects;

(iv) **aortic stenosis**—a form of chronic valvular disease of the heart in which the aortic orifice becomes narrowed as a result of atheroma involving the valve cusps;

(v) **renal artery stenosis** (see p 163).

Pathological calcification is common in atheromatous lesions, frequently to an extent which renders them visible on radiographs.

Various forms of angiography (e.g. peripheral, cerebral, renal, and coronary angiography, aortography) are extensively employed in the investigation of clinical disorders resulting from atheroma. The presence of atheromatous plaques may be shown by areas of irregularity in vessel walls, and thrombosis by narrowing or complete blockage of their interiors, and an interventional radiological technique, called transluminal angioplasty, may be used to dilate narrowed segments. Information regarding collateral circulation (see p 68) may also be obtained.

There is no specific treatment for atheroma. In certain sites the continuity of an artery occluded by thrombosis may be restored by the surgical operations of **disobliterative endarectomy** or **arterial grafting**. **Amputation** (i.e. cutting off a limb) is the treatment for established gangrene.

Syphilitic disease of arteries—syphilitic infection in the walls of the thoracic aorta is a fairly common feature of tertiary syphilis. This condition is called **syphilitic aortitis**. It causes dilatation of the aorta which may lead to stretching of the aortic valve ring, resulting in an inability of the valve cusps to close completely; a condition termed **aortic incompetence** or, alternatively, **aortic regurgitation**. Aneurysm formation is a not uncommon complication of syphilitic aortitis.

The arteries of the central nervous system may also be the site of syphilitic inflammation in the disorder called **meningovascular syphilis**, another manifestation of tertiary syphilis. Arteries supplying the meninges, brain and spinal cord may be affected and various different clinical conditions produced according to the site of the inflammatory lesions.

Aneurysm formation—as noted when discussing atheroma, an aneurysm is a localised dilatation of a vessel usually resulting from undue stretching of a diseased area in its wall. The commonest cause of arterial aneurysm nowadays is atheroma, although aneurysms may also be due to syphilis or trauma, and in the cerebral circulation they may be of a congenital origin.

The stretching of a diseased area in the vessel wall produces a bulge which may enlarge into a rounded or fusiform swelling, producing in the first instance a **saccular aneurysm**, and, in the second, a **fusiform aneurysm**. Saccular and fusiform aneurysms occur both in the aorta and peripheral arteries. Angiography plays an important part in their diagnosis. Aneurysms tend to rupture causing severe and often fatal haemorrhage. Surgery is thus the treatment of choice when practicable.

Of a different type to the above aneurysms is the **dissecting aneurysm**, which originates in the thoracic aorta, but which may extend to include the abdominal aorta. It is formed when a tear in the intima (innermost coat) of the aorta permits blood to seep into the media and spread along this coat. This can only occur, however, when the media itself is the subject of degenerative arterial disease called **cystic medionecrosis**. The presence of a dissecting aneurysm is characterised by a tearing pain in the chest or abdomen. Plain X-ray films, followed by aortography, are important procedures in diagnosis. Treatment is surgical whenever possible.

Acute arterial block—this is caused by blockage of an artery by an embolus from the heart, or by rapidly developing thrombosis in an atheromatous artery. The causal embolus or thrombus may in many instances be surgically removed; the operation being called **embolectomy**.

Raynaud's syndrome— a condition of spasm in the arteries of the fingers due to a variety of different causes, among which may be mentioned cervical ribs and atheroma. Maurice Raynaud was a French physician of the nineteenth century.

Some other arterial disorders—these include conditions with the following names:
(i) **arteriovenous fistula**—a communication between an artery and a vein due to trauma, or of congenital origin;

(ii) **frostbite**—due to exposure to severe cold;

(iii) **chilblains, erythrocyanosis, acrocyanosis, erythromelalgia**—all of which are various forms of abnormal response to cold;

(iv) **Buerger's disease**—(thromboangiitis obliterans), **polyarteritis nodosa, temporal arteritis**—terms which denote uncommon inflammatory conditions of unknown cause.

Note: the term **arteritis** means inflammation of arteries, and **phlebitis** means inflammation of veins. The prefix **angio-** refers to vessels, usually blood vessels, and the term **angiitis** refers to inflammation of arteries, veins and capillaries, as does the synonymous term **vasculitis**.

Diseases of Veins

Thrombophlebitis—this is a disorder in which inflammation in the walls of affected veins (phlebitis) leads to clot formation (thrombosis) in their interiors. Slowing of blood flow, injury to vein walls and infection are considered to be factors in causation. Severe infection can sometimes result in pus formation in the clot, the condition then being described as suppurative thrombophlebitis and it may lead to pyaemia (see pylephlebitis p 136).

Clinically, thrombophlebitis is seen most commonly in the form of **superficial vein thrombosis** occurring as a complication of varicose veins or of intravenous therapy.

Phlebothrombosis—is a common condition, referred to more usually as **deep vein thrombosis** (DVT). It occurs most frequently in veins of the pelvis and lower limbs after surgical operation or childbirth, or sometimes in those taking contraceptive pills and may result in pulmonary embolism through detachment of a fragment of clot (see p 105).

The presence and extent of deep vein thrombosis may be demonstrated by phlebography, thermography, ultrasound (using Doppler techniques) or by techniques using radioactive isotopes (e.g. ^{125}I-fibrinogen).

Deep vein thrombosis is treated by giving anticoagulants (e.g. heparin, phenindione—Dindevan—and warfarin) and, if these are unsuccessful in preventing spread of the disorder, by surgical measures.

Varicose veins—the word **varix** means crooked. Varicose veins are dilated venous channels which pursue a tortuous course. They frequently occur in the legs and are seen less commonly in the form of varicocele (see p 174) and of oesophageal varices (see p 139).

Varicose veins in the legs appear to be caused by a number of factors, among which are congenital weakness of the vein walls and prolonged standing. They are usually found in the superficial circulation, but the deep veins may be affected. Pregnancy may also be a factor in their development.

Before starting treatment for varicose veins, it is often necessary to demonstrate the deep venous circulation by venography (phlebography).

In a region where varicosity of the veins is pronounced, the circulation may be interfered with to such an extent that it impairs the nutrition of the surrounding tissues. This may lead to the development of a skin disorder called **varicose dermatitis**. Ulceration, known as **varicose ulceration**, may also result, and infection of the ulcerated area may produce localised periostitis in an underlying bone.

Non-suppurative thrombophlebitis is another complication of varicose veins.

Note: **Haemorrhoids** (piles), formerly described as varicose veins in the region of the anus and anal canal are no longer regarded as such. According to Taylor and Cotton (5) internal haemorrhoids are thickenings of fibromuscular tissue lying close to the submucous venous plexus in the anal canal, and external piles are swellings related to the subcutaneous perianal plexal veins.

Haemorrhoids are prone to bleeding, thrombosis and prolapse.

REFERENCES

(1) Duthie, J. J. R. (1966). *The Principles and Practice of Medicine*, 8th Edn. (Davidson S., ed.) Edinburgh: Livingstone.

(2) Brimblecombe, F. and Barltrop, D. (1978). *Children in Health and Disease*. London: Baillière Tindall.

(3) Report of a Joint Working Party of the Royal College of Physicians of London and the British Cardiac Society (1976). *Journal of the Royal College of Physicians*; **10**; 213.

(4) Turner, R. W. D. (1971). *The Principles and Practice of Medicine*, 10th Edn. (Davidson, S., Macleod, J., ed.) Edinburgh: Churchill Livingstone.

(5) Taylor, S., Cotton, L. (1982). *A Short Textbook of Surgery*, 5th Edn. London: Hodder and Stoughton.

RESPIRATORY SYSTEM

Some Anatomical and Physiological Considerations

The respiratory system is concerned primarily with providing the blood with oxygen from inspired air, and with the removal of carbon dioxide from the blood and excretion of this waste product in expired air. This exchange of gases is affected in the lungs. Certain organs of the system have other functions also, e.g. voice production in the larynx, olfactory functions of the nose (**olfactory** refers to the sense of smell).

The respiratory system includes the following.

The upper respiratory system, consisting of the *nasal cavities* and *nasopharynx*, *oropharynx* and upper part of the *laryngopharynx* (structures common to both the respiratory and digestive systems), and *larynx*. The *accessory nasal sinuses* open into the nasal cavities and infection of these structures is frequently associated with other respiratory disease.

The lower respiratory system, consisting of the *trachea*, *bronchi*, *lungs* and *pleurae*.

The lungs and pleurae are contained in the thoracic cavity and between them is the space called the *mediastinum*. This latter contains numerous important structures, among which are the following: the heart and origins of the great vessels; the greater part of the oesophagus; portions of the vagus, phrenic and left recurrent laryngeal nerves; the lower part of the trachea and the origins of the two main bronchi; the thoracic duct and numerous lymph glands and lymphatic vessels; and the thymus gland.

In several diseases of the lower respiratory system, associated pathological changes are found affecting structures in the mediastinum.

The right lung contains three major subdivisions known as *lobes*, and the left lung has two lobes. Each lobe is divided further into *bronchopulmonary segments*, composed of large numbers of small structures called *acini* or *primary lobules*, each of which contains several *respiratory bronchioles*, small air passages called *alveolar ducts*, which lead into small air spaces termed *atria*, and large numbers of minute air sacs called *alveoli*.

The alveoli are the principal elements of the functional tissue, or *parenchyma*, of the lungs and are surrounded by a network of connective tissue referred to as the *interstitial tissue* of the lungs.

The regions on each side where the main bronchi, and main branches of the pulmonary artery enter the lungs are known as the *hila* (singular: hilum). Situated in the hila are the *hilar lymph glands*, into which drain lymph from the lungs. Efferent vessels from these glands pass to the *mediastinal lymph glands*. Enlargement of hilar and mediastinal lymph nodes is a frequent concomitant of some lung diseases.

Some prefixes used with reference to the respiratory system are: **rhino-** pertaining to the nose; **laryngo-** pertaining to the larynx; **tracheo-** pertaining to the trachea; **broncho-** pertaining to a bronchus or bronchi; **pleuro-** pertaining to the pleura; and **pneumono-** pertaining to lung.

Some General Aspects of Respiratory Diseases

Diseases affecting the respiratory system may be congenital, traumatic, infective, neoplastic, or due to a variety of other causes, or idiopathic (of unknown causation).

Among those with the highest incidence are different forms of upper respiratory tract infection, bronchitis, asthma, pleurisy, traumatic lesions of the lung, pneumonias, neoplasms of the bronchi and pleura, dust diseases of the lung, and a degenerative disorder called emphysema.

Among the clinical symptoms and signs which may be associated with respiratory disease are **rhinorrhoea** (running from the nose), **epistaxis** (bleeding from the nose), sore throat, hoarse voice, pain on swallowing and breathing, cough, **haemoptysis** (coughing of blood), **stridor** (a harsh sound produced on breathing in or out), **cyanosis** (blue skin and mucous membrane), **dyspnoea** (difficulty in breathing), **tachypnoea** (abnormally rapid respirations).

Certain diseases of the respiratory system fall within the province of the ear, nose and throat specialist, others within that of the general physician or of the chest physician. Diseases of the lower respiratory tract that require surgical treatment are generally referred to a specialist in chest surgery termed a thoracic surgeon.

It is to be noted that a serious lack of adequate oxygenation of the blood, developing either in acute or chronic form, may occur in certain lung disorders causing **respiratory failure** (**ventilatory failure**). Complete cessation of respiratory function is termed **respiratory arrest**.

The occurrence of heart disease secondary to disease of the lungs or pulmonary vessels has already been noted (see under chronic pulmonary heart disease).

Special Methods of Investigation

Radiological investigation—this is extensively used in the investigation of chest diseases. Plain films and fluoroscopy may be supplemented by methods such as (i) **tomography** (layer radiography), a method which produces radiographs of selected thin layers within the interior of the body, and blurs out the images of structures in layers other than the one selected, (ii) **bronchography**—contrast radiography of the bronchial tree, (iii) **pulmonary angiography**—contrast radiography of the blood vessels of the lungs, (iv) radioisotope scanning, e.g. in the diagnosis of pulmonary embolism, (v) CT e.g. to show mediastinal masses and metastases.

Visual inspection with special instruments—inspection of the interior parts of the respiratory passages by the procedures called **rhinoscopy** (nose); **pharyngoscopy** (pharynx); **laryngoscopy** (larynx); **bronchoscopy** (trachea and main bronchi); **mediastinoscopy** (upper mediastimum); **pleuroscopy** (pleural cavity).

The termination **-scopy** denotes a visual examination; and the termination **-scope**, the instrument with which such examination is performed.

Examination of sputum—by the naked eye, and by microscopic and bacteriological methods.

Respiratory function tests—these include various tests designed to estimate the efficiency of the respiratory organs. They use methods such as **spirometry** (i.e. estimations of volumes of inspired and expired air) e.g. estimations of vital capacity; forced expiratory volume, i.e. the amount of air that can be forcibly exhaled from the lungs in 1 second (FEV1); peak expiratory flow rate (PEFR) determined by the Wright peak-flow meter); **blood gas analysis** (i.e. measurements indicating amounts of oxygen and carbon dioxide in the blood); and other tests.

Lung biopsy—i.e. removal of a very small amount of lung tissue for microscopic examination. This may be done at open operation or during bronchoscopy, or using a special needle or drill by **needle biopsy** or **drill biopsy**.

Diseases of the Upper Respiratory Tract

Congenital Disorders

Deviation of the nasal septum—in this disorder the nasal septum is bent and may cause obstruction of one or both nasal passages. It is treated surgically if it causes symptoms. Besides being due to congenital causes, this abnormality can also result from trauma.

Choanal Atresia—a rare disorder in which developmental failure results in blockage of one or both *choanae*, i.e. the posterior openings of the nasal cavities into the nasopharynx.

Traumatic Disorders

Among these may be mentioned the introduction of extraneous objects into the body, which become lodged in the nasal cavities, pharynx or larynx. Such objects are termed **foreign bodies**, and when they become immovably fixed in a certain site they are said to be **impacted**. Children not infrequently push small objects into their noses.

Infective Diseases

These provoke inflammatory reactions which, according to their sites, are termed **rhinitis**, **sinusitis**, **pharyngitis** and **laryngitis**. Among these diseases are the following.

Coryza (common cold)—a virus infection causing inflammation of the mucous membranes lining the nose and nasopharynx. During the course of the infection the mucous membranes may become further infected by pathogenic bacteria, which are then referred to as **secondary invaders**. Such secondary invasion may result in the spread of infection to other parts of the upper and lower respiratory tracts, and also via the Eustachian tube to the middle ear on one or both sides.

Accordingly sinusitis, otitis media, laryngitis and bronchitis are not uncommon complications.

The name coryza derives from the running nose which is the most prominent clinical feature of this condition.

Influenza—a virus infection causing fever, inflammation of the upper respiratory tract, and severe aching in the back and limbs. Secondary infection with pathogenic bacteria during the course of this disease, may cause **pneumonia** (inflammation of the lungs).

Sinusitis—inflammation of the accessory nasal sinuses. This occurs most frequently in the maxillary sinuses (maxillary antra) but may develop in any of the other nasal sinuses in acute or chronic form.

Infective material from diseased sinuses frequently descends into the lower respiratory tract, where it may lead to infection in the bronchi or lungs.

Sinusitis is not always caused by pathogenic micro-organisms. It quite frequently occurs as an allergic manifestation and may complicate hay fever.

In radiographs, an inflammatory reaction, due to infection or allergy, may be evidenced by an appearance called mucosal thickening due to swelling of the lining mucosa of affected sinuses; or by opacity resulting from inflammatory exudate within their interiors. In a sinus in which appreciable quantities of fluid exudate and air are both present a fluid level may be demonstrable because the air will rise above the heavier fluid.

Adenovirus infections—due to viruses called the *adenovirus group*, which cause inflammatory conditions in the upper respiratory tract.

Enlarged adenoids—swellings of collections of lymphatic tissue in the nasopharynx. Such swellings develop as a result of chronic infection and are usually associated with chronic tonsillitis. If surgical treatment (adenoidectomy) is required, tonsillectomy is usually performed at the same time.

Enlarged adenoids are a common cause of mouth-breathing and may cause deafness by blocking the pharyngeal opening of the Eustachian tubes.

Soft tissue swelling produced by adenoidal enlargement can be shown in soft-tissue lateral radiographs of the nasopharynx.

Tonsillitis—the tonsils are masses of lymphoid tissue covered by mucous membrane and lying between the pillars of the fauces in the lateral walls of the oropharynx. They are frequently the site of acute or chronic infection and in the latter instance may require surgical removal.

Streptococcal infection is a common cause of acute tonsillitis and may lead to serious complications in the form of acute nephritis or acute rheumatism. Streptococcal tonsillitis is sometimes difficult to differentiate from faucial diphtheria.

Scarlet fever is a manifestation of a special type of streptococcal tonsillitis.

Acute infection of the tonsils may sometimes lead to the formation of a **peritonsillar abscess** commonly known as a **quinsy**, characterised by a large swelling of the soft palate on the affected side, difficulty in swallowing and severe pain in the throat.

Laryngitis—the word denotes inflammation of the larynx. **Acute laryngitis** is frequently of infective origin but may result from other causes, e.g. inhalation of irritant fumes. **Chronic laryngitis** is sometimes caused by a tuberculous or syphilitic infection but develops much more often as a result of excessive use of the voice or heavy tobacco smoking.

Hoarseness and loss of voice are prominent features in both acute and chronic laryngitis.

Acute laryngitis in childhood may be associated with stridor (harsh respiratory sounds) due to spasm of laryngeal muscles; the condition then being described as **spasmodic croup**.

Retropharyngeal abscess—the prefix **retro-** means behind and the term describes an abscess in the soft tissues behind the pharynx. It usually occurs in infancy as a result of infection of retropharyngeal lymph glands consequent upon a throat infection.

> The condition commonly gives rise to marked soft tissue swelling and this may be readily demonstrated by soft tissue lateral X-ray films of the neck.

Neoplasms

These may occur in any part of the upper respiratory tract and include the following.

Benign—the most common of these is a tumour called a **papilloma of the vocal cords**, which arises from mucous membrane covering the cords. It causes hoarseness of the voice and, if it attains a large size, may also cause dyspnoea.

Note: The localised soft tissue swellings found in the nose, and called **nasal polypi** are regarded as tissue overgrowth and are not considered to be truly neoplastic in nature.

Malignant—carcinomas of the **maxillary antrum**, **ethmoid cells**, **pharynx** and **larynx**. Taylor and Cotton (1) classify laryngeal tumours as 'supraglottic (includes epiglottis), glottic (vocal cords), subglottic (cricothyroid region)'.

A high degree of malignancy is a usual feature of malignant tumours of the nasopharynx, some of which are carcinomas, while others belong to the other great class of malignant tumours termed sarcomas, e.g. **nasopharyngeal lymphosarcoma**.

CT is often a great help in showing the extent of malignant disease in the upper respiratory tract. Surgery and radiotherapy, either singly or in combination, are extensively employed in the treatment of malignant neoplasms of the upper respiratory tract.

Other Diseases

Hay fever, an allergic disorder of the upper respiratory tract, so-called because it is produced as a result of hypersensitivity to various types of pollen, most of which are grass pollens. The principal clinical features are rhinorrhoea (running nose) and conjunctivitis.

Allied to hay fever, but resulting from sensitivity to other substances, is another allergic disorder called **perennial rhinorrhoea** or **perennial rhinitis**.

Diseases of the Trachea

The only common disease of the trachea is an acute inflammatory disorder called **acute tracheitis**. This may accompany various inflammations of the upper respiratory tract. It also not infrequently occurs in association with acute bronchitis when the condition is described as **acute tracheobronchitis**.

Diseases of the Bronchi

Bronchitis—this term denotes the presence of inflammatory changes in the mucous membrane lining the bronchi. The description **bronchiolitis** is applied to inflammation of the smallest branches of the bronchial tree which are known as *bronchioles*. Acute bronchiolitis occurs fairly frequently in early childhood, the commonest cause being a virus called the *respiratory syncytial virus*.

- **Acute bronchitis**—this is usually due to infection but may develop as a result of exposure to irritating dust and gases. Common clinical features are cough, fever and a tight feeling in the chest. The disease frequently follows an infection of the upper respiratory tract and may progress to bronchopneumonia. It is also a common complication of measles.
- **Chronic bronchitis**—is an extremely common disease in middle and old age. It may be a sequel to acute bronchitis or may be chronic in type from the start. In many instances there is no apparent cause but, in others factors such as exposure to fumes and dust, tobacco smoking and chronic sinusitis appear to play some part.

  The chief symptoms are cough and **expectoration** (spitting) and, in advanced cases, shortness of breath. In early cases symptoms often disappear in the summer but recur each winter. Many sufferers from chronic bronchitis develop a lung disorder called **emphysema** (see later). The combination of these two conditions is frequently referred to as **chronic obstructive airways disease**.

Attacks of acute bronchitis and bronchopneumonia are frequent complications of chronic bronchitis and the disease may eventually lead to respiratory failure and to pulmonary heart disease.

Neither acute nor chronic bronchitis produce specific X-ray appearances, but radiographs are usually needed at some stage of these disorders to exclude other conditions which could cause similar symptoms or to investigate suspected complications and associated emphysematous changes.

Bronchiectasis—the name of this disorder signifies the presence of abnormally dilated bronchi, or bronchioles, in the lungs, the ending **-ectasis** indicating a state of widening or expansion.

Such dilatation of bronchi is liable to develop in areas of lung which, as a result of bronchial obstruction, become the site of persistent **collapse**. This latter condition is described in more detail on p 95.

Among the many causes of bronchial obstruction, those associated with the subsequent development of bronchiectasis include inflammatory exudates and plugs of mucus in acute pulmonary infections, impacted foreign body in a bronchus, pressure from enlarged tuberculous glands, pulmonary fibrosis and bronchial carcinomas.

Abnormal strain on bronchial walls in collapsed areas of lung, distension of the bronchi beyond an obstruction by infective secretions, and weakening of bronchial walls as a result of infective processes, have all been postulated as factors in the development of different varieties of bronchiectasis.

Bronchial dilatation may be reversible in its early stages if the bronchial obstruction responsible for its development can be effectively relieved.

The main clinical feature in bronchiectasis is the coughing up of purulent sputum. Haemoptysis is fairly common and the fingers often show an abnormality called **clubbing**, i.e. they show expansion of their ends and abnormal curvature of the nails. Clubbed fingers also occur in some other lung diseases, including bronchial carcinoma, and in certain heart disorders.

The presence of bronchiectasis is proved by demonstration of dilated bronchi by bronchography (contrast radiography of the bronchial tree).

Surgical removal of portions of lung affected by bronchiectasis is carried out in younger subjects when the disease is localised.

Bronchial asthma—this disease is usually referred to as **asthma**, its name indicating the gasping for breath which is the most prominent clinical feature and results from spasm of plain muscle in the walls of the smaller bronchi. (See also cardiac asthma, p 79).

The disorder is frequently familial (i.e. occurring in members of the same family) and often first appears in childhood. It is often associated with chronic bronchitis and the development of emphysema.

The cause is usually obscure and factors which may operate in different cases include hypersensitivity (allergy) to various substances (e.g. dusts, pollens, face powders, eggs, milk, certain drugs); psychological disturbances and bronchial infection.

Sufferers from asthma are frequently subject to other allergic disorders such as hay fever and eczema. Asthmatic attacks are usually of fairly short duration. Rarely, however, a single attack may persist for longer than 24 hours, producing a condition termed **status asthmaticus**.

Recurrent attacks of bronchitis and bronchopneumonia are common in sufferers from asthma.

Like chronic bronchitis, asthma produces no specific X-ray changes but radiographic examination may be required to show complicating lung infection or to investigate associated emphysema.

The combination of asthma and chronic bronchitis is sometimes referred to as **chronic asthmatic bronchitis**.

Drugs used for treating asthma include salbutamol (Ventolin), sodium cromoglycate (Intal), aminophylline, hydrocortisone and other steroids. When hypersensitivity to a known agent appears to be a factor, an attempt may be made to counteract this by process called **desensitisation**.

Breathing exercises are of considerable value to asthmatic patients.

Bronchial neoplasms—bronchial adenoma and bronchial carcinoma are discussed later (see p 106).

Diseases of the Pleura

Most diseases of the pleura are secondary to disease in the lungs or elsewhere in the body. Primary disorders of the pleura are uncommon.

Pleural effusion—this term indicates the presence of fluid within the pleural cavity, resulting from (i) transudation of oedema fluid, e.g. due to heart failure or to nephritis; (ii) exudation of fluid as a result of an inflammatory reaction in the pleura produced in response to injury to the chest wall, infection of the lungs or subphrenic space, infarction in underlying lung, or pleural involvement by metastases or primary neoplasms.

If the inflammatory exudate is thick and scanty the condition may be referred to as one of **dry pleurisy**; if it is of fluid consistency it may be described as **pleurisy with effusion**. The term **pleuritis** is synonymous with pleurisy.

During the course of pleurisy-with-effusion, the fluid may become walled off in a localised part of the pleural cavity, as a result of the development of fibrous adhesions. A pleural effusion which is thus confined is known as an **encysted effusion**.

Both dry pleurisy and pleural effusion produce well-marked clinical features. Pain, due to pleurisy, must among other conditions be distinguished from that due to pain in the thoracic muscles from a virus disease called **Bornholm disease (epidemic myalgia)**.

The term *hydrothorax* is also used to describe the presence of fluid in the pleural cavity. A mixture of fluid and air in the cavity is called a **hydropneumothorax**.

Pus in the pleural cavity constitutes a **pyothorax** or **empyema**, and bleeding into the cavity produces a **haemothorax**.

> X-ray examination may yield no evidence of a dry pleurisy, but is impor-
> tant in showing the site and extent of a pleural effusion, and the presence or
> absence of associated lesions within the chest. The nature of the fluid present
> in the pleural cavity is not, however, revealed by radiology.

Pathological examination of a sample of fluid obtained by aspiration through a needle is an essential investigation in many cases of pleurisy with effusion. With large effusions, **chest aspiration** may also be necessary as a therapeutic measure. Aspiration of the chest is also called **paracentesis thoracis**.

Pneumothorax—this is a condition in which air or other gas is present in the pleural cavity. It may result from rupture of the lung through disease, when it is called a **spontaneous pneumothorax**; from injury to the lung or chest wall; from accidental puncture of the lung during aspiration of a pleural effusion; or from the operation of **thoracotomy**, in which an opening is made into the thorax.

An **artificial pneumothorax** used to be widely used as a form of treatment of pulmonary tuberculosis.

Pleural effusion frequently occurs in cases of pneumothorax, the condition then becoming one of hydropneumothorax.

> A pneumothorax of any appreciable size is readily shown on a
> conventional PA chest radiograph taken on inspiration. A very small
> pneumothorax may, however, only be demonstrable on an expiratory film.

The commonest causes of spontaneous pneumothorax is rupture of an emphysematous bulla (see p 103).

Pleural Neoplasms

See p 106.

Diseases of the Lung

These may be congenital; traumatic, infective; neoplastic; due to cyst formation; due to the inhalation of harmful gases or dusts; allergic; or idiopathic. Pathological changes in the lungs often develop as a secondary result of heart disease.

Before proceeding to discuss terms relating to individual lung diseases and groups of such diseases, it will be useful to indicate the nature of three pathological processes which occur in various different types of pulmonary (lung) disorder.

Pulmonary collapse—a condition in which a portion of lung, or sometimes a whole lung, becomes airless and thus collapses down, as a result of obstruction of the bronchus which supplies it with air. According to the site of the bronchial obstruction, the collapse may be lobar, segmental or lobular in type.

The term **atelectasis** which means a condition of incomplete expansion is frequently used as a synonym for pulmonary collapse, but in the stricter sense indicates lung tissue which has failed to expand normally, e.g. as in congenital atelectasis. (*Note:* the derivation of atelectasis is from a- meaning without and -ectasis meaning expansion.)

Pulmonary consolidation—a condition in which the area of lung acquires a solid or semisolid consistency owing to the air in its alveoli being replaced by material such as an inflammatory exudate (e.g. in pneumonia) or a mass of tumour cells.

Pulmonary fibrosis—a condition in which areas of lung tissue become replaced by overgrowth of fibrous connective tissue. It may be localised or diffuse and occurs in areas where the pulmonary tissues have been severely damaged by disease, e.g. severe pneumonias, pulmonary tuberculosis. It may also develop as a manifestation of radiation damage (**radiation fibrosis**), as a reaction to the presence of various harmful dusts in the lungs in certain of the diseases called pneumoconioses and also may be caused by certain poisons and drugs.

Areas of pulmonary collapse and consolidation and pleural effusions all produce abnormal densities on chest radiographs. It is, however, often possible for the experienced observer to say which of these three is responsible for a particular area of opacity, or, when varying combinations of the three processes occur together, indicate which predominates in the radiological picture.

Pulmonary fibrosis may be indicated on radiographs by evidence of a diminished size of a lung or of one or more of its lobes (shrinkage), displacement of normal structures (e.g. trachea, heart, diaphragm on side of lesion) towards the fibrotic area, and sometimes abnormal linear opacities of varying thickness.

Congenital Disorders

Congenital abnormalities of clinical significance are not very common in the lungs. They include conditions such as (*a*) **pulmonary hamartoma**—described by Kerley (2) as a 'tumour-like malformation in which there is an abnormal mixing of normal tissue components of the lung'. Its name is derived from a Greek work meaning to err; (*b*) **congenital cystic disease of the lungs**; (*c*) **agenesis of the lung**—a condition in which there is a failure of development of the whole of a lung or part of a lung.

Traumatic Disorders

The lungs may be damaged in both what are termed **penetrating** (open) and **non–penetrating** (closed) **chest injuries**, this distinction being made according to whether or not the injury causes an open wound which penetrates into the interior of the thoracic cavity and hence may permit the entry of external air into the thorax.

Chest injuries may result in **lung contusion** (bruising of the lung) and sometimes in a localised collection of effused blood called a **haematoma of the lung**. Sometimes they may also cause laceration of the pleura and lung tissue, with the development of a haemothorax or pneumothorax, particularly if one or more ribs are fractured by the trauma.

Multiple rib fractures may result in the deformity called **stove-in-chest**, or the condition known as **flail chest**.

> A haematoma may show on a chest X-ray film as an opacity which, on account of its roundness, is described as a coin lesion. It then, as pointed out by Lodge and Darke (3), has to be differentiated from a carcinoma and other lesions causing round or oval opacities in radiographs of the lungs.

Development of a pneumothorax may be associated with leakage of air into the neighbouring soft tissues causing a condition called **surgical emphysema**.

Penetrating and non–penetrating chest injuries may be associated with tears of the diaphragm.

Severe chest injuries may require surgical treatment (e.g. tracheostomy, drainage of a haemothorax, thoracotomy) and oxygen administration. In some cases what is termed **intermittent positive pressure ventilation** (IPPV) may be administered with a mechanical respirator.

Infective Diseases

Pneumonias—the term pneumonia indicates an inflammation of lung tissue. The word **pneumonitis** has a similar meaning but is used much less frequently.

Pneumonias include a group of infective lung diseases which result from either infection of lung tissue by specific pathogenic bacteria, viruses, rickettsiae, chlamydiae, fungi, or, rarely, protozoa, or from infection of non–specific type.

Bacterial pneumonias include those due to infection with pneumococci, staphylococci, streptococci, tubercle bacilli, *Klebsiella pneumoniae* (*Friedlander's bacillus*) and *Legionella pneumophila*, the causal organism of **Legionnaire's disease**, a condition in which lung infection may be accompanied by mental confusion and gastrointestinal disorder.

Virus pneumonias include influenzal pneumonia, measles

pneumonia, chickenpox pneumonia and pneumonia due to respiratory syncytial virus.

Pneumonia due to rickettsiae occurs in **Q (Query) fever**.

Pneumonia due to chlamydial infection occurs in **psittacosis** (ornithosis), a disease contracted from infected parrots, budgerigars and other birds.

Pneumonia due to fungi—e.g. *Aspergillosis fumigatus*.

Pnuemonia due to protozoa occurs in a rare type of lung infection, seen chiefly in debilitated infants and due to a protozoan organism called *Pneumocystis carinii*.

Note: Pneumonias due to fungi and protozoa are examples of **opportunistic infections**, i.e. infections due to micro-organisms which are normally not disease-producing but can be pathogenic in patients whose resistance to infection is lowered by treatment with immunosuppressive drugs, cytotoxic drugs, or because of malignant disease, other severe illnesses or exposure to high doses of radiation.

Aspiration Pneumonias—due to inhalation into the lungs of infective material from the upper respiratory tract (e.g. from infected paranasal sinuses), or from infected bronchi, or due to the inhalation of food or vomit. Infection is often of non-specific type.

The basic pathological feature of pneumonia is the occurrence of pulmonary consolidation (see p 95). This may include the whole of one or more lobes, or segments, or may involve numerous lobules in one or both lungs in a patchy manner. Clinically, pneumonia is often described according to the type of consolidation encountered, as **lobar**, **segmental** or **lobular pneumonia**. Lobular pneumonia is also called **bronchopneumonia**.

The consolidation in pneumococcal pneumonia is generally of lobar type, and that of aspiration pneumonia generally lobular in distribution.

Pneumonia can occur at any age, but is seen most commonly in children and elderly subjects. Common clinical features are cough and shortness of breath, together with raised temperature and pulse rate. Dry pleurisy is a frequent accompaniment and causes pain in the chest.

Complications of pneumonia occur much less frequently since the advent of anitbiotics. They include (i) heart failure (ii) pleural effusion (iii) empyema (iv) suppuration in the lung causing **lung abscess** (v) pulmonary collapse which may persist and lead eventually to bronchiectasis (vi) failure of resolution of the consolidation and the development of pulmonary fibrosis in the affected area of lung (vii) spread of infection by the bloodstream, causing infective lesions in other structures, e.g. pneumococcal arthritis and meningitis in pneumococcal pneumonia.

The diagnosis of pneumonia is usually made on clinical evidence. Sputum examination may show the nature of the infecting organism and the sensitivity of the latter to various antibiotic drugs may be investigated when desirable.

X-ray examination is of value both in demonstrating the extent and distribution of the pulmonary consolidation, and also in the assessment of progress under treatment and the investigation of complications.

Numerous scattered punctate calcified opacities may be seen, dispersed widely in the lungs of patients who have suffered from chickenpox pneumonia. The X-ray appearances in such instances bear a strong resemblance to those seen in healed miliary tuberculosis, or as a result of a fungus disease called **histoplasmosis**, which occurs mainly in the USA.

Treatment is rest, sedation and the administration of drugs such as penicillin and other antibiotics. Oxygen may be necessary in severe cases.

Note: In addition to pneumonia in infective causation there is another type of lung inflammation called **chemical pneumonia** which can be caused by inhalation of irritant gases or mineral oils (e.g. paraffin).

Lung abscess—an abscess is a cavity containing pus and results from infection of tissues by pyogenic bacteria.

Abscess cavities in lung tissue may be single or multiple. They may develop as a result of pneumonia, particularly staphylococcal pneumonia, or arise from a number of other causes. Among these are inhaled foreign body and the lodgement in the lungs of septic emboli from septic infective lesions in other parts of the body.

At an early stage of its development a lung abscess usually develops a communication with a bronchus and the patient then starts to cough up purulent sputum.

The bronchial communication also enables air to enter the cavity, and rising above the pus within the cavity causes the formation of a fluid level which may be readily demonstrated by X-ray films, taken with appropriate positioning.

Treatment of a lung abscess is generally by postural drainage and antibiotics. Surgery is sometimes necessary when conservative measures fail.

Pulmonary Tuberculosis

● **Primary pulmonary tuberculosis**—as noted in Part III, the lung is a common site for primary tuberculous infection. The initial lesion in lung tissue is termed a **primary focus** or **Ghon focus**, after a pathologist called Anton Ghon.

The presence of the primary focus characteristically results in associated, and often pronounced inflammatory changes in draining lymph glands at the hilum of the affected lung. This combination of primary focus and hilar adenitis (lymph gland inflammation) is called a **primary tuberculous complex**, and in later years its site may be rendered evident as a result of pathological calcification in both the lung and gland lesions.

In most cases primary pulmonary tuberculosis does not produce any recognisable clinical effects. However, it sometimes can present as a severe infection and it can also sometimes produce serious complications. These include: pulmonary collapse (due to pressure of enlarged hilar glands on a bronchus and sometimes leading to bronchiectasis); pleural effusion; tuberculous bronchopneumonia; metastatic lesions in other structures (e.g. bone and joint tuberculosis, tuberculous meningitis); miliary tuberculosis.

A skin condition called **erythema nodosum** may rarely occur in association with primary lung tuberculosis, as may an uncommon eye disorder called **phlyctenular conjunctivitis**.

The treatment of primary pulmonary tuberculosis and its complications is primarily by chemotherapy with antituberculous drugs.

• **Post-primary pulmonary tuberculosis** (adult type pulmonary tuberculosis, adult phthisis)—this condition is thought to occur as a result of reactivation of a dormant tuberculous infection, or less commonly a reinfection, with tubercle bacilli in an individual who has previously had primary tuberculosis in the lung or in some other site.

This disease can start in childhood or in old age. Most cases, however, first develop in adolescence or early adult life.

The inflammatory reaction, produced by the infection, is chronic in nature. In some cases it produces much exudation. In others it is associated with considerable fibrosis. Tissue destruction is marked in many of the severer types of disease producing air-containing cavities within the lungs. Involvement of the pleura by the inflammatory process may result in either dry pleurisy or pleural effusion.

Some degree of fibrosis occurs during the healing of all types of tuberculous lung lesions and pathological calcification is common in areas of healed disease.

Occasionally the disease is seen in acute form, giving rise to a pneumonic type of inflammation termed **tuberculous pneumonia**.

Common symptoms and signs of post-primary tuberculosis are cough, haemoptysis, loss of weight, loss of energy, night sweats, evening pyrexia and amenorrhoea (absence of menstrual periods).

Radiological examination is essential in both investigating suspected cases and in assessing the progress under treatment of diagnosed cases. Examination of the sputum for *tubercle bacilli* and frequently sputum culture are also highly important investigations.

The **Mantoux** and **Heaf skin tests** are positive in nearly all patients with active or healed tuberculous lesions.

In radiographs the exudative lesions of pulmonary tuberculosis commonly produce an appearance of mottling. The fibrotic lesions are often seen in the form of abnormal linear shadows and sites of healed foci of disease as calcified opacities. Cavities may be demonstrated in plain films but often tomography is necessary to outline them clearly.

In many instances the X-ray changes are fairly characteristic, but in others they may be difficult to differentiate from those produced by other lung disorders (e.g. pneumonias, neoplastic disease).

When sputum tests for tubercle bacilli are negative, serial radiographs at intervals are frequently necessary before a diagnosis can be made.

In the more developed countries, improved hygiene and nutrition, together with the extensive use of antituberculous drugs, have led to a considerable decrease in the incidence of pulmonary tuberculosis and also diminished the incidence of complications in sufferers from the disease.

Some of the complications of post-primary pulmonary tuberculosis which may result from direct spread of tubercle bacilli were referred to in Part III, where it was noted this type of infection may also produce metastatic tuberculous lesions as a result of spread of tubercle bacilli via blood vessels and lymphatic channels.

The treatment of pulmonary tuberculosis is by rest and measures to improve the general health and, in all patients with active disease, chemotherapy with **antituberculosis drugs** e.g. ethambutol, rifampicin, isoniazid, streptomycin. In occasional cases, areas of diseased lung may be removed surgically, this procedure being termed **lung resection**.

Other pulmonary infections—these are all rare. They include:

- **Pulmonary mycoses** (i.e. fungus infections of the lungs) among which are **aspergillosis** (due usually to infection from pigeons), **candidiasis**, **histoplasmosis**, **pulmonary blastomycosis** (European and N. American types).
- **Pulmonary hydatid disease**—see p 137.
- **Pulmonary amoebiasis**—see p 309.
- **Pulmonary syphilis**.

Neoplasms

Neoplasms of the lung will be discussed later, together with bronchial and other intrathoracic new growths.

Cysts

Cysts are cavities with a lining membrane and contain fluid, semifluid material or air. They may form in the body as a result of either developmental error in infective disease.

Congenital cysts may occur in the lung in an uncommon disorder called **congenital cystic disease of the lungs** which in some of its forms has to be distinguished from a type of bronchiectasis known as **cystic bronchiectasis**.

Cyst formation may result from some pulmonary infections and may sometimes complicate pneumonia, especially when due to staphylococci. Infective cysts due to hydatid disease may sometimes occur in lung tissue.

Very large cysts known as **pneumatoceles** (pneumoceles) or **giant air cysts** may be found in the lungs.

Multiple small cysts, with widespread distribution occur in **honey-comb lung** (cystic lung), an uncommon acquired disorder of unknown basic causation. It may be seen in association with uncommon disorders such as sarcoidosis, xanthomatosis, scleroderma, and a rare familial disorder called tuberose sclerosis. It may also develop in a type of fibrosis of the lungs called **fibrosing alveolitis** (see p 105).

Occupational Diseases of the Lungs

These are a group of pulmonary diseases caused by inhalation of harmful dusts or gases in the course of the sufferer's daily work. Those produced by mineral dusts are called pneumoconioses (from the Greek word konis meaning dust) and include **asbestosis** (from asbestos fibres), **berylliosis** (from berryllium-containing dust), **coal workers' pneumoconiosis** (from coal dust), **siderosis** (from iron-containing dust), **silicosis** (from silica-containing dust), **aluminium fibrosis**, **graphite pneumoconiosis**, **kaolin workers' pneumoconiosis**, **stannosis** (from dust containing tin), **suberosis** (from cork dust).

Three important types of pneumoconioses are given below.

Coal workers' pneumoconiosis—a condition due to the inhalation of a coal dust in high concentration and especially prevalent in the South Wales coalfields. Aggregations of coal dust form nodules within the lung and the condition may lead to the development of pulmonary fibrosis of varying degree. In severe cases this latter may take the form of **progressive massive fibrosis** (PMF) where large areas in the upper parts of the lungs become replaced by masses of fibrous tissue which may later break down with the formation of cavities.

Chronic bronchitis, emphysema, and eventually pulmonary heart disease, leading to right-sided heart failure, are common complications of coal-workers' pneumoconiosis.

This disease produces characteristic appearances on X-ray films with reticulation, nodular shadowing and, in advanced cases, appearances of pulmonary fibrosis, together with large opacities when progressive massive fibrosis has developed.

Silicosis—an occupational disorder due to the inhalation of dust containing a high proportion of fine silica particles. It may develop in those engaged in occupations such as rock drilling, sand-blasting, stonemasonry, pottery, metal grinding and quarry working.

Continued inhalation of fine silica particles into the lungs results eventually in widespread pulmonary fibrosis. The main clinical feature is breathlessness.

Radiographs show first mottling caused by nodules of silica and later also demonstrate abnormal appearances resulting from the fibrosis.

Asbestosis—Asbestos fibres contain magnesium silicate and have considerable heat-resistant and anticorrosive properties and are widely used as a heat insulating material and for other purposes. Long continued inhalation of high concentrations of asbestos dust by occupationally exposed people can lead to the development of asbestosis. The main pathological feature of this disease is a diffuse pulmonary fibrosis, mainly affecting the lower parts of the lungs. This is often accompanied by pleural thickening and pleural calcifications.

Clinically there is shortness of breath and cough, and aggregations of asbestos fibres of typical dumb-bell shape may be demonstrated by microscopic examination of the sputum.

Sufferers from asbestosis are particularly liable to develop bronchial carcinoma, or less commonly, a tumour called a **mesothelioma of the pleura**.

Occupational lung diseases due to inhalation of organic dusts also occur and include **Farmer's lung** (due to fungi in mouldy hay), **bagassosis** (due to dust from sugar cane) and **byssinosis** (due to cotton dust).

Farmer's lung and bagassosis produce an allergic reacton within the lungs of a type called **allergic alveolitis**, and byssinosis an allergic inflammation of small bronchi.

Idiopathic Diseases

Pulmonary emphysema—the term **emphysema** means inflation, and, used without qualification, indicates several different lung conditions, some diffuse and others localised, in which there is enlargement of small air spaces contained within the pulmonary acini (primary lung lobules, see p 86). Such enlargement results from either dilation of the air spaces or destruction of their walls, or a combination of both.

Two principal types of diffuse pulmonary emphysema are described, although the distinction between them is not always clear cut.

- **Panacinar emphysema**—in which there is general involvement of air spaces within affected acini. The lungs generally become enlarged, the diaphragm is pushed down, and the chest wall is pushed outwards with consequent development of a so-called barrel chest.

- **Centriacinar (centrilobular) emphysema**—a type seen frequently in association with chronic bronchitis. Pathological changes are confined chiefly to the central parts of the acini. The lungs do not usually develop the considerable enlargement seen with the panacinar emphysema.

Dyspnoea is the cardinal symptom of both these types of emphysema. In the panacinar type cyanosis is not a feature and sufferers are sometimes referred to as 'pink puffers'. Centriacinar disease, however, often leads to pulmonary hypertension, and ultimately to right-sided heart failure. Cyanosis is therefore common leading to sufferers being called 'blue bloaters'.

There is no specific treatment for emphysema but in less advanced cases considerable benefit may be derived from breathing exercises.

Spontaneous pneumothorax is not uncommon in emphysematous subjects. In severe cases of emphysema rupture of dilated alveoli may result in the formation of cyst-like spaces of varying size within lung tissue. Such spaces are called bullae; the word **bulla** meaning a bubble.

Emphysema of panacinar type often produces characteristic X-ray appearances. The lungs appear larger than normal causing flattening of both sides of the diaphragm, which are low in position. The small vascular markings within the lungs appear, as emphasised by Pierce and Grainger (4), to be diminished in size and number, a feature best seen in the middle and outer thirds of the lungs.

In localised form, emphysema may develop as a result of partial obstruction of a large bronchus (e.g. by a foreign body)—**obstructive emphysema**, or as a compensatory mechanism when there is shrinkage or loss of normal lung tissue—**compensatory emphysema**.

It should also be noted that the term **surgical emphysema** is used to describe conditions in which, as a result of injury or surgical operation, air finds its way into superficial or deep soft tissues, e.g. surgical emphysema of chest wall due to traumatic pneumothorax, mediastinal emphysema due to perforated oesophagus.

Pulmonary sarcoidosis—is a chronic inflammatory disease of unknown cause, classified as a granuloma. The characterictic lesions, when examined under the microscope, bear some resemblance to the chronic inflammatory foci found in tuberculosis. They occur in sites such as the skin, *uveal tract* (i.e. the iris diaphragm, ciliary body and choroid coat of the eye), lungs, hilar and other lymph glands, bones, and in other organs and tissues. In bones they cause a condition called **osteitis multiplex cystoides**.

In the individual patient, sarcoid lesions may be limited to one particular organ or widespread throughout the body. The disease usually begins in adults under 40 years of age.

The term **sarcoid** means flesh-like and has the same derivation as the name of the malignant neoplasm of connective tissues called a sarcoma. These two conditions are, however, otherwise unrelated.

Sarcoidosis of the lungs sometimes follows on sarcoidosis of the hilar lymph glands, a condition frequently associated with a skin disorder called **erythema nodosum**. In the majority of cases the intrathoracic lesions clear up completely but sometimes the lung changes lead to widespread pulmonary fibrosis and eventually to pulmonary heart disease.

Both the enlarged hilar glands and lung lesions produce abnormal appearances in chest radiographs. Rarely, films of the hands and feet may show cysts in the phalanges.

A skin test called the **Kveim test** is positive in most subjects with sarcoidosis. Another diagnostic investigation is measuring the amounts of *angiotensin-converting enzyme* (SACE) in the blood serum. In patients who have lesions in the skin or in superficial lymph glands the presence of the disease may be confirmed by biospy.

A large proportion of patients with the disease show a negative Mantoux test, although some authorities regard the disorder as being a manifestation of an atypical type of tuberculous infection.

There is no specific treatment for sarcoidosis but many patients benefit greatly from steroids.

Hyaline membrane disease—a condition in which difficulty in breathing is caused in newly born premature babies owing to the presence of abnormal material, referred to as **hyaline membrane**, lining the alveoli of the lungs and the terminal air passages. It is thought that the basis of this condition is a deficiency of **surfactant** (a substance containing the lipids lecithin and sphingomyelin) which is secreted by the alveoli, and by lowering surface tension, permits their expansion and protects their walls.

Radiographs of the chest often show a fine mottling throughout both lungs, sometimes accompanied by small areas of consolidation.

Treatment is directed to relief of symptoms, there being no specific therapy.

Hyaline membrane disease is frequently referred to as **respiratory distress syndrome** (RDS).

Other idiopathic lung diseases—among these are the following.

- **Idiopathic pulmonary haemosiderosis**—a condition in which haemosiderin (an iron-containing pigment derived from the haemoglobin of the blood) is deposited in the lungs.
- **Loeffler's syndrome**—a condition, thought to have an allergic basis, in which transient areas of consolidation in the lungs are accompanied by **eosinophilia**, i.e. a rise in the circulating blood of white cells of the variety called eosinophil leucocytes (eosinophils).

- **Pulmonary lesions in connective tissue disease**—see p 307.
- **Fibrosing alveolitis**—an uncommon condition characterised by the usually slow development of a diffuse fibrosis in the interstitial tissue of the lungs and the walls of the alveoli. The basal parts of the lungs are particularly affected and the disease causes a progressive shortness of breath. It may arise from completely unknown causes, as a sequel to allergic alveolitis (p 102), or in association with connective tissue diseases.

Pulmonary Embolism

As mentioned when discussing general pathological processes in Part II, the process of clot embolism consists of the detachment of a fragment of a thrombus from its original position within the lumen of a vein or artery, and its carriage in the bloodstream until it becomes arrested (the detached fragment of clot constitutes the **embolus**).

Venous emboli are very much commoner than arterial emboli. A fragment of blood clot detached from a thrombus in a vein will be carried through venous channels to the right side of the heart. From its origin from some site of **deep vein thrombosis**, such as a leg or pelvic vein, during the course of its carriage to the right ventricle, the embolus will progress through successively larger blood vessels. Once it is pumped out of the right ventricle into the pulmonary circulation, however, it will traverse arterial blood vessels of progressively diminishing calibre, so unless it is minute, it will eventually enter an artery or arteriole which is too small for it to pass through and become impacted therein.

The seriousness of pulmonary embolism varies in accordance with the size of the detached fragment of thrombus which becomes arrested within the pulmonary circulation. Thus a large thrombus may occlude the pulmonary artery itself or one of its two main branches (massive pulmonary embolism) causing sudden death or death within a few hours. If smaller, it may deprive an area of lung of its arterial blood supply, causing death of the tissue cells therein, the dead tissue being referred to as a **pulmonary infarct** and the causal process being termed **pulmonary infarction**. A very small embolism may cause only slight clinical signs and symptoms and produce negligible lung damage.

The occurrence of pulmonary embolism is often evidenced by sudden pain in the chest. Such pain frequently persists owing to the development of pleurisy over the area of the infarct. Haemoptysis is also a frequent feature of the condition and if a large infarct is produced there is often shortness of breath.

Infected emboli may cause abscess formation in the lungs.

Suspected pulmonary embolism may be investigated by plain radiography (often using a ward mobile unit), isotope lung scanning, or pulmonary angiography—or often by a combination of these methods.

Signs looked for in plain films include elevation of the diaphragm on the affected side, dilated pulmonary artery proximal to an impacted embolus, translucency of an area of lung because of elimination of its supply of blood from the pulmonary circulation, and lung opacities resulting from areas of infarction.

Lung emboli may be single or multiple.

In cases of so-called massive pulmonary embolism, **embolectomy**, surgical removal of the impacted thrombus may be considered. Less severe cases are treated with rest, antibiotics, and anticoagulants or by streptokinase, a drug which dissolves fibrin and is therefore referred to as a **fibrolysin**. (*Note:* **fibrin** is a protein substance which forms the framework of all thrombi.) This last type of treatment is referred to as **thrombolytic therapy**.

Measures to prevent the occurrence of **deep vein thrombosis** (e.g. physiotherapy, getting of patients out of bed at an early stage after surgical operation) are of value in diminishing the incidence of pulmonary embolism and infarction.

Intrathoracic Neoplasms

Intrathoracic neoplasms may arise from the pleural membranes, bronchi, lungs or structures within the mediastinum.

Pleural Neoplasms

Primary pleural neoplasms are rare, but a malignant tumour called a **mesothelioma of the pleura** is occasionally encountered. Pleural metastases from carcinomas elsewhere in the body, especially from the lung and breast, are frequent and are a common cause of pleural effusion.

Bronchial and Pulmonary Neoplasms

Benign tumours of the lung and bronchi are uncommon, but do occasionally occur, that with the highest incidence being a tumour of the lining epithelium of a bronchus called a **bronchial adenoma**.

Primary and secondary malignant neoplasms are common. Most of the former are bronchial carcinomas, often incorrectly referred to as lung carcinomas.

Bronchial carcinoma—this is a tumour which has been much in the news for many years because of its frequent incidence, and the strong probability that heavy cigarette smoking is often a factor in its causation.

It occurs much more often in men than in women and shows its maximum incidence in middle age.

Bronchial carcinoma usually arises in one of the larger bronchi near the hilum of the lung. It may, however, develop in a small peripheral bronchus. The growth starts in the bronchial mucosa and may grow so as to block the bronchial lumen, thus causing collapse of a segment or lobe or of the whole lung, according to the size of the blockage. Outward spread may also occur through the bronchial wall into the lung.

Spread of the disease by the lymphatics, first to the hilar and then to the mediastinal lymph glands, is often a fairly early feature in the disease. Glandular metastases may involve the phrenic nerve and cause paralysis and elevation of the diaphragm on the affected side. Pleural effusion is a common complication as is bronchopneumonia. Blood-borne spread is usually a late feature, but when it occurs the bones, the brain and other parts of the lungs are common sites for metastases.

Cough and haemoptysis are the most frequent early symptoms.

Radiological appearances are diverse in nature according to the site, size of the growth, its mode of spread and the presence, or absence, of intrathoracic complications such as spread to the hilar glands, pneumonic changes and pleural effusion. A rounded opacity, with an irregular outline, and often situated close to the hilum of the lung is a common form of presentation. Conventional and computerised tomography are both of value in the demonstration of early primary lesions, and of metastatic lesions in the lung, pleura and mediastinum. Inclined frontal plane tomograms (IFPTs), as indicated by Peace and Price (4), are particularly useful in demonstrating or excluding metastases in the mediastinal lymph nodes.

Bronchoscopy is an important investigation in suspected early cases of bronchial carcinoma. When the tumour is accessible, a biopsy is carried out. It is also sometimes possible to confirm the diagnosis by microscopic examination of cancer cells in the sputum, or in the fluid obtained by aspiration of a pleural effusion.

Thoractomy (surgical opening of the chest) is sometimes necessary as a diagnostic measure.

Treatment is by surgical removal of the tumour and surrounding area of lung, either lobectomy or pneumonectomy being performed, when the diagnosis is made before the growth has spread outside the lung. More advanced growths are treated by radiotherapy or cytotoxic drugs.

Pulmonary metastases—the lungs are the commonest site of the body for the occurrence of bloodborne metastases from malignant neoplasms, other than from those neoplasms arising in the area of drainage of the portal vein. Primary tumours arising in this latter area, as might be expected, produce their first bloodborne metastases most commonly in the liver.

Pulmonary metastases are usually multiple. Their presence is evidenced clinically by symptoms such as cough, haemoptysis and shortness of breath. Sometimes, however, they may be demonstrated on routine radiographs before they produce any clinical signs or symptoms. Metastases in the lungs frequently spread to involve the overlying pleura. Such involvement frequently results in pain in the chest and the formation of a pleural effusion.

On radiographs, metastases produce opacities which are generally rounded. These opacities may be very large and produce the picture of 'cannon-ball metastases' or very small and numerous, causing a widespread mottling in both lungs characteristic of as **miliary cacinomatosis**.

Carcinomatous metastases can also permeate lymphatic vessels in the lungs, causing a condition called **lymphangitis carcinomatosa**.

Mediastinal Neoplasms

Various types of neoplasm may occur within the mediastinum but, with the exception of carcinomatous metastases, none of them are very common and some are very rare.

Some of the principal neoplasms and related disorders which affect mediastinal structures (other than the oesophagus and trachea) are given below.

Benign
   (i) Arising from the nervous system: **neurofibroma**—a tumour of the sheath of a spinal nerve; **ganglioneuroma**—a tumour of the sympathetic nervous system.
   (ii) Arising from abnormally persisting embryonic tissue— **dermoid; benign teratoma**.

Malignant
   (i) Occurring in lymph glands: **carcinomatous metastases; malignant lymphomas** (Hodgkin's and non-Hodgkin's types); **leukaemic deposits** in lymph glands.
   (ii) Arising in abnormally persisting embryonic tissue—**malignant teratoma**.
   (iii) Arising in the thymus gland—**malignant thymoma**.

Mediastinal tumours are frequently demonstrable on X-ray films of the chest. Enlargement of the mediastinal shadow due to a benign or malignant neoplasm must, however, be differentiated from enlargement due to certain non-neoplastic disorders, such as; tuberculous mediastinal lymph glands; aneurysm of the thoracic aorta; retrosternal goitre (enlargement of the thyroid gland downward behind the sternum); mediastinal cysts; and simple enlargements of the thymus gland.

Some Surgical Operations on the Respiratory System and Chest

Adenoidectomy and tonsillectomy—surgical removal of the

adenoids and the tonsils. These two operations are frequently combined.

Antral puncture—puncture of the maxillary antrum through the nasal cavity by means of a trochar and cannula. A **trochar** is a pointed metal rod, used as a perforator. It is enclosed, except for its point, in a hollow metal tube called a **cannula**. When the antral wall has been perforated, the trochar is removed and fluid or pus in the antrum can then be aspirated through the cannula and the antrum can be washed out.

Caldwell-Luc operation—an operation for making an opening into the maxillary antrum through the vestibule of the mouth. The incision is made through the alveolar process of the maxilla in the molar region.

Decortication of the lung—an operation in which diseased and thickened pleura is stripped off underlying lung. It is one form of treatment for chronic empyema.

Drainage operations for empyema—these include **drainage by rib resection**, wherein access to the abscess cavity, in order to institute drainage of pus, is obtained by removing an overlying portion of rib, and **intercostal drainage** wherein drainage is accomplished by inserting a large catheter, into the abscess through an intercostal space (i.e. a space between two ribs). A trochar and cannula are employed to insert the catheter.

Laryngectomy—removal of the larynx.

Laryngofissure—an operation to give access to the interior of the larynx, by splitting the thyroid cartilage vertically in the midline.

Lung resection—removal of a part of a lung, or the whole of one lung. The latter procedure is termed **pneumonectomy**. Removal of a lobe is called **lobectomy** and removal of a bronchopulmonary segment is termed **segmental resection**.

Pharyngotomy—the making of an opening into the pharynx.

Phrenic crush—crushing the phrenic nerve in the neck to effect a temporary paralysis on one side of the diaphragm.

Reconstruction of the pharynx—involves the creation of an artificial pharynx from a segment of colon or stomach. The pharynx and larynx are removed and a tracheostomy made during the course of this operation.

Rib resection—removal of a rib. Partial rib resection may be undertaken in order to drain empyema cavities.

Thoracoplasty—an operation in which portions of a varying number of ribs were removed, thus permitting the chest wall to fall in. It used to be much employed in cases of chronic pulmonary tuberculosis with the object of effecting partial collapse of lung tissue, thereby limiting the functional activity of diseased areas.

Thoracotomy—making an opening into the thoracic cavity.

Tracheostomy—making an opening into the trachea to relieve respiratory obstruction, arising in the upper respiratory system, and inserting a tube to maintain the airway.

REFERENCES

(1) Taylor, S., Cotton, L. (1982). *A Short Textbook of Surgery*, 5th Edn. London: Hodder and Stoughton.

(2) Kerley, P. (1973). *A Textbook of X-Ray Diagnosis*, 4th Edn. (Shanks, C. S., Kerley, P., eds.) Vol. III. London: Lewis.

(3) Lodge, T., Darke, C. S. (1964). *Recent Advances in Radiology*, 4th Edn. (Lodge, T., ed.) London: Churchill.

(4) Pierce, J. W., Grainger, R. G. (1980). *Textbook of Radiology and Imaging*, 3rd Edn. (Sutton, D., ed.) Edinburgh: Churchill Livingstone.

(5) Peace, P. K., Price, J. L., (1973). Preoperative tomographic assessment of the mediastinum in bronchial carcinoma. *Thorax*; **24**: 367–70.

DIGESTIVE SYSTEM

Anatomical and Physiological Considerations

The digestive system includes (a) the *alimentary canal* which consists of the *mouth*, *oropharynx*, *laryngopharynx* (*hypopharynx*), *stomach*, *small intestine* (*duodenum*, *jejunum* and *ileum*) and *large intestine* (*caecum*, *vermiform appendix*, *colon*, *rectum*, and *anal canal*), and (b) the *accessory digestive organs*, namely the *teeth*, *salivary glands*, *liver*, *pancreas*, *gall bladder* and *bile ducts*.

The term **digestion**, from which the system is named, indicates the processes by which foodstuffs are broken down into substances which can be absorbed from the intestines and used for tissue building and repair. The digestive system is concerned with the digestion of foodstuffs, the absorption into the body of digested food and of water, and the excretion of undigested food in the faeces.

Ingested food is propelled through the alimentary canal chiefly by a type of muscular action referred to as **peristalsis**.

Digestion is effected by the action of substances called digestive *enzymes* (see p 75) which act on specific classes of foodstuffs and are secreted by the salivary glands, by glands in the walls of the stomach and small intestine, and by the pancreas, e.g. *pepsin* which is secreted in the stomach and acts on proteins, and by *amylase*, a pancreatic secretion which acts on starches.

The digestion of fatty foodstuffs is aided by the action of *bile*, which is secreted by the liver and is concentrated in the gall bladder. Besides secreting bile, the liver has a number of highly important functions concerned with the metabolism of proteins, carbohydrates and fats, and also with the inactivation of toxic substances.

The following are among the word components referring to organs of the digestive system: **gloss–** tongue; **gastr–** stomach; **enter–** intestine, particularly the small intestine; **sigmoid–** sigmoid colon; **proct–** rectum; **hepat–** liver; **chole–** bile; **cholecyst–** gall bladder; **cholangi–** bile ducts. **Cheilo–** means pertaining to the lips and **labio–** has a similar meaning.

The adjective **oral** means pertaining to the mouth; and **buccal** pertaining to the cheek.

General Aspects of Diseases of the Digestive System

Diseases affecting this system may be congenital, traumatic, infective, neoplastic, due to cyst formation, metabolic, due to chemical poisons, allergic or idiopathic—all of which are associated with structural changes, i.e. **organic diseases**.

So-called **functional diseases**, i.e. diseases in which the symptoms and signs appear to arise as a result of functional disorder without demonstrable structural changes, are especially frequent in the digestive system and may produce symptoms which closely resemble those of organic diseases such as peptic ulceration, chronic appendicitis, and the milder types of colonic inflammation.

Disorders of the digestive system may give rise to various signs and symptoms according to the part of the system affected. Some of these are as follows: pain arising from various parts of the system and including cramp-like pains in the abdomen, due to spasm of plain muscle, described as **colic** (e.g. intestinal colic, biliary colic, appendicular colic); sore mouth and throat, **dysphagia** (difficulty in swallowing), heartburn, nausea, flatulence, **anorexia** (loss of appetite), vomiting, abdominal discomfort, abdominal distention, **haematemesis** (vomiting of blood), **melaena** (passage of stools which are black owing to presence of altered blood), diarrhoea, constipation, rectal bleeding, **jaundice** (yellow colouration of the skin and mucous membranes), **steatorrhoea** (passage of stools containing excessive amounts of fat).

Symptoms such as flatulence, anorexia, vomiting, intestinal colic, and abdominal discomfort, are frequently referred to as being due to **indigestion**, a term of ill-defined usage indicating disordered digestion. The term **dyspepsia** is a synonym for indigestion.

Disorders affecting the stomach and intestine are often referred to as **gastrointestinal disorders**.

Special Methods of Investigation

Radiological investigation—this may take the form of plain X-rays or contrast radiography or other forms of diagnostic imaging.

The commoner types of contrast radiography of the digestive system and the parts of this system they are designed to demonstrate are: **barium swallow**—oesophagus; **barium meal**—stomach and duodenum; **barium meal 'follow-through'**—jejunum, ileum and, sometimes, also, large intestine; **barium enema**—large intestine; **cholecystography**—gall bladder; **cholangiography** (peroperative, postoperative, and transhepatic)—bile ducts; **intravenous cholangiocholecystography** (IVC)—bile ducts and gall bladder.

Information regarding certain lesions of the liver and pancreas may be obtained by various forms of angiography and also by ultrasonic methods, radioisotope scanning and CT.

A combination of endoscopy and contrast radiology may be used to demonstrate the biliary and pancreatic ducts in the procedure generally referred to as **ERCP**, initials indicating **endoscopy with retrograde cholangiopancreatography**.

Pathological Investigations—these are very diverse. Included among them are (i) **gastric analysis**, i.e. analysis of gastric secretions obtained by aspiration of the stomach contents through a Ryle's gastric tube, and often performed after giving a test meal of gruel or after injection of histamine; (ii) **examination of the faeces for occult blood** by chemical tests or tests involving the use of radioactive isotopes. The word occult means concealed, and **occult blood** is blood which is not evident to the naked eye; (iii) **bacteriological examination of the faeces** in suspected gastrointestinal infections; (iv) **estimation of the fat content of the faeces** in suspected malabsorption syndromes (see p 133); (v) **biopsy**—this may be performed under direct vision in the mouth and through special instruments (see below) in the oesophagus, stomach, colon and rectum. **Small intestine biopsy** may be performed by specially designed biopsy tubes or by means of a small hollow capsule, containing a spring-loaded knife-blade and called a **Crosby capsule**. **Liver biopsy** may be performed by inserting a biopsy needle through the lower chest wall directly into the liver; (vi) investigation of pressure within the bowel and the pH of the intestinal contents given by swallowed **telemetry capsules** which contain small transmitters designed to provide information at a distance from the body; (vii) **liver function tests**—used to investigate some of the many functions of the liver. There are a great many of these tests. The names of just a few of them are: **estimation of serum bilirubin**; **bromsulphthalein test** (BSP); **estimation of serum alkaline phosphatase**; **estimation of serum proteins**; **estimation of the serum aminotransferase**; (viii) **pancreatic function tests**, e.g. **estimation of the blood amylase** (a pancreatic enzyme).

Visual inspection by special instruments—the interiors, or parts thereof, of the following organs may be examined visually by procedures using special instruments: the pharynx—by **pharyngoscopy**; the oesophagus—by **oesophagoscopy**; the stomach—by

gastroscopy; the duodenum by **duodenoscopy**; the colon—by **colonoscopy**; and the rectum by **proctoscopy**. The instruments employed have similar names to the procedure, their names ending with the suffix **-scope**, e.g. proctoscopy is performed with a proctoscope. The visual examination of the oesophagus, stomach, duodenum and colon has been greatly extended since the introduction of instruments of a type termed **fibreoptic endoscopes** (the term **endoscopy** is used with reference to the visual inspection of the interior of any hollow organ in the body).

Gastric photography—this may be accomplished by passing a specially designed gastric camera into the interior of the stomach, which may then be photographed using a special colour film. The position of the gastric camera during the taking of the various exposures, may be controlled by fluoroscopy (X-ray screening).

Diseases of the Mouth and Tongue

Congenital Disorders

The most important of these are gaps along normal lines of developmental fusion in the upper lip and palate, giving rise to the conditions called **cleft lip** (hare lip) and **cleft palate**. The reasons for the occurrence of developmental defects of this type are unknown.

Cleft lip and cleft palate may occur independently or both be present in the same patient. Both interfere with feeding and cleft palate causes defective speech. The treatment of both conditions is surgical.

Inflammatory Conditions

Inflammation of the mouth is called **stomatitis**, and of the tongue **glossitis**. **Gingivitis** means inflammation of the gums.

Among the various types of stomatitis are: (a) **candidiasis** (moniliasis), known popularly as **thrush**, a fungus infection, seen most often in infants but in adults may follow antibiotic treatment, (b) **aphthous ulcers**—small painful recurrent ulcers, of unknown causation which may develop in any part of the mouth, and (c) **Vincent's infection** (trench mouth) which is usually seen in debilitated subjects, is ascribed to a mixed infection with spirochaetes and bacteria called fusiform bacilli.

Glossitis is of various types and chronic inflammatory changes in the mucosa of the tongue may result in the development of a pre-cancerous condition called **leucoplakia**. The prefix **leuco-** or **leuko-** means white and this name is descriptive of the white patches which constitute the earlier lesions of the disorder.

Neoplasms

Benign tumours are not common in the mouth and tongue. Carcinomas are of fairly frequent occurrence and may arise in the mucous membrane covering the lip, cheek, tongue, floor of mouth and the gums. The great majority of these are of the type of growths known as **epitheliomas** or, alternatively, **squamous-cell carcinomas** as they arise from epithelium of the squamous type. (*Note:* The external surface of the body is covered by, and all its internal cavities are lined by, cellular tissue called **epithelium**.)

Early spread by the lymphatics is often seen in these carcinomas, but bloodborne metastases are not common. Pneumonia is a frequent complication in advanced cases.

Surgery and radiotherapy, singly or in combination, are employed in the treatment of carcinomas of the mouth and tongue and their metastases in the cervical lymph glands. In suitable cases, however, these latter may be removed by a surgical operation called a **block dissection of the neck**.

Cysts

Among these are the condition called **ranula**, a cyst in the floor of the mouth below the tongue, and **thyroglossal cyst**, a cyst of congenital origin found in the midline of the tongue or neck arising from remnants of an embryonic structure called the thyroglossal duct.

Diseases of the Salivary Glands

These include the formation of calculi (stones) called **salivary calculi**, inflammatory conditions referred to as **sialitis**, and neoplasms. The virus disease called mumps is one form of acute sialitis. Chronic sialitis may lead to dilatation of the terminations of small ducts in a salivary gland. This disorder is termed **sialectasis**, and in the parotid and submandibular (submaxillary) salivary glands it may be demonstrated by a form of contrast radiography called **sialography**.

Chronic inflammation of the parotid gland, together with an eye disorder called iridocyclitis, may occur as an uncommon manifestation of sarcoidosis.

Lesions in the salivary glands are also prominent features in two rare disorders called **Mikulicz's syndrome** and **Sjogren's syndrome**.

The most important neoplasm in the salivary glands is the so-called mixed tumour which usually occurs in the parotid gland.

Mixed parotid tumour (parotid adenoma)—this is a benign neoplasm of epithelial origin. Formerly it was thought to belong to the class of mixed tumours which contains several different types of tissue (cf dermoids and teratomas), and it has retained its old name. It may, rarely, develop malignant changes.

The tumour is slow growing. Treatment is by complete surgical removal of the growth.

Diseases of the Pharynx

The nasopharynx is part of the upper respiratory tract. The oropharynx and upper part of the laryngopharynx are common to the respiratory and digestive systems. Some reference has already been made to diseases of the pharynx (i.e. pharyngitis, adenoids, tonsillitis, quinsy, and certain carcinomas have already been referred to when discussing diseases of the upper respiratory system).

Among the disorders found in the lower part of the laryngopharynx are impaction of swallowed **foreign bodies** (especially meat and fish bones), pharyngeal pouch, and post-cricoid carcinoma.

Pharyngeal Pouch (Pharyngeal Diverticulum)

This condition is thought to arise as a result of the presence of a small area of congenital weakness between muscles in the lower part of the pharynx. With advancing years a bulge of mucous membrane through this weak area develops. At first this forms a small pouch, which tends to increase in size gradually, until ultimately it may become very large. Large pouches cause **dysphagia**, i.e. difficulty in swallowing, as a result of their pressing on nearby portions of the lower pharynx and upper oesophagus. The presence of a pharyngeal pouch is readily demonstrable by barium swallow.

An alternative name for the condition is **pharyngeal diverticulum**. It is to be noted that pouches, or diverticula, may arise in other parts of the alimentary canal and occur fairly frequently in the colon.

Neoplasms of the Oropharynx and Laryngopharynx

Benign tumours are uncommon in the pharynx. Carcinomas may affect any part of this structure, the opening of the larynx into the pharynx, the pyriform fossa, the lateral wall of the laryngopharynx and the postcricoid region.

Post-cricoid carcinoma is chiefly a disease of women showing its maximum incidence in middle age. Early lymphatic spread is often a feature of this tumour. The growth frequently develops as a sequel to Plummer-Vinson syndrome (see p 208). Dysphagia is the cardinal symptom.

Pharyngoscopy with biopsy, and barium swallow, are important diagnostic investigations.

Treatment is mainly by radiotherapy, few patients being suitable for surgery.

Diseases of the Oesophagus

These include congenital abnormalities, foreign body in the oesophagus, rupture of the oesophagus as a result of trauma or disease, burns from hot or corrosive liquids, an inflammatory condition called reflux oesophagitis, diverticula, carcinoma, and a disorder called achalasia of the cardia.

Congenital Abnormalities

The oesophagus is a hollow muscular tube. In rare instances, as a result of development error during early intrauterine life, the upper and lower portions of the oesophagus may be separated by an area, of varying length, where the interior lumen is absent or narrowed. If absent the condition is described as **oesophageal atresia**; if narrowed as **oesophageal stricture**.

In cases of atresia the patent part of the lumen of either the upper segment, or more often the lower segment of the oesophagus is connected to the trachea by a fistula (a track with two open ends). The disorder is then described as a **tracheo–oesophageal fistula**. Affected infants vomit their first feed and all subsequent feeds. The diagnosis may be confirmed by failure to pass a soft rubber catheter down the oesophagus and further established radiologically by giving an opaque swallow using a bronchographic contrast medium, e.g. propyliodone (Dionosil) instead of barium. Treatment is by urgent surgery.

Congenital oesophageal strictures are much less common than acquired oesophageal strictures. The latter may result from burns from corrosive liquids, trauma, neoplasms, etc., but more often develop as a result of reflex oesophagitis (see later).

Another type of developmental error may result in the oesophagus being abnormally short. In patients with **congenital short oesophagus**, the junction between the oesophagus and stomach lies within the thorax and hence there is a **congenital hiatus hernia**.

A **hernia** is a protrusion of a structure through the wall of the cavity in which it is normally contained. A protrusion of the stomach through the oesophageal hiatus of the diaphragm is called a **hiatus hernia**.

Hiatus hernia is a fairly common condition. In most cases, however, whether presenting in childhood or in adult life, the disorder is thought to be acquired (see below). Both the congenital and acquired sliding varieties are demonstrable by barium swallow but are indistinguishable radiologically.

Reflux Oesophagitis and Hiatus Hernia

Reflux oesophagitis is a disease in which inflammation of the mucosa of the oesophagus results from gastro–oesophageal reflux, i.e. reflux of acid gastric juice from the stomach into the oesophagus. Its basis is inefficiency of the sphincter mechanism at the cardia (i.e. the opening at the joint of junction of the oesophagus and stomach), this latter condition being known as **incompetence of the cardia** or as **lax cardia**. Reflux oesophagitis occurs most frequently in childhood, during middle and old age, and during pregnancy.

Heartburn is the commonest symptom. There may also be pain behind the sternum, which may mimic anginal pain, when it is called **pseudoangina** (see p 74). Vomiting, dysphagia and haematemesis may also be features of the disease. As described by Pracy, Siegler and Stell (1) many patients said to have **globus hystericus** (a persistent feeling of a lump in the throat unaccompanied by other symptoms) have reflux oesophagitis.

The oesophageal inflammation may lead to mucosal ulceration and may also cause a localised spasm of the circular muscle coat of the oesophagus, resulting in a spastic narrowing in the lower part of the lumen of this organ. When inflammation is severe, fibrosis may occur in the oesophageal wall and an initially spastic narrowing may develop into a permanent fibrous **oesophageal stricture**.

Reflux oesophagitis is often associated with the presence of a **sliding hiatus hernia**, an acquired condition in which a portion of stomach of varying size protrudes intermittently or permanently through the oesophageal hiatus in the diaphragm and, as a result, the cardiac orifice of the stomach lies intermittently or permanently within the thorax. The anatomical abnormality in this disorder is thus similar to that of a congenital short oesophagus with associated partial intrathoracic stomach (congenital hiatus hernia).

Laxity of the oesophageal hiatus, spasm of oesophageal musculature consequent upon resultant reflux, and raised intra-abdominal pressure are thought to be factors in the causation of sliding hiatus hernia.

Note: In addition to the congenital and sliding varieties of hiatus hernia, a third type of hiatus hernia, known as a **rolling hiatus hernia** or **paraoesophageal hernia** sometimes occurs. This is an acquired condition in which the oesophagus is of normal length and the cardia lies below the diaphragm.

> Gastro-oesophageal reflux and the presence of hiatus hernia are demonstrable by barium swallow. In some instances they are readily shown. In others special methods, such as examination during bending, tipping into the Trendelenburg position, swallowing in the supine position, have to be employed for their demonstration. An opaque swallow will also demonstrate stricture formation in the oesophagus.

In addition to contrast radiology, oesophagoscopy is also frequently indicated.

Treatment is medical in most patients with both conditions; surgery is indicated, however, when medical treatment does not relieve the severe symptoms of oesophagitis or when there is a large hiatus hernia or an oesophageal stricture. This latter complication may also be treated by dilatation of the stenosed area by cylindrical rods called **bougies**.

Carcinoma of the Oesophagus

Carcinoma may originate anywhere in the oesophagus, but occurs most frequently at the extreme upper and lower ends, and in the middle third of this viscus. It is predominantly a disease of old age and much commoner in men than in women.

Dysphagia is the chief symptom and results from narrowing of the oesophagus. Barium swallow, oesophagoscopy and biopsy are all important diagnostic procedures in suspected cases.

Surgical excision may be practicable with early growths, particularly with carcinomas of the lower end of the oesophagus. Most cases are unsuitable for surgery and are treated by radiotherapy. In some cases a **Celestin tube** may be inserted into the stenosed area to maintain a patent channel through which the patient may be fed. Alternatively, it may be necessary to perform a bypass operation, anastomosing a loop of jejunum to the oesophagus above the growth.

Achalasia of the Cardia (Cardiospasm)

This is a condition of narrrowing of the lower end of the oesophagus, caused by spasm of circular muscle fibres in this region. The spasm is thought to result from degeneration of certain nerves in the oesophageal wall, and causes a failure of normal relaxation of the cardiac sphincter during swallowing. This gives the disease its name of **achalasia**, this term meaning a failure to relax. The cause of the condition is unknown.

Solids and fluids are held up above the spastic area and, as a result, the oesophagus above this area becomes dilated and lengthened.

Dysphagia is the chief symptom and usually develops in middle age, although the condition sometimes presents in childhood.

Oesophagitis and bronchopneumonia are common complications. The condition produces characteristic appearances at barium swallow.

Treatment may be by instrumental or pneumatic dilatation of the spastic area or by surgery. (See Heller's operation.)

Diseases of the Stomach and Duodenum

Congenital Abnormalities

Congenital pyloric stenosis—in this condition, as indicated by its name, there is a stenosis (narrowing) of the pylorus (the opening between the stomach and duodenum) due to hypertrophy of the circular muscle fibres in the region of the pyloric sphincter. The stenosis produces a varying degree of obstruction to the passage of gastric contents from the stomach into the duodenum. The disease is much commoner in male than in female children. The cardinal symptom is vomiting which, however, does not usually occur until about three weeks after birth and is projectile. There is often a palpable swelling in the abdomen caused by the thickened muscle at the pylorus, and peristaltic waves passing from left to right may often be observed in the upper abdomen after a feed.

Barium meal is a valuable investigation when the clinical diagnosis is in doubt.

Some cases are treated with antispasmodic drugs but in most patients treatment is surgical division of the thickened pyloric muscle (**Ramstedt's operation**).

Congenital duodenal atresia—a condition in which developmental error results in the presence of an area where the lumen of the duodenum is absent. As a result of this there is vomiting from birth. The vomitus (vomited material) is bile-stained because the atresia occurs below the level where the common bile duct enters the duodenum.

Inflammatory Diseases

Gastritis—this term means inflammation of the stomach and is used to describe a group of acute and chronic inflammatory disorders with rather ill-defined signs and symptoms, but in some instances producing clinical pictures that bear a similarity to those of either peptic ulceration or carcinoma of the stomach.

The simple type of acute gastritis is extremely common and may be caused by overindulgence in alcohol, dietary indiscretion, food poisoning, the action of certain drugs, or acute infective conditions such as influenza. It is evidenced by clinical features such as nausea, anorexia, vomiting and abdominal pain and discomfort.

Peptic ulceration—An ulcer has already been defined as an open sore caused by an inflammatory process breaking through the skin or a mucous membrane. In sites where *pepsin*, an enzyme found in gastric juice, comes in contact with mucous membranes, a type of ulcer called a peptic ulcer may develop.

Peptic ulcers are therefore found mainly in the stomach and duodenum and are referred to respectively as gastric and duodenal ulcers. The commonest site for their occurrence is the first part of the duodenum. They may also occur in the jejunum, usually as a sequel to certain types of operation which establish a direct communication between the stomach and jejunum (i.e. certain forms of partial gastrectomy and gastrojejunostomy). Rarely, also, peptic ulceration may be found in the lower oesophagus.

Peptic ulcers are common and may be acute or chronic. They are sometimes seen in children but their greatest incidence is in middle-age. Their cause is unknown. Occasional cases of acute peptic ulceration are associated with steroid therapy (e.g. for rheumatoid arthritis), sensitivity to aspirin, or severe burns.

Acute gastric and acute duodenal ulcers may cause symptoms of indigestion but, sometimes, first reveal their presence as the result of the ulcerative process producing either severe bleeding or causing perforation of the overlying wall of the stomach, or duodenum, with resultant leakage of gas and fluid into the peritoneal cavity, i.e. a condition of **perforated peptic ulcer**.

Chronic gastric and duodenal ulcers may also cause bleeding or perforation but these complications are rarely the first evidence of their presence. Dyspepsia and pain after meals are usually the chief symptoms and vomiting is a feature in some cases.

An appreciable degree of bleeding from a peptic ulcer will result in **melaena** (the passage of stools, coloured black owing to the presence of altered blood). Haemorrhage from a gastric ulcer frequently also causes **haematemesis** (vomiting of blood). Haematemesis can occur also from a duodenal ulcer but much less frequently.

Perforation of an acute or chronic peptic ulcer is characterised by the sudden onset of severe abdominal pain and by shock.

Chronic peptic ulceration may result in the development of fibrosis in and around the ulcerated area. With ulcers in the region of the pylorus, contraction of fibrous tissue may lead in time to narrowing of the pylorus. This complication is called **pyloric stenosis** and is of serious import because it impedes gastric emptying, thus leading to vomiting of the stomach contents with consequent dehydration and loss of weight.

Occasionally a carcinomatous growth may develop in a chronic gastric ulcer but this happens infrequently. (*Note:* carcinoma does not develop in connection with chronic duodenal ulceration.)

Fibreoptic endoscopy is of great value in demonstrating peptic ulceration in both the stomach and duodenum and is generally the investigation of choice identifying the site of a bleeding ulcer.

Acute gastric and duodenal ulcers are often difficult to demonstrate radiologically because they tend to be small and shallow. A high proportion of chronic peptic ulcers may, however, be shown by a barium meal examination. This investigation can also reveal complications such as pyloric stenosis and neoplastic change. The use of a double-contrast technique is frequently of considerable advantage when performing barium studies.

When perforation has occurred, plain radiographs, taken with appropriate positioning, will frequently reveal gas that has escaped through the perforation into the peritoneal cavity. The diagnosis may also be established by giving a water-soluble iodine contrast medium and demonstrated by subsequent radiographs that it has leaked into the peritoneal cavity.

In many instances of chronic peptic ulceration information of value may also be obtained by performing a test meal and gastric analysis. Treatment of an uncomplicated peptic ulcer may be medical or surgical. Usually medical treatment is given an adequate trial to begin with. Liquorice preparations and bismuth compounds are often of considerable therapeutic value in gastric ulceration, and a drug called cimetidine (Tagamet) in duodenal ulceration. Most cases of haematemesis are treated medically in the first instance, but surgical intervention may be necessary if the bleeding does not stop within a reasonable period. Perforated ulcers may be treated either by immediate operation or by gastric suction and administration of fluids through an intravenous drip. Surgical treatment is necessary in cases of pyloric stenosis.

Duodenitis—means inflammation of the duodenum. This condition may be demonstrated either by duodenoscopy or by barium meal.

Gastroenteritis—food poisoning has been referred to as a cause of gastritis. When inflammation of the stomach is due to this cause, concomitant inflammatory changes are frequently produced in the bowel. These are referred to as enteritis and the disorder is thus called **gastroenteritis**.

Food poisoning may result from ingestion of food or drink contaminated by pathogenic bacteria, or from the ingestion of certain chemical poisons (e.g. arsenic). It may also occur as a manifestation of hypersensitivity to certain foods (e.g. shellfish) in individuals with food allergy.

Important causes of bacterial food poisoning are bacilli of the *Salmonella* and *Campylobacter* groups, certain strains of staphylococci, and a bacillus called *Clostridium welchii*. An uncommon causal organism, but one which causes a serious and often fatal illness is the *Clostridium botulinus* which is responsible for the infection known as **botulism**.

Acquired pyloric stenosis—narrowing of the pylorus, with resultant obstructive signs and symptoms, may be due to fibrosis caused by the inflammatory changes of gastric or duodenal ulceration.

By no means, however, are all cases of this condition of inflammatory origin. As already noted, it may be due to developmental error as in congenital pyloric stenosis, and as will be indicated later, it may be produced by a carcinoma arising in the distal part of the pyloric antrum of the stomach.

Pyloric stenosis is also seen in an idiopathic disorder of adults called **chronic hypertrophic pyloric stenosis**.

Neoplasms

Benign neoplasms of the stomach are rare the commonest being a tumour of smooth muscle called a **leiomyoma**. Any type of duodenal new growth is exceedingly uncommon. On the other hand, gastric carcinoma has a high incidence in males and occurs fairly frequently in females.

Carcinoma of the stomach—the maximum incidence of this disease is in middle age and the commonest site for its origin is in the mucosa of the pyloric antrum. It can, however, develop in the mucosal lining in any other part of the stomach. It may arise as a sequel to a chronic gastric ulcer but this does not often happen.

As it progresses, the growth may either infiltrate the stomach wall around its site of origin, produce a large tumour which projects into the lumen or the stomach, or cause malignant ulceration of the gastric mucosa.

According to the site of the growth, complications such as obstruction of the cardia, 'hour-glass' deformity of the body of the stomach, and pyloric stenosis may develop as local spread of the malignant processes takes place. Perforation sometimes occurs but is not common.

Lymphatic metastases are often an early feature in the disease and when they occur in the cleft in the undersurface of the liver, known as the *porta hepatis*, they may cause jaundice by pressing on and obstructing the bile ducts. (*Note:* **jaundice** is yellow colouration of the skin and mucous membranes due to excess of bilirubin, a bile pigment, in the circulation.)

A gastric carcinoma causes symptoms and signs such as anorexia, loss of weight, pain in the epigastrium, vomiting, anaemia, and sometimes haematemesis and melaena. In advanced cases there may be a palpable mass in the epigastrium.

Barium meal examination is an important diagnostic measure. The radiological detection of the disease in its earlier stages is extremely difficult but may be facilitated by using a double contrast technique, which may be helped by the preliminary intravenous injection of either hyoscine butylbromide (Buscopan) or glucagon to cause a temporary relaxation of the gastric muscles and permit an adequate degree of distension of the stomach.

Gastroscopy combined with biopsy is another important investigation. However, sometimes, **diagnostic laparatomy** (the opening of the abdomen by surgical incision, as a diagnostic procedure) may be advisable when, in spite of negative radiological and gastroscopic findings, there is a strong suspicion on clinical evidence that a carcinoma of the stomach is present.

The treatment of a gastric carcinoma, diagnosed in an operable stage, is by radical surgery, and in advanced cases some form of palliative surgery is often advocated to relieve vomiting.

Other Gastric and Duodenal Diseases

These include: (*a*) **foreign bodies** in the stomach and duodenum—an uncommon but interesting type of foreign body, seen usually in the stomach, is the **bezoar**. This results from the gradual accumulation within the viscus of small ingested amounts of material such as the patient's hair forming a **trichobezoar** (hairball), or of fruit or vegetable fibres forming a **phytobezoar**; (*b*) gastric and duodenal **diverticula** (pouches); (*c*) **volvulus of the stomach**—a condition in which the stomach becomes twisted around one of its axes, the word volvulus indicating a twisting, but being originally derived from a Latin word meaning to roll; (*d*) **acute dilatation of the stomach**—a rare post-operative condition; (*e*) **chronic duodenal ileus**—a condition of chronic partial duodenal obstruction resulting from pressure of the superior mesenteric artery (and its containing fold of mesentery) on the third part of the duodenum, and consequently also termed **chronic arteriomesenteric obstruction** or **vascular compression of the duodenum**; (*f*) duodenal obstruction associated with **malrotation of the gut** (see p 124).

Diseases of the Small and Large Intestine

The intestine is referred to also as the bowel or the gut. The small intestine is composed of the duodenum, jejunum and ileum, but, for purposes of description, it is convenient to consider disorders of the duodenum together with those of the stomach, as has been done here. The ensuing descriptions will thus refer more particularly to diseases of the jejunum, ileum and large intestine.

Congenital Abnormalities

Various developmental abnormalities may affect the intestines. Some of the more important are given below.

Meckel's diverticulum—is a narrow tube, which communicates with the lower ileum and arises from a failure of closure of a duct (the vitelline duct), which is present at a certain stage of fetal life. This abnormality is fairly common but rarely causes trouble. Sometimes, however, the diverticulum may become inflamed producing an illness similar to an attack of acute appendicitis. Also, there may be bands, attached to the diverticulum, which can cause intestinal obstruction through pressure on an adjacent loop of small bowel.

Hirschsprung's disease (congenital megacolon)—a condition in which a narrowed segment of bowel is found in the pelvic colon. This forms a partial obstruction to normal downward passage of faeces into the rectum. As a result, the bowel above the narrowing becomes dilated owing to the accumulatation of faeces within it. It is this dilatation which is responsible for the word **megacolon**, meaning large colon, in the alternative name of the disease.

The condition is, however, more frequently referred to as Hirschsprung's disease, after H. Hirschsprung, who was a Danish physician.

The narrow segment results from a failure of development of nerve ganglion cells in the affected part of the colon.

Constipation from birth and increasing abdominal distension are the main clinical features. Acute intestinal obstruction is a common complication.

> The narrowed segment and the dilated bowel behind it may both be demonstrated by barium enema. Describing a technique for demonstrating such a narrow segment, Ward (2) many years ago stressed the importance of observing (during screening) the initial filling of the rectum and rectosigmoid region, stopping filling at various stages and taking films in various positions to show abnormalities, and the rectosigmoid region.

Treatment is surgical, the narrow segment and dilated portion of the colon being resected.

Congenital megacolon must be differentiated from another variety of colonic dilation of unknown causation, called **idiopathic megacolon** (acquired megacolon) and also from a condition called the **small left colon syndrome**.

Idiopathic megacolon, which is treated medically, is also characterised by chronic constipation and abdominal distension. There is, however, no narrowed segment of bowel and the rectum is dilated as well as the colon.

Imperforate anus—this is a condition in which, as a result of developmental error, the rectum does not open normally into the anal canal. The two may merely be separated by a thin membrane or the rectum may terminate blindly at some distance from the anus.

> The extent of the gap may often be shown by radiography. Films are taken with a metal marker placed at the anus and the child is held upside down, in order that gas in the bowel may rise and outline the terminal portion of the rectum.

Treatment is surgical.

Malrotation of the gut—during fetal life the developing intestines undergo a considerable degree of rotation in order to reach the positions in the abdomen which they normally occupy after birth. An upset in these processes constitutes malrotation of the gut, an uncommon condition that includes major and minor abnormalities.

The most important major abnormality of this type is called **situs inversus partialis**, wherein the small bowel lies in the right side and the colon in the left side of the abdomen, the caecum being found near the midline.

Twisting of the intestine in the region of the duodenojejunal flexure and resultant duodenal obstruction is a not infrequent complication of malrotation.

Meconium ileus—this term indicates blockage of the small intestine by thick meconium, a disorder which occurs as a result of **mucoviscidosis** (see p 144).

In a newly born infant the faeces are at first dark green and at this stage are referred to as **meconium**. Any type of intestinal obstruction may be termed an **ileus**.

Traumatic Disorders

The bowel may be contused or ruptured by injuries to the abdomen of non-penetrating type. Penetrating wounds may also cause contusion of the intestine, traumatic perforation, or sometimes complete division of a segment of bowel.

Inflammatory Diseases

It is to be noted that while **enteritis** means inflammation of the intestine, it is sometimes used to indicate inflammation of the small bowel only.

Inflammation of the colon is called **colitis**; inflammation of the caecum, **typhlitis**; and inflammation of the rectum, **proctitis**.

Inflammation of the small bowel with concomitant inflammatory changes in the colon is sometimes described as **enterocolitis**.

Among the inflammatory disorders that occur in small and large bowel are the following.

Gastroenteritis due to food poisoning—see p 121.

Regional enteritis (Crohn's disease, granulomatous enterocolitis)—this is a chronic inflammatory disorder, classified as a non-infective granuloma, so-called because the changes affect one or more regions of bowel rather than being generalised in distribution. It is, however, perhaps more widely referred to as **Crohn's disease** after B. B. Crohn, an American physician. Its cause is unknown. Its maximum incidence is chiefly in young adults but it is not very common.

The disease affects principally the terminal portion of the ileum, but may occur elsewhere in the small or large bowel (including the anorectal region, where it may be a cause of **fistula-in-ano**, see later) and rarely in the stomach or oesophagus. When the lesions are confined to the ileum it is sometimes referred to as **regional ileitis**.

In an affected area the chronic inflammatory lesions cause considerable fibrosis with thickening of the bowel wall and consequent narrowing of its lumen. They also produce ulceration of the intestinal mucosa and perforation of ulcerated areas may lead to the formation of multiple small abscesses around the bowel. Such abscesses may eventually produce internal fistulae which communicate with other loops of bowel, or external fistulae which lead from the bowel and discharge faeces and pus through the abdominal wall. Those which discharge faecal matter externally are called **faecal fistulae**.

Other complications include intestinal obstruction and malabsorption syndrome.

The principal clinical features of regional enteritis are pain and diarrhoea and palable abdominal swelling develops in many patients. There is usually loss of weight and general debility.

> Narrowing areas of the small bowel may be shown radiologically by a barium small bowel meal or enema, and colonic changes, when present, by a barium enema. These latter changes may sometimes be difficult to distinguish from those of another inflammatory colonic disorder called ulcerative colitis.

Nowadays, in uncomplicated cases, medical treatment is generally advised to begin with surgical measures usually being reserved for certain complications of the disease.

Intestinal tuberculosis—the intestine, as noted in Part II, may be the site of primary tuberculosis and infection in this site may lead to inflammatory changes in draining lymph glands in the mesentery, i.e. **tuberculous mesenteric adenitis**.

> Evidence of this latter infection, which is generally mild, may be seen subsequently on X-ray films in the form of pathological calcification in old healed infective foci within the glands.

Rarely, **tuberculous ileitis** may occur as a complication of advanced post-primary tuberculosis, and another rare type of tuberculous infection. termed **hyperplastic caecal tuberculosis**, may develop in the caecum. Tuberculosis, also, is an uncommon cause of **fistula-in-ano** (see later).

Typhoid fever (enteric fever)—see p 52 and **cholera**, see p 310.

Appendicitis—this term means inflammation of the appendix and includes inflammatory conditions such as **acute appendicitis** (catarrhal appendicitis), **recurrent appendicitis**, **subacute appendicitis**, **chronic appendicitis**, and **grumbling appendix**.

Infection appears to be an important factor in provoking the inflammation. In the type of disorder termed **acute obstructive appendicitis**, the infection appears to be a secondary result of obstruction of the lumen of the appendix.

Obstructive appendicitis may result in **perforation of the appendix** with either the formation of a localised **appendix abscess** in the region of the perforated organ, or in the discharge of infective material into the peritoneal cavity producing a condition called **general peritonitis**.

The clinical features vary considerably with the type of inflammation present but in most instances pain and tenderness in the right iliac fossa are cardinal features of an attack of the disease. Inflammation of mesenteric lymph glands due to the condition known as **non-specific mesen-**

teric adenitis, or rarely caused by bacterial infection of a type called **yersinia infection** can sometimes present a similar picture to that of acute appendicitis.

The diagnosis of acute appendicitis is made on the clinical features.

In the less acute forms of appendicitis, radiological investigation may be necessary to exclude other diseases which might produce similar signs and symptoms e.g. carcinoma of caecum or colon, diverticular disease, Crohn's disease, ureteric calculus, gall stones.

Treatment is by appendicectomy (removal of the appendix) but, according to the nature of the case, this may have to be an emergency operation or, in other instances, delayed until after the subsidence of an active phase of the disease.

When the disease is complicated by diffuse peritonitis, drainage of the infected peritoneal cavity is necessary in addition to appendicectomy. This is effected by inserting a rubber tube or strip of corrugated rubber to provide a channel for the escape of infective material to the exterior. The outer end of the **drain** (i.e. the tube or corrugated rubber) is brought out through a small 'stab' incision in the abdominal wall in order not to interfere with the main abdominal incision required for the appendicectomy. Some cases of appendix abscess also require surgical drainage.

Dysentery—colitis caused by bacillary dysentery and amoebic dysentery will be referred to in Part V.

Ulcerative colitis—is an inflammatory disease of the large bowel which frequently leads to widespread ulceration of the colonic mucosa and fibrosis of the walls of the colon. The rectum is also usually affected by the disease and quite often the caecum as well.

The cause is unknown and the condition is sometimes referred to as non-specific ulcerative colitis to distinguish it from other causes of colonic ulceration (e.g. amoebic and bacillary dysentery).

The inflammatory changes result in diarrhoea, often with blood and mucus in the stools. The disease pursues a chronic course but periodic remissions (i.e. periods during which the symptoms diminish in intensity or subside) are a common feature. Sometimes, however, the disease may present initially in acute form.

The early lesions are usually seen in the distal part of the sigmoid colon and may be visualised through a sigmoidoscope.

Complications include the development of severe anaemia, stricture formation in the bowel, carcinoma of the bowel, perforation, and occasionally a type of arthritis called **colitic arthritis**. This latter condition has some similarity to ankylosing spondylitis.

Double-contrast barium enema examination is useful to show the extent of the disease and to reveal complications such as stricture of the bowel and the development of a carcinoma in a diseased area of colon.

This examination can show changes in the mucosa, evidence of ulceration during active stages of the disease and evidence of fibrosis in the colonic walls during its later stages.

Medical treatment is extensively used in ulcerative colitis and this often controls the disease. Some patients, however, sooner or later need surgery and in these it is now generally the practice to perform **total colectomy** (removal of the whole colon) with or without concomitant **proctectomy** (removal of the rectum).

Irritable bowel—this is an ill-defined disorder, also called **spastic** or **irritable colon** or **colospasm**. In many cases the condition appears to be due to a mild inflammation of the colon, but in others it seems to be a functional disorder in which psychological factors may play a part.

Clinical features include attacks of both diarrhoea and constipation and cramp-like abdominal pains.

Diverticular disease of the colon—it has already been noted that pouches called diverticula (singular: diverticulum) may be found in the pharynx, oesophagus, stomach and duodenum. They may also occur in the jejunum and less commonly in the ileum. The commonest site for their occurrence is, however, in the large bowel—especially in the sigmoid part of the colon.

The presence of diverticula constitutes **diverticulosis** and if inflammatory changes develop in the walls of the pouches the condition may then be referred to as **diverticulitis**.

Diverticula may be congenital or acquired. In diverticulosis, the diverticula are, in the great majority of instances, of the acquired type and consist of small pouches of colonic mucosa which protrude through weak areas in the bowel wall. The formation of such pouches is thought to occur secondary to a primary disorder of colonic musculature, resulting in irregular thickening of the circular muscle of the colonic wall in affected areas. An important factor in the causation of this muscle disorder is thought to be the absence of adequate amounts of natural fibre in the diet of highly civilised communities.

Stagnation of faecal matter readily occurs within diverticula and may lead to infection and the resultant inflammatory changes of diverticulitis.

Diverticulitis is a common disease in middle-aged and elderly subjects of both sexes and produces a variety of clinical features according to whether the inflammation is acute or chronic.

Acute diverticulitis may resemble an attack of acute appendicitis, except that the signs are referable to the left iliac fossa. Perforation of an acutely inflamed diverticulum may result in the formation of a **paracolic abscess** or general peritonitis. An abscess may burst into the bladder or vagina, forming either a **vesicocolic fistula** or a **vaginocolic fistula**. (*Note:* **vesico-** means pertaining to the urinary bladder.)

Chronic diverticulitis causes pain in the left iliac fossa and constipation, often interrupted by intermittent attacks of diarrhoea. The stools often contain blood. Intestinal obstruction may develop in severe cases.

Colonic diverticula and evidence of muscle thickening in the bowel wall are demonstrable by barium enema examination. Opaque enemas, with a water-soluble contrast medium (e.g. Gastrografin), are useful to demonstrate complicating fistulae.

Treatment in mild and uncomplicated cases is by diet and laxatives. Complicated and severe cases frequently require surgical treatment.

Ischiorectal abscess—this is the name given to an abscess that develops in the ischiorectal fossa (i.e. an area in each side of the perineum, lying between the anal canal and the side wall of the bony pelvis). The initial cause of the infection is often not obvious but it is thought that in most cases pathogens gain access to this fossa through some lesion in the wall of the anal canal or lower part of the rectum. An ischiorectal abscess may burst and cause a fistula-in-ano.

Perianal abscess—this condition results from the development of infection in an anal gland or thrombosed haemorrhoid. The abscess lies close to the anal margin and may result in the formation of a fistula-in-ano.

Fistula-in-ano—this is an infective condition in which a fistula is formed opening at one end into the anal canal, and at the other on the skin surface near the anal margin. As already noted it may result from bursting of an ischiorectal or perianal abscess, or be due to Crohn's disease or, rarely tuberculous infection.

Fissure-in-ano (anal fissure)—a common and painful disorder in which a longitudinal ulcer develops in the mucous membrane lining the anal canal. It may occur in acute or chronic form and it is thought to be of initially traumatic causation, resulting from tearing of the mucosa.

Neoplasms

Benign and malignant neoplasms are rare in the small bowel and, with the exception of a tumour called a **solitary adenoma**, benign neoplasms are also rare in the large bowel. Carcinoma arising from the mucosa of the large bowel is, however, fairly frequent in older people.

An adenoma sometimes grows so that its main part becomes rounded and is connected to the mucous membrane from which it arises by a stem-like process, referred to as a **pedicle**. It may then be referred to as a **polyp** or **polypoid adenoma**.

Some important types of neoplastic disease are given below.

Multiple familial polyposis (polyposis coli)—multiple adenomas, many with polypoid form, are found in this rare but interesting hereditary disease. The tumours are small but often widespread in the large bowel and bleed easily. Rectal haemorrhage is the cardinal feature of the disease, often appearing in childhood. Carcinomatous changes in the polyps are frequent and accordingly removal of the whole of the large bowel is frequently carried out in this disorder.

Double-contrast enemas, using barium and air inflation, are of particular value in demonstrating polyps of the large bowel.

Carcinoid tumours—this name describes certain uncommon tumours which occur in the appendix or more rarely, in the ileum. They are slow growing, but in the course of time some of those that arise in the small bowel develop malignant properties; hence the name **carcinoid**, which means cancer-like. They are also called **argentaffinomas** or **chromaffinomas** from the names of the cells from which they arise. Measuring the amount of 5HIAA (5-hydroxy indole acetic acid) excreted in the urine is a useful diagnostic investigation.

Carcinoma of the large intestine—the cause of carcinoma of the large intestine is unknown, but pre-existing polyps and changes due to ulcerative colitis are sometimes predisposing factors in its development. Both sexes show an equal incidence of this disease. It may occur in any site between the tip of the caecum and the anal canal but is seen most frequently in the rectum and sigmoid colon.

Intestinal obstruction is a common complication of advanced growths.

Metastases in lymph glands usually occur much earlier than blood-borne metastases do. The liver is the commonest site for the latter.

The growth, when advanced, may spread through the bowel wall and involve organs such as the bladder, small intestine or stomach. Peritoneal involvement results in **malignant ascites** (i.e. effusion into the peritoneal cavity), and involvement of other hollow organs in fistula formation, e.g. **vesicocolic fistula** when the bladder is involved, and **gastrocolic fistula** when a growth of the colon extends through the wall of the stomach.

Clinical features vary considerably according to the site of the carcinoma. In the left half of the colon alteration in bowel habit is often an early symptom. In the right half of the colon, pain is often an early feature. In the rectum, passage of blood in the stools may be the first sign of the disease. Not infrequently a colonic carcinoma produces little in the way of clinical signs and symptoms until those of intestinal obstruction develop.

In investigating a suspected case of carcinoma of the large intestine, radiology plays a major role except with growths of the rectum. In the rectum digital examination and visual inspection through a **proctoscope** are essential diagnostic methods. In the distal part of the sigmoid colon, it is emphasised that radiological examination is complementary to **sigmoidoscopy**. **Colonoscopy** using a fibreoptic endoscope is now also widely employed diagnostic procedure. When indicated, biopsies may be taken during the course of proctoscopy, sigmoidoscopy or colonoscopy.

Barium enema is the radiological method of choice in the investigation of all patients who are fit enough to undergo this examination. When a carcinoma is present it may show as a filling defect in the barium-filled bowel, or produce an area of narrowing—usually with an irregular outline.

The treatment of carcinoma of the large bowel is surgical whenever practicable, often supplemented by radiotherapy in rectal carcinomas, or by cytoxic drugs in carcinoma of the colon.

If the disease recurs after treatment this may be detected at an early stage by periodically estimating the amount of an antigen called carcinoembryonic antigen in the blood.

Intussusception

In this condition a portion of the bowel wall invaginates into the lumen of the portion of the bowel immediately distal to it.

Cochrane Shanks and Young (3) describe an intussusception as consisting of three concentric tubes, i.e. an entering tube, a returning tube and a receiving tube or sheath.

The invaginating process tends to be progressive once it has started, and the blood vessels which supply the bowel are dragged into the intussusception. As the condition advances, interference with the blood supply may be such as to cause gangrene of the affected parts of the bowel wall.

Intussusception occurs most commonly in the first two years of life but is occasionally seen in older children and adults.

The main clinical features are intermittent attacks of colic and the passage of blood and mucus per rectum. A sausage-shaped tumour may be palpable in the abdomen. Later there is vomiting due to intestinal obstruction.

The diagnosis can usually be made clinically, but a barium enema may be required to demonstrate the nature of the condition when the clinical signs are not clear-cut. In some centres, reduction of intussusceptions by barium enema is practised as a therapeutic measure. In the UK, however, surgical reduction is generally the treatment of choice.

Volvulus of the Intestine

This is a condition in which a segment of the intestine becomes twisted around its long axis. It can occur in either the small or large intestine, but in most cases it is seen in the pelvic colon of elderly people. The twisting of the bowel results in intestinal obstruction.

Valuable evidence regarding the presence of volvulus may be obtained from plain radiographs, and barium enema examination may also be requested if the patient is fit enough.

Treatment is surgical.

Intestinal Obstruction

The name of this condition is self-explanatory. In intestinal obstruction the normal onward passage of faeces and **flatus** (i.e. intestinal gas) is markedly delayed, or completely prevented, according to whether the lumen of the bowel is partially or totally blocked. The obstruction may result from causes in the intestinal wall, external pressure on the intestinal wall, or causes in the lumen of the bowel.

As regards the first cause: changes in the bowel wall resulting from diverticulitis, carcinoma, regional enteritis, and tuberculosis of the small intestine may all result in intestinal obstruction, as may fibrous strictures due to colitis, volvulus and intussusception.

Among the external causes of intestinal obstruction are constriction of the bowel wall by peritoneal adhesions, pressure from a pelvic tumour, and pressure on the bowel walls by the edges of a hernial orifice (see p 134).

A mass of inspissated faeces resulting from severe chronic constipation, is one factor in the actual lumen of the bowel which may cause blockage of the intestinal canal.

In newly born infants intestinal obstruction may be due to atresia of the duodenum or less commonly other sites in the bowel, malrotation of the gut, meconium ileus, a condition called the **inspissated milk curd syndrome**, Hirschsprung's disease, and **meconium plug syndrome**.

All the above causes of intestinal obstruction are mechanical in nature. There is also another important type of intestinal obstruction which is of nervous origin, and is due to paralysis of the musculature of the bowel wall. This type is called **paralytic ileus** and usually only affects the small bowel. It may occur as a complication following a major operation, in the course of **peritonitis** (inflammation of the peritoneum lining the abdominal cavity and covering the abdominal organs), as a sequel to injuries which cause haemorrhage into the retroperitoneal tissues, and after childbirth.

Intestinal obstruction may present as a acute, subacute or chronic condition. The chief clinical features are colicky pain, constipation, increasing distention of the abdomen and vomiting. There is also accompanying toxaemia, due to absorption of toxins from the stagnant intestinal contents, and, in acute cases, often pronounced shock.

Plain radiography is often of great value in cases of intestinal obstruction as distended loops of bowel can be demonstrated, and also **fluid levels** due to separation of gas and fluid layers in the stagnant contents of the intestine above the obstruction. Distended loops of jejunum, ileum and colon produce differing radiographic appearances. It is thus frequently possible to obtain approximate location of the site of an obstructing lesion from supine views. Films taken erect, or in lateral decubitus with horizontal ray projection, are essential for showing fluid levels. When the patient is fit enough and the obstruction is in the large bowel, the causal lesion may be demonstrable by a barium enema. Barium meal examination is often inadvisable in cases with suspected intestinal obstruction, but may be warranted in certain circumstances. An opaque meal using a water-soluble contrast medium (e.g. Gastrografin) which carries no risk of converting a partial obstruction into a complete obstruction is often a preferable alternative.

The treatment of mechanical intestinal obstruction is in most cases surgical.

Vascular Lesions of the Colon

Samuel and Laws (4), under the heading of **ischaemic colitis**, give a classification of these lesions which result from obstruction of either the arterial or venous blood supply of the colon, and have described their radiological appearances. Laws (5) also gives an account of primary vascular lesions affecting the small bowel.

Malabsorption Syndromes

The malabsorption syndromes include a great many different disorders which possess the common characteristic of causing defective absorption of various minerals, vitamins and essential foodstuffs from the bowel into the bloodstream.

The defective absorption may be due to: damage to the mucosa of the small intestine, as occurs in certain intestinal diseases (e.g. coeliac disease, idiopathic steatorrhoea, tropical sprue); Crohn's disease; digestive disorder arising from disease of the biliary system or pancreas; and effects such as intestinal hurry which may sometimes result from certain operations on the alimentary canal (e.g. total or partial gastrectomy, small bowel resection).

Chronic diarrhoea is a usual feature of malabsorption syndromes and in some excessive amounts of fat are present in the stools. This latter condition is called **steatorrhoea**. It causes an abnormal appearance of the stools and biochemical testing of these will establish the presence of an abnormally high fat content.

Other common features of these syndromes are anaemia, debility and loss of weight and in some a bone disorder called **osteomalacia** (see p 238) may develop owing to a defective absorption of vitamin D and calcium.

Biochemical and haematological tests are important in assessing the state of nutrition of the patient, e.g. measuring concentrations of calcium, iron, alkaline phosphatase and haemoglobin in the blood.

Radiological investigation is of help in many cases and peroral biopsy of the jejunal mucosa may yield information of considerable value in patients with disease of the small bowel mucosa.

In some types of malabsorption, notably those associated with steator-rhoea, a small bowel barium meal may show widening of small bowel loops, thickening of mucosal folds and flocculation of barium suspension, changes sometimes described as producing a deficiency pattern.

Coeliac disease is a disease of infancy and childhood in which there is steatorrhoea, anaemia and retardation of growth. Absorption of fats, vitamins, minerals and carbohydrates is deficient. A type of bone disease called **coeliac rickets** may develop as a result of vitamin D deficiency.

Coeliac disease is thought to be due to an abnormal sensitivity to gluten, a substance found in wheat flour and other cereals and has therefore been given the alternative name of **gluten-induced enteropathy**.

Idiopathic steatorrhoea (non-tropical sprue) is a condition allied to coeliac disease but occurring in adults. It is thought also to be due to gluten sensitivity.

Tropical sprue—bears some similarity to idiopathic steatorrhoea. It is associated with deficiency of folic acid (a vitamin belonging to the vitamin B complex) and sometimes vitamin B_{12} deficiency also. It is a disease of warm climates, and steatorrhoea is one of its main features.

Among the many other causes of malabsorption syndromes may be mentioned **blind loop syndrome**—a condition in which features of malabsorption develop as a result of the presence of a blind loop of bowel (in most instances due to surgery) in which there is stasis of bowel contents and infection; **lactose intolerance**—in which because of deficiency of the enzyme *lactase*, a fatty diarrhoea results from taking milk or milk products; and **Whipple's disease**—a rare condition in which steatorrhoea is associated with chronic polyarthritis (inflammatory changes in many joints) and widespread enlargement of lymph glands.

Hernias

The term **hernia** describes a protrusion of any structure through the wall of the cavity in which it is normally contained.

The opening through which a hernia protrudes is known as a **hernial orifice** and may be:

(i) an opening which is normally present, e.g. hiatus hernia—a projection of stomach through the oesophageal hiatus in the diaphragm;

(ii) an opening due to developmental defect, e.g. hernia through a developmental defect in the diaphragm;

(iii) an acquired opening, e.g. an **incisional hernia** where the herniated structures protrude through an area of weakness caused by a surgical incision.

In the abdomen hernias which project through the walls of the abdominal cavity are called **external hernias**, and the most important of these are: (i) **inguinal hernia**, in which the hernia protrudes through the inguinal canal, or through part of this canal. An inguinal hernia may form a bulge in the groin, or in a male may descend into the scrotum (scrotal hernia) and in a female into the labium majus (labial hernia); (ii) **femoral hernia**—the hernia protrudes through the femoral canal in the upper part of the thigh; (iii) **umbilical hernia**—the hernia in children protrudes through the umbilicus or, in adults, just above or to the side of the umbilicus.

Abdominal hernias which protrude through some opening, congenital or acquired, in the interior of the abdominal cavity are called **internal hernias**. They are uncommon but may cause intestinal obstruction.

Hernias are described as **reducible** or **irreducible** according to whether or not the hernial contents can be returned back through the hernial orifice through which they are protruding. When, as is frequently the case, a portion of the small or large intestine is present in an irreducible hernia, pressure of the margins of the hernial orifice on the bowel frequently results in the development of intestinal obstruction. Such pressure may also deprive the hernial contents of their normal blood supply and eventually result in necrosis and gangrene. A hernia, in which there is such impairment of blood supply is known as a **strangulated hernia**.

Diseases of the Liver

Congenital abnormalities are rare in the liver.

As regards traumatic disorders, **rupture of the liver** not infrequently occurs as a result of the more severe types of injury to the upper abdomen and lower thorax, especially in crush injuries. The liver being a very vascular organ, tears in its substance may cause much bleeding into the peritoneum. The presence of blood in the peritoneal cavity is termed **haemoperitoneum**.

The liver may be the site of certain infective diseases, of infestation with worms and other parasites and of primary and secondary neoplasms. Among its other disorders several types of disease associated with permanent damage to liver cells, resulting from infection, poisoning, and deficiencies in diet are of considerable interest.

As the portal vein carried venous blood from the stomach, intestine, spleen and pancreas to the liver, it will also be convenient to refer here to certain terms relating to disorders of the portal circulation.

Infective Diseases

Viral hepatitis—this term indicates acute inflammation of the liver due to virus infection. The main types are (i) **infective hepatitis**, wherein sufferers and carriers of the disease excrete the causal virus, *hepatitis A virus*, in their faeces and spread of the disease usually occurs as a result of faecal contamination of food and water; (ii) **serum hepatitis** (syringe hepatitis) which is transmitted by injection of whole blood, serum or plasma containing the causal virus, *hepatitis B virus*, or by using syringes and needles contaminated by infected blood and imperfectly sterilised; (iii) **non-A, non-B hepatitis**, which is commonly caused by faecal contamination of food.

Clinically, the types of viral hepatitis show a marked similarity; although serum hepatitis has a longer incubation period and infective hepatitis may produce large epidemics under conditions in which hygienic standards are low. Both take the form of a febrile illness accompanied in most cases by jaundice and **hepatomegaly** (enlargement of the liver). An antigenic substance called **Australia antigen** (hepatitis B antigen) is detectable in the blood of many of the patients suffering from serum hepatitis.

Complete recovery occurs in most cases, but occasionally chronic inflammatory changes may develop, leading to **chronic hepatitis** or permanent damage to liver cells may result, causing some form of liver necrosis or cirrhosis (see later).

There is no specific treatment for viral hepatitis. Inoculation with immunoglobulin can afford temporary protection against hepatitis of A or B type. Subjects at special risk can now be given a vaccine which affords long-term protection against hepatitis B.

Bacterial infections—multiple hepatic abscesses may form in the course of general septicaemia when pyogenic bacteria are present in the systemic circulation and reach the liver via the hepatic artery. They may also develop as a result of a disorder of the biliary system called **infective cholangitis**. This infection may develop in conditions in which there is some obstruction to the flow of bile and occurs most commonly as a sequel to impaction of a gallstone in the common bile duct.

Multiple abscesses may also result from the carriage of pyogenic bacteria in the portal vein from a septic focus in the area of drainage of this vein (e.g. a suppurating appendix). The presence of pus-producing bacteria in the portal circulation, together with the production of multiple liver abscesses, constitutes the disorder known as **portal pyaemia**. This condition is often associated with septic inflammatory changes of spreading type in the veins of the portal system associated with clot formation, i.e. a septic thrombophlebitis which is referred to as **septic pylephlebitis**. Inflammation of veins is called **phlebitis**, and the prefix **pyle-** means pertaining to the portal vein.

Amoebic hepatitis (hepatic amoebiasis)—is a term describing inflammatory changes in the liver resulting from infection with *Entamoeba histolytica*, a protozoon which is the causal pathogen of amoebic dysentery. This infection may lead to the formation of an abscess within the liver known as an **amoebic liver abscess** or **tropical abscess**.

Other hepatic infections—among these are (i) **hepatitis due to actinomycosis**, (ii) **Weil's disease** (leptospirosis), a spirochaetal disease of worldwide distribution which is carried by infected rats who excrete the causal spirochaetes in their urine. It is characterised by a febrile illness accompanied by jaundice in many patients, kidney damage and various types of haemorrhage (see p 61); (iii) **yellow fever**—a virus disease of the tropics carried by a mosquito called the *Aedes aegypti*. The name of this disease derives from the jaundice resulting from the inflammatory changes in the liver; (iv) **visceral leishmaniasis**—(kala-azar) an infection of the cells of the mononuclear phagocyte system in which lesions occur in the liver, spleen, other organs and lymph glands. It is due to a protozoon called *Leishmania donovani*, and transmitted by sandflies.

Diseases due to Parasitic Worms and Flukes

These diseases are more properly referred to as **infestations** than as infections, because they are caused by parasitic organisms which consist of more than one cell. (*Note:* infections are caused by pathogenic micro-organisms, i.e. bacteria, viruses, rickettsiae, fungi and protozoa, all of which are single-celled organisms).

Among the diseases of this type in which clinical signs and symptoms result from infestations of the lever are: **hydatid (echinococcus) disease** of the liver; **clonorchiasis**, a tropical disease caused by Chinese liver fluke; and **fascioliasis**, infestation with the sheep liver fluke.

Hydatid disease (Echinococcus disease)—is due to *Taenia echinococcus*, a small tapeworm which is a parasite of dogs, which most commonly acquire the infestation from feeding on infected meat from sheep or cattle. The dogs then excrete the tapeworm ova in their faeces. If these ova are ingested by man they may develop into larvae and, after penetrating the intestinal wall, settle in some site such as the liver or less commonly in tissues such as the lungs, spleen and bone. A larva that survives may then develop into a hydatid cyst.

Hydatid cysts occur most frequently in the liver, and in this organ usually only one cyst develops in any one individual. It may, however, become large and require surgical treatment. Cysts may also be found in sites such as lung, kidney and bone and in these may produce radiological evidence of their presence.

Suspected cases of hydatid disease are investigated by a blood test of the type called a complement fixation test and a skin test called the **Casoni intradermal test**. A blood count will frequently show **eosinophilia**, i.e. increased numbers of circulating eosinophil leucocytes (white blood cells).

Neoplasms

The liver is a common site for metastases from primary carcinomas arising within the area of drainage of the portal vein (e.g. carcinomas of the stomach and large bowel) and metastases from other primary carcinomas (e.g. lung and breast) also frequently occur in this organ.

There is also a rare primary tumour of liver cells called a **malignant hepatoma** also called a **hepatocellular carcinoma**, and an even rarer neoplasm, a **cholangiocarcinoma** which arises from the bile ducts.

Hepatic angiography, isotope scanning, ultrasonography and CT may all be employed to detect hepatic neoplasms and other space-occupying lesions (e.g. abscesses and cysts) in this organ.

Other Hepatic Diseases

Included among these are several diseases whose clinical manifestations are the result of serious damage to liver cells. Such damage may be due to causes such as infective processes (e.g. viral hepatitis), alchoholism, toxic agents of various types (e.g. certain drugs, chemical poisons, toxic substances present in the toxaemia of pregnancy called eclampsia), and to deficiencies in diet and other factors.

The damage to the liver cells may develop rapidly and where extensive may produce a condition termed **acute massive liver necrosis** (see below).

Damage to liver cells of slower onset is associated with the presence of fibrosis and areas of regenerated liver cells resulting in the development of various forms of cirrhosis of the liver. (*Note:* the liver is one of the organs whose specialised cells retain their powers of multiplication throughout life and can thus to some extent undergo the form of repair called regeneration.)

Some of the clinical disorders occuring as a result of acute or chronic liver damage are as follows.

Acute massive liver necrosis (acute yellow atrophy)—this uncommon disease occurs as a result of extensive and rapidly developing damage to liver cells and may follow hepatic infections or poisonings, or may rarely develop as a complication of eclampsia.

It produces features such as jaundice, haemorrhage and also mental changes which, in this condition, are manifestations of **hepatic failure** (hepatocellular failure). Severe cases may end fatally with a form of coma termed **hepatic coma** preceding death. Less severe cases may result in a type of hepatic cirrhosis called **post-necrotic cirrhosis**.

Cirrhosis of the liver—this is a disorder caused by damage to hepatic cells, and fibrosis is one of its principal features. Excess fibrous tissue gives the liver a harder consistency than normal, and the word cirrhosis has thus come to indicate hardening or fibrosis, although its correct meaning is yellowish red from the colour the organ may acquire in some forms of this disorder.

(i) **Portal cirrhosis** (Laennec's cirrhosis) is the commonest form of hepatic cirrhosis and is so called because the fibrosis usually starts around small branches of the portal vein. Previous infective diseases of the liver, deficiencies in diet and chronic alcoholism are factors which can operate in its causation. When it occurs in chronic alcoholics it may be referred to as **alcoholic cirrhosis**. (*Note:* this condition represents severe damage to liver cells. Less severe damage associated with excessive intake of alcohol occurs in the conditions called **fatty liver** and **alcoholic hepatitis**. According to Thomson and Cotton (6) both these conditions are reversible if the consumption of alcohol stops.)

Cirrhosis of portal type also develops in a rare disorder of copper metabolism called Wilson's disease (see p 285).

The extensive and widespread fibrosis which develops in portal cirrhosis causes narrowing of many of the intrahepatic branches of the portal venous system, causing a rise in venous pressure through this system spoken of as **portal hypertension**.

One effect of the obstruction to the passage of portal blood through the liver is to cause dilatation of anastomotic (communicating) channels which connect the portal and systemic veins. One site for such channels is the mucosa at the lower end of the oesophagus, where the dilated veins are called **oesphageal varices**. They frequently bleed, causing haematemesis and melaena which lead to the development of anaemia. Another effect of portal hypertension is to cause **ascites** (exudation of fluid from the blood into the peritoneal cavity).

Other clinical features seen in portal cirrhosis are due to impairment of various liver functions and the disease leads slowly, but ultimately, to hepatic failure.

Portal vein thrombosis occasionally develops as a complication of cirrhosis and also of a number of other conditions (e.g. pylephlebitis).

Oesophageal varices are in many instances demonstrable by barium swallow, and portal vein thrombosis by portal venography.

There is no specific treatment for cirrhosis but medical measures (e.g. appropriate diet, administration of diuretics) may arrest deterioration of the disease for a long time. Emergency surgery may be necessary for haemorrhage and, in selected patients, surgical measures may be employed to reduce the portal venous pressure, e.g. portocaval anastomosis.

(ii) **Other types of hepatic cirrhosis**—these include **obstructive biliary cirrhosis**, associated with obstructive jaundice and resulting from long-standing obstruction to the biliary system;

haemachromatosis (bronze diabetes), a disease in which there is an error of iron metabolism; and **postnecrotic cirrhosis** which has already been mentioned as a sequel to the less severe forms of acute liver necrosis.

Diseases of the Biliary System

The biliary system consists of the *gall bladder* and the *intrahepatic* and *extrahepatic bile ducts*. Bile is formed in the liver and carried through the bile ducts into the duodenum, being concentrated in the gall bladder on its way through the biliary system.

The pigment called *bilirubin* is formed from the haemoglobin of red cells whose life in the circulation is finished. It is carried to the liver and excreted by hepatic cells in the bile. If excessive bilirubin accumulates in the circulating blood, the skin and mucous membranes acquire a yellowish tinge and **jaundice** is then said to be present. Alternatively, but less commonly, the condition may be called **icterus**.

The word jaundice derives from the French word jaune, meaning yellow.

Excessive bilirubin in the blood results principally from: (i) excessive breakdown of red cells as in **haemolytic jaundice**; (ii) failure of normal excretion of bilirubin in the bile as a result of damage to liver cells—**hepatic jaundice** (hepatocellular jaundice); (iii) obstruction to the flow of bile into the duodenum—**obstructive jaundice**.

Various radiological methods can be used while investigating suspected biliary disease and during the treatment of confirmed cases of such disease. Some are alternatives and others complementary procedures, and their use varies according to the nature of the problem. These methods include plain radiography; oral cholecystography; intravenous cholegraphy (cholangiocholecystography); ultrasonic investigation of the gall bladder and bile ducts; examination of the bile ducts by percutaneous transhepatic cholangiography (PTC) and endoscopic retrograde choledochopancreatography (ERCP), and CT of the bile ducts, operative and postoperative cholangiography, and treatment methods of interventional radiology.

The two commonest disorders affecting the biliary system are cholecystitis and gall stones, and these often coexist in the same patient.

It should be appreciated that as regards X-ray investigations, oral cholecystography is usually contraindicated in acute cholecystitis, and the majority of most gall stones are not radio-opaque.

Cholecystitis

Chole—means bile, **cyst** means a bladder. The name of this condition thus indicates inflammation of the gall bladder. The word **gall** is a synonym for bile.

Cholecystitis may present an acute or chronic form and both forms are often associated with gall stones.

The inflammatory changes are usually due to infection with a mixture of pathogenic microbes, i.e. a so-called **non-specific infection**, except in those uncommon cases when cholecystitis occurs as a complication of typhoid or paratyphoid fever and is due to a **specific infection** with typhoid or paratyphoid bacilli.

The infection of **acute cholecystitis** frequently develops as a secondary result of blockage of the cystic duct (i.e. the duct that leads from the gall bladder and joins the common hepatic duct to form the common bile duct), by an impacted gall stone. A patient with **acute cholecystitis** is usually very ill with pain in the upper right side of the upper abdomen and sometimes also in the right shoulder-blade, or tip of the right shoulder and has a fever and increased pulse rate.

Chronic cholecystitis may develop insidiously, or may be the sequel to an attack of acute cholecystitis. It is much commoner in women then in men and uncommon before middle age. Common symptoms are indigestion, flatulence, intolerance to fatty foods, pain in the right side of the upper abdomen and sometimes also in the right shoulder-blade or tip of the right shoulder, and periodic attacks of vomiting.

Acute cholecystitis is usually treated medically until the acute inflammation has subsided. Surgical treatment is then carried out. Chronic cholecystitis may be treated either medically or surgically; surgical treatment is usually advised in patients suitable for operation.

Gall Stones (Cholelithiasis)

Gall stones are formed as a result of precipitation from the bile of one or more of its main constituents. They are of three main types: (*a*) **cholesterol stones**; (*b*) **bile pigment stones**; (*c*) **mixed stones** consisting of a mixture of cholesterol, bile pigment and calcium. (*Note:* **cholesterol** is a lipid substance normally present in the bile—see p 73.)

They are frequently found in association with cholecystitis, and are commoner in women than in men. Their maximum incidence occurs in middle age. They are occasionally seen in children who suffer from an uncommon blood disease known as **acholuric jaundice**.

Gall stones which remain confined in the gall bladder may be symptomless. If, however, one or more stones pass out of this organ and lodge in either the cystic or common bile ducts, severe cramp-like pains called **biliary colic** may be caused.

Impaction of a stone in the common bile duct may block the duct and cause jaundice of the obstructive type. Persistence of this condition may in the course of time lead to the liver disease called **obstructive biliary cirrhosis**. Impaction of a stone in this site may also lead to an ascending infection of the bile ducts termed **infective cholangitis**. As noted when discussing hepatic infections, infective cholangitis can result in the formation of multiple liver abscesses.

As also noted when discussing intestinal obstruction, gall stones occasionally ulcerate through the gall bladder wall into the bowel. A large gall stone may then cause obstruction of the lumen of the bowel. Treatment of gall stones, causing symptoms, is usually by surgery.

When operation is contraindicated, suitable patients may be given a course of chenodeoxycholic acid in an attempt to dissolve the stones.

Other Diseases of the Biliary System

Among these are the following.

Carcinoma of the gall bladder—an uncommon type of carcinoma. Irritation of the mucosa by gall stones is thought to play a part in the causation of some cases.

Cholangitis—this term means inflammation of the bile ducts. **Infective cholangitis** is a not uncommon complication when a gall stone becomes impacted in the common bile duct.

Biliary fistula—uncommonly a fistula may develop in connection with the biliary system either as a result of disease, or after surgery. Biliary fistulae, according to their cause, may open on the surface of the body or into the stomach, duodenum, small intestine or colon, e.g. **cholecystogastric fistula**—connecting the gall bladder and stomach; **choledochoduodenal fistula**—connecting the common bile duct and duodenum.

Carcinoma of the extrahepatic bile ducts—a rare condition but important as an occasional cause of obstructive jaundice.

Diseases of the Pancreas

The pancreas contains cells, arranged in lobules, which produce digestive enzymes (*exocrine pancreas*) and collections of endocrine cells (*endocrine pancreas*), the so-called *islet cells* which constitute the *islets of Langerhans* and secrete the hormones *insulin* (B cells), *glucagon* (A cells), *somatostatin* (D cells), and *gastrin* (G cells).

The digestive enzymes are dischared into the duodenum through the main and accessory pancreatic ducts, and the hormones are secreted directly into the bloodstream.

With the exception of diabetes mellitus, diseases of the pancreas are uncommon and, apart from this disease, the most important are certain inflammations, pancreatic carcinoma, pancreatic cysts, and fibrocystic disease of the pancreas.

Diabetes mellitus is generally classified as an endocrine disorder, and will therefore be discussed under the endocrine system.

Inflammations

Acute pancreatitis (acute haemorrhagic pancreatitis, acute pancreatic necrosis)—an acute inflammatory disorder, the cause of which is unknown. In some cases there appears to be some association with alcoholism, gall stones or infection of the bile ducts. In others a bloodborne infection has been suggested as a likely cause of the inflammation.

The inflammatory changes are generally severe and may result in haemorrhages within the gland, necrosis of its cells, and digestion of pancreatic tissue by its own enzymes which are set free by the disease processes. Self-digestion of this type is called **autolysis** or **auto-digestion**.

Acute pancreatitis rarely occurs before middle age. Its onset is usually sudden with severe abdominal pain, shock and vomiting. Mild jaundice develops in many patients and, in a few, bruising appears in the loins. This latter is due to extravasation of blood from the inflamed pancreas, and its spreading through the soft tissues. (*Note:* **extravasation** means an escape of fluid from the vessel, space or cavity in which it is normally contained.)

The pancreatic enzyme concerned with carbohydrate digestion is called *amylase* and in acute pancreatitis this substance may be shown in greatly increased amounts in blood serum during the early stages of the disease.

Acute pancreatitis is difficult to diagnose clinically, and the nature of the condition is frequently first discovered at operation. If, however, a strong presumptive diagnosis of this condition can be made without diagnostic laparotomy (p 149), conservative, i.e. non-operative treatment, is usually advocated.

Subacute pancreatitis—a relatively mild form of inflammation which may sometimes complicate mumps and certain other infective diseases.

Chronic pancreatitis—a chronic inflammatory condition which may occur as a sequel to acute pancreatitis or chronic alcoholism and in many instances is associated with the presence of gall stones. It produces diffuse fibrosis and may cause abdominal pain and steatorrhoea, and also diabetes mellitus if the endocrine cells in the organ are involved in the disease processes.

Obstructive jaundice may be a serious complication as a result of compression by fibrous tissue of the lower part of the common bile duct where it lies in its groove on the posterior aspect of the head of the pancreas.

Various surgical procedures may be used in treatment, e.g. partial pancreatectomy.

Neoplasms

Carcinoma of the pancreas—this is not a very common type of malignant neoplasm in the UK. The most usual site for its origin is in the head of the gland and here it may grow and cause blockage of the common bile duct and result in obstructive jaundice.

Pain is a usual feature of the disease and signs of disordered pancreatic function such as glycosuria (sugar in the urine) and steatorrhoea (excess of fat in the stools) are frequent.

Pancreatic carcinomas often displace or infiltrate the stomach and those arising in the head of the pancreas may cause deformity of the duodenum, thus producing signs which may be detectable by barium meal examination. It may, however, be possible to detect pancreatic carcinomas at an earlier stage by endoscopic retrograde pancreatography or by angiography. Ultrasonic examination, radioisotope scanning and CT are also employed to demonstrate these tumours.

Islet-cell tumours—these are all rare. They comprise: (i) **insulinomas**—arising from B cells, associated with over production of insulin, and usually benign; (ii) **glucagonomas**—arising from A cells, associated with diabetes mellitus and a skin rash and often malignant; (iii) **gastrinomas**—arising from G cells, associated with gastric hyperacidity, increased secretion of pepsin and peptic ulceration, and producing the so-called **Zollinger—Ellison syndrome**.

Cysts

Various types of **true pancreatic cysts** may occur, e.g. retention cysts, neoplastic cysts, hydatids, and may become large. There also arise in connection with this gland what are called **pancreatic pseudocysts**, i.e. false cysts.

A pseudocyst usually forms within a recess in the peritoneal cavity, called the *lesser sac*, and contains fluid which has leaked from the pancreas as a result of traumatic injury or severe inflammation of the gland.

Other Diseases

Mucoviscidosis (fibrocystic disease of the pancreas). This uncommon inherited disorder is a generalised disease of glands which secrete mucus throughout the body. When affected by mucoviscidosis these glands produce an abnormally viscid secretion. This results in obstruction of ducts and secondary effects of a serious nature in the intestinal tract and the lungs.

Duct obstruction may lead to fibrosis and cyst formation in the pancreas, hence the name of **fibrocystic disease** or **cystic fibrosis of the pancreas**.

Clinical signs of mucoviscidosis may appear during the first few days after birth when absence of mucus from the stools may result in solidification of the intestinal contents, and resultant intestinal obstruction which is often fatal. The intestinal contents of a newly born baby are known as **meconium**, and this manifestation of the disease is called **meconium ileus**.

In older infants the disease may take the form of steatorrhoea (fatty diarrhoea). This results from a deficiency of digestive enzymes normally secreted by the pancreas and constitutes one variety of malabsorption syndrome.

Mucus secreting glands in the mucosa of the bronchi are frequently involved in mucoviscidosis, and many of the infants with fatty diarrhoea subsequently develop recurrent lung infections which lead eventually to permanent lung damage. The lung changes are demonstrable radiologically.

Measurement of sweat electrolytes is an important diagnostic test, the sweat in mucoviscidosis being highly concentrated and showing increased concentrations of sodium and chloride.

Subphrenic Abscess

This condition is conveniently discussed here as it is a complication of certain diseases of the digestive system and it may also follow certain abdominal operations.

The term **subphrenic** means under the diaphragm and **subdiaphragmatic abscess** is another name for this condition. A subphrenic abscess can be caused by a bloodborne infection. It is usually due, however, to infective material reaching the area below the diaphragm from some intra-abdominal lesion, such as a perforated peptic ulcer or perforated appendix, or as a result of certain surgical operations on the stomach, duodenum, or elsewhere on the intestine or biliary tract.

Pleural effusion or pneumonitis (inflammation of lung tissue) or a mixture of both frequently develop in the region of the base of the lung on the affected side when a subphrenic abscess is present.

A subphrenic abscess causes fever, increased pulse rate and general malaise, together with pain in the region of the abscess, and often pain in the shoulder blade on the affected side. Examination of the blood shows a pronounced increase in the numbers of circulating polymorphs.

Radiological examination frequently helps in diagnosis, particularly if the abscess cavity contains a fluid level or, if on screening, restriction or abscence of diaphragmatic movement is demonstrated on the side of the suspected abscess. It is often possible to locate the site of a subphrenic abscess by ultrasound examination or by CT.

Pneumoperitoneum

The presence of air or other gas in the peritoneal cavity is called **pneumoperitoneum**.

This condition occurs as a result of **laparotomy** (i.e. the surgical operation of making an opening into the abdominal cavity). It is also produced by perforation of the stomach or intestine as a result of disease or trauma. Perforation of a peptic ulcer is a common cause.

Some Operations on the Digestive System

Mouth and Pharynx

Glossectomy—excision of the tongue, total or partial.
Pharyngectomy—excision of part of the pharynx.

Oesophagus

Heller's operation (cardiomyotomy)—An operation performed for relief of achalasia of the cardia, a longitudinal incision being made in the muscles around the narrow area at the lower end of the oesophagus and the mucous membrane being allowed to bulge through the gap.

Oesophagectomy—Partial or complete removal of the oesophagus; operations which also involve accompanying procedures to restore the continuity of the gastrointestinal tract, e.g. oesophagojejunostomy (see below).

Stomach and Duodenum

Gastrectomy

(i) **Partial gastrectomy**—removal of part of the stomach. This operation is mainly performed for peptic ulceration and for early carcinoma in the distal part of the stomach. This gastric remnant is made to open into either the duodenum, as in the **Billroth I** type of operation, or into the upper jejunum, as in the **Billroth II** and **Polya** types of partial gastrectomy. The new opening is termed a **stoma**.

(**Stomal ulceration**, i.e. peptic ulceration at the stoma is a rare sequel to partial gastrectomy but occurs rather more frequently after gastrojejunostomy (see later). Other undesirable sequelae which may sometimes follow partial gastrectomy are referred to as **postgastrectomy syndromes**.)

(ii) **Total gastrectomy**—in this operation which is mainly performed for carcinoma of the stomach, the whole of the stomach is removed. The oesophagus is then made to open into the duodenum—**oesophagoduodenostomy**, or the cut end of the duodenum is closed and the oesophagus is made to open into the side of a loop of upper jejunum—**oesophagojejunostomy**.

Vagotomy—In this operation the lower parts of the right and left vagus nerves are divided (truncal vagotomy), or the main trunks of the vagi are left intact and either all (selective vagotomy) or some of their gastric branches are divided (highly selective vagotomy), with the object of removing vagal nerve influences from the stomach and so reducing the secretion of acid.

As the vagus supplies motor fibres to the stomach, some form of drainage operation, in the form of gastrojejunostomy or pyloroplasty (see below), is generally performed at the same time as the vagotomy to facilitate gastric emptying. Vagotomy, together with a drainage operation such as pyloroplasty, is widely employed in the surgical treatment of chronic peptic ulcers, especially those occurring in the duodenum.

Gastrojejunostomy (gastroenterostomy)—in this operation no tissue is removed but an opening is made between the stomach and one of the upper loops of the jejunum. A short circuit is thus provided whereby food can pass direct from the stomach into the upper part of the small intestine, without passing through the pylorus and duodenum. This operation is extensively used in cases of pyloric obstruction, due to either peptic ulceration or carcinoma. As in a partial gastrectomy, the new opening between the stomach and the intestine is called a **stoma**.

Gastrojejunostomy may also be used as an alternative to partial gastrectomy in certain cases of peptic ulceration uncomplicated by pyloric stenosis.

Pyloroplasty—this is a reconstructive operation designed to enlarge the pylorus and facilitate emptying of the gastric contents into the duodenum. It is most often performed in association with vagotomy (see above).

Ramstedt's operation—an operation, for the relief of congenital pyloric stenosis in infants, where the thickened muscles around the narrowed pyloric canal are incised longitudinally and the mucosa of the pyloric canal allowed to bulge through the gap.

Fundoplication— an operation for hiatus hernia involving the wrapping of gastric fundus around the lower ends of the oesophagus, to prevent recurrent herniation.

Intestine

Appendicectomy—removal of the vermiform appendix.

Intestinal resection—this terms means removal of a portion of the intestine and includes:

(i) **partial enterectomy**—removal of part of the small bowel;
(ii) **partial colectomy**—removal of part of the colon;

(ii) **total colectomy**—removal of the whole colon;

(iv) **proctectomy**—excision of the rectum. This operation is usually performed through incisions made both into the abdominal cavity and perineum and is then termed **abdominoperineal resection of the rectum**.

After intestinal resection, **intestinal anastomosis** or, alternatively, **ileostomy** or **colostomy** are performed (see below).

Intestinal anastomosis—an operation of joining one portion of the bowel to another. It may be employed to join the cut ends of the intestine immediately after an intestinal resection, or at a later stage when it is desired to close a temporary colostomy, or ileostomy, which has been made in conjunction with an intestinal resection. Alternatively, it may be used to short-circuit an inoperable lesion which is causing obstruction of the bowel.

According to the manner in which the two portions of the bowel are joined, an anastomosis may be described as an **end-to-end, end-to-side**, or **lateral anastomosis**.

Examples of intestinal anastomosis are: (i) **ileocolic anastomosis**, where the terminal ileum is joined to the left half of the transverse colon after removing the right half of the colon and the caecum, and (ii) **ileorectal anastomosis** following the total colectomy.

Stapling techniques may be used to join the cut ends of the bowel in certain types of intestinal anastomosis operations.

Colostomy and **ileostomy**—These are two types of operation where a portion of bowel is made to open on the anterior abdominal wall, thus providing a permanent or temporary artificial anus through which the faeces are discharged. If the portion of bowel used in this manner is part of the colon the operation is called **colostomy**, or if part of the ileum **ileostomy**.

Operations of this type are mainly performed in cases of intestinal obstruction. Ileostomy may also be used to rest the inflamed bowel in ulcerative colitis.

Liver

Hepatectomy—removal of the liver, partial or total. The latter operation must be followed by **liver transplantation**.

Portal Vein

Portocaval anastomosis—an operation for the relief of portal hypertension where the distal part of the portal vein is made to open into the inferior vena cava.

Biliary Tract

Cholecystectomy—Removal of the gall bladder.

Operative cholangiography is frequently performed during this operation to investigate the presence or absence of stones in the common bile duct and also to demonstrate the patency of this structure.

Cholecystostomy—opening and drainage of the gall bladder.

Choledochotomy—opening of the common bile duct. Usually employed in order that the interior of the duct may be explored for the presence of gall stones.

Choledochostomy—drainage of the common bile duct. Postoperative cholangiography is performed by injection of contrast medium through the drainage tube inserted at this operation.

Cholecystoduodenostomy—the making of an opening between the gall bladder and duodenum. Used to short circuit a lesion which is obstructing the common bile duct.

Pancreas

Pancreatectomy—total or partial removal of the pancreas.

Diagnostic Laparotomy

An operation where the abdominal cavity is opened in order to inspect the organs of the digestive system or other structures. This operation may be indicated as a diagnostic measure when other investigations have failed to establish a cause for abdominal symptoms.

Operations for Hernia

These consist of **herniotomy** (surgical removal of a hernial sac); and repair operations called **hernioplasty** and **herniorrhaphy**.

REFERENCES

(1) Pracy, R., Siegler, J., Stell, P. M. (1974). *A Short Textbook of Ear, Nose and Throat*. London: English Universities Press.

(2) Bodian, M., Stephens, F. D., Ward, B. C. H. (1949). Hirschsprung's disease and idiopathic megacolon. *Lancet*; **1**: 6–15.

(3) Shanks, S. C., Young, A. C. (1969). *A Textbook of X-Ray Diagnosis*. Vol. IV. (Shanks, S. C., Kerley, P., eds). 4th edn. London: Lewis.

(4) Samuel, E., Laws, J. W. (1980). *A Textbook of Radiology and Imaging*, 3rd edn. (Sutton, D., ed.). Edinburgh: Churchill Livingstone.

(5) Laws, J. W. (1980). *A Textbook of Radiology and Imaging*, 3rd edn. (Sutton, D., ed.). Edinburgh: Churchill Livingstone.

(6) Thomson, A. D., Cotton, R. E. (1983). *Lecture Notes on Pathology*, 3rd edn. Oxford: Blackwell.

URINARY SYSTEM AND MALE REPRODUCTIVE SYSTEM

Some Anatomical and Physiological Considerations

The **urinary system** consists of the *kidney*, *ureters*, the *urinary bladder* and the *urethra*. *Urine* is secreted by the kidneys, these organs being concerned with the excretion of the waste products of metabolism and of foreign substances from the body, the retention of various essential substances (by tubular reabsorption—see later) and the maintenance of a normal water balance and normal balance of *electrolytes* (i.e. inorganic ions such as sodium, potassium, calcium, bicarbonate, chloride, phosphate) in the blood and tissue fluids. In the exercise of this latter function the kidneys are thus concerned with the maintenance of a normal reaction (*acid-base balance*) in the blood and tissue fluids.

The **male reproductive system** includes the *testes* and *epididymes*; the *vasa deferentia*, the *seminal vesicles* and *ejaculatory ducts*; the *prostate gland*; the *penis* and the greater part of the *urethra*. Throughout most of its length this last-named structure is, in the male, common to both the reproductive system and the urinary system. (*Note:* in the female the two systems are entirely separate as far as the point where the lower end of the urethra opens into the vulva.)

The testes are the reproductive glands of the male and produce the male germ cells, called *spermatozoa*, and secrete the male sex hormone, *testosterone*. The testes occupy the *scrotum*.

The prefixes **reno-** and **nephro-** both mean pertaining to the kidney, **pyelo-** pertaining to the pelvis of the kidney, and **cysto-** and **vesico-** pertaining to the bladder. **Orchi-** and **orchid-** mean pertaining to the testis.

General Aspects of Diseases of the Urinary and Male Reproductive Systems

Both these systems may be affected by congenital abnormalities, traumatic conditions, infective and other inflammatory conditions, neoplasms and other types of acquired disease.

Among the clinical signs and symptoms of these diseases may be mentioned **albuminuria** (the passage of the protein called albumen in the urine), **dysuria** (difficulty in passing urine), **haematuria** (blood in the urine), **pyuria** (pus in the urine), **retention** (inability to void urine from the bladder), **anuria** (suppression of the excretion of urine from the kidneys), **incontinence of urine** (inability to control the emptying of urine from the bladder), **oliguria** (passing of urine in amounts which are much less and more concentrated than normal), **polyuria** (passing excessive amounts of dilute urine), painful micturition (i.e. pain on passing urine), scalding micturition; **bacteriuria** (presence of bacteria in the urine); palpable swellings of the kidney, prostate gland, testes and epididymis; pain in the loin, bladder region or testis; pain of the type termed **renal colic** (see p 159).

It should also be noted that high blood pressure may be a sign of kidney disease (see hypertension of renal origin).

The branch of medicine concerned with diseases of the urinary system is called **urology**.

Surgical disorders of the urinary system in both sexes and the male reproductive system fall within the province of the branch of surgery called **genitourinary surgery**, whereas surgical disorders of the female reproductive system are the concern of the gynaecologist.

Certain infective diseases which affect the reproductive system are of venereal origin and reference has already been made to these in Part III. (See Sexually Transmitted Diseases.)

Special Methods of Investigation

Urine examination—investigations under this heading include naked eye examination of the urine for abnormal colour, presence of threads, etc., determination of reaction and specific gravity of the urine; microscopic examination for blood cells, pus cells, crystals, and abnormal structures formed under certain disease conditions in the kidney tubules and called **urinary casts** (renal casts); bacteriological examination and culture to determine the nature of infective organisms excreted in the urine; and chemical tests to investigate the presence of abnormal substances such as albumen and blood in the urine. Chemical examination of the urine may also be employed in certain tests of renal function (see later) and quantitative examinations may be carried out to determine whether normal urinary constituents such as chlorides and calcium are present in normal or abnormal amounts.

Blood examinations—in a number of urinary diseases, damage to renal cells may diminish the ability of the kidneys to excrete waste products of metabolism. Substances such as urea and creatinine, which are breakdown products of protein metabolism, may then be shown to be present in the circulating blood in amounts above the normal, by various forms of quantitative chemical tests. The best known of such tests is the **blood urea estimation**.

Renal function tests—reference was made to the various functions of the kidneys on p 150.

Urine is formed in these organs by filtration through capillary tufts called *renal glomeruli*. This filtrate then passes through structures in the solid part of the kidney called *renal tubules* before being collected in the renal calyces and pelvis and passed down the ureters. In the tubules, according to the current needs of the body, the urine is concentrated by reabsorption of water and electrolytes (e.g. sodium, potassium, calcium) and various other substances (e.g. glucose, urea) are also reabsorbed. These proceses are referred to as *selectice tubular reabsorption*.

Renal function tests may be designed to investigate either the function of the glomeruli (e.g. blood urea estimation, urea clearance test, creatinine clearance test) or of the tubules (e.g. urine concentration test, estimation of amounts of various electrolytes in the blood plasma or urine).

Note: the prefixes **hyper-** and **hypo-** are used to indicate respectively the presence of abnormally high or abnormally low amounts of various normal constituents of the blood plasma, e.g. **hypernatraemia**—an excessive amount of sodium in the blood; **hypokalaemia**—a deficiency of blood potassium. An abnormal increase in the total amount of circulating blood itself is termed **hypervolaemia**.

Radiological investigations—certain information about the urinary system can be obtained from plain X-rays but many patients with suspected urinary diseases require some form of **contrast urography**. This term includes the examination generally described as **intravenous pyelography** (IVP), but more correctly termed **intravenous urography** as the investigation is not confined to demonstration of the renal pelvis, but also produces films to show the ureters and bladder. Radiological investigation also includes the examinations of **retrograde urography** (retrograde pyelography), **antegrade pyelography**—as indicated by Sherwood (1) this examination can be of considerable value in urinary tract obstruction problems, **conventional** and **micturating cystography** (contrast-radiography of the bladder) and **urethrography** (contrast-radiography of the urethra).

In selected cases it may be desirable to demonstrate the renal blood vessels by performing **aortography** or **selective renal angiography**.

Radioactive isotopes may be used in **isotope renography** to investigate renal function and may also be used to demonstrate renal tumours and cysts.

Ultrasonic investigation and CT are also being increasingly used in kidney disorders and in the investigation of bladder tumours and prostatic disease.

Visual inspection by special instruments—the interior of the urethra may be inspected by a panendoscope and that of the bladder by a cystoscope, these procedures being termed respectively **urethroscopy** and **cystoscopy**.

Biopsy of lesions in the bladder may be carried out during cystoscopy.

Renal biopsy—the taking of a minute fragment of renal tissue for microscopic examination.

Diseases of the Kidney and Ureter

Congenital Abnormalities

A large number of developmental abnormalities may occur in the kidneys and ureters. Many are of a minor nature and the more marked of them are not very common. They include the following.

Congenital absence of one kidney—a serious disability if the patient's only kidney becomes diseased.

Ectopic kidney—the term **ectopic** means abnormally placed or displaced. As a result of developmental error an ectopic kidney lies in the pelvic cavity or lower abdomen.

Congenital hypoplastic kidney—a kidney which fails to develop normally both in size and in the development of its internal structure.

Horseshoe kidney—a condition in which there is a partial fusion of the two kidneys. The fusion is usually between the lower poles, which are joined by a band of renal tissue which lies in front of the spine.

Duplex kidney (duplication of the renal pelvis)—in this anomaly, which may be present on one or both sides, the renal pelvis consists of two partial or complete divisions. In the latter case there is usually an associated partial or complete duplication of the ureter.

Congenital polycystic kidneys—in this condition the kidneys are enlarged and contain numerous thin-walled cysts. It is caused by inherited developmental error and, although present at birth, symptoms do not usually appear until adult life is reached. Haematuria is a common symptom. Hypertension (high blood pressure) may develop as a complication of the disease.

The cysts cause deformity of the renal pelvis and calyces which is demonstrable by urography.

Medullary sponge kidney—a congenital abnormality of the kidneys in which there is widespread dilatation of renal tubules and associated cyst formation. There is often some accompanying degree of **nephrocalcinosis**, i.e. deposition of calcium salts in the solid part of the kidneys.

Ureterocele—a localised dilatation of the lower end of the ureter. It is sometimes associated with an abnormally placed opening of the ureter (i.e. an **ectopic ureteric orifice**) which may be into the bladder, the urethra, the vagina or elsewhere.

Traumatic Conditions

Injuries in the region of the loin (e.g. blows, kicks, crushing injuries) may result in bruising referred to as **contusion of the kidney**; tearing of kidney substance when the condition is referred to as **ruptured kidney**; or, rarely, tearing through of the renal pedicle with separation of the kidney from its ureter and renal artery and veins. This is termed **total avulsion of the kidney**, the word avulsion meaning tearing off and being sometimes also used to describe certain fractures and injuries elsewhere in the body.

Haematuria is a usual feature of renal trauma.

Intravenous urography is indicated in all suspected cases, not only to try to obtain information regarding kidney damage but also to assess the state of the uninjured kidney, this being of considerable importance if the case is one in which surgical treatment is required.

Kidney damage may be evidenced by absent or defective concentration of contrast medium on the injured side, by abnormality of renal outline and, if a tear involves the pelvicalyceal system, by leakage of contrast medium out of this system.

Investigation of the renal blood supply by angiography is also desirable in a proportion of cases.

Infective Diseases

Pathogenic micro-organisms may reach the kidney by the bloodstream or by ascending the ureter from the lower part of the urinary tract.

Important factors in many cases of kidney infection are, firstly, obstruction and, secondly, **vesicoureteric reflux**, i.e. reflux of urine from the bladder up one or both uteters, an abnormality which may or may not be associated with lower urinary tract obstruction.

Obstructive lesions that affect the urinary system result in **urinary stasis** of varying degree, i.e. delay in the passage of urine through this system, a condition predisposing to infection because stagnant urine is a good medium for bacterial growth.

Vesicoureteric reflux affords a ready means for bacteria to be carried up from bladder to kidney in cases of bladder infection; a very common disorder in the female sex, both in childhood and adult life.

Renal disease secondary to reflux of this type is termed **reflux nephropathy**.

The principal infective diseases found in the kidney are given below.

Pyelonephritis—this term indicated that both the renal pelvis and its calyces (i.e. the hollow part of the kidney) together with the solid part of the kidney are affected by inflammatory changes resulting from an infection (other than a tuberculous infection), i.e. there is **pyelitis** (inflammation of the renal pelvis and calyces) plus **nephritis** (inflammation of the renal substance).

Acute pyelonephritis is predominantly a disease of females. Pregnancy appears to be a predisposing factor but this infection can occur at any age. It sometimes occurs in males, generally as a complication in disorders causing urinary stasis.

The most frequent causal pathogen is a bacterium called the *Escherichia coli*, which is a normal inhabitant of the human intestinal tract.

The infection usually affects only one kidney but may be bilateral. Common symptoms are pain in the loin, frequent and painful micturition, pyrexia, tachycardia and **rigors**, i.e. shivering attacks.

The infecting micro-organisms may be cultured from the urine and, when the acute attack has subsided, radiological investigation may be requested to exclude associated abnormalities in the urinary system.

Chronic pyelonephritis—this disease, which may also be unilateral or bilateral, may develop as a sequel to acute pyelonephritis or may be of chronic nature from its outset. It is often associated with some pre-existing disease, congenital or acquired, in the urinary system and, as described by Hodson and Edwards (2), with vesicoureteric reflux (see p 154). Radiological examination is therefore an important procedure in this disease.

Intravenous urography may show evidence of renal scarring and an appearance called calyceal clubbing in affected kidneys. Micturating cystography may demonstrate vesicoureteric reflux.

Common long-term results of chronic pyelonephritis are scarring of affected kidneys, the development of hypertension (high blood pressure) and renal failure.

Treatment is by sulphonamides or antibiotics.

Pyonephrosis—a condition in which the renal pelvis and its calyces are dilated and filled with pus (cf hydronephrosis in which the dilated pelvis and calyces are filled with urine). The dilatation is caused by some form of obstuction to the outflow of urine from the renal pelvis, e.g. by a calculus (stone) impacted in the ureter, and the pus is produced as a result of supervening infection with pyogenic bacteria.

Renal carbuncle (carbuncle of the kidney)—a carbuncle is an inflammatory mass that breaks down to form multiple small abscess cavities. Renal carbuncle is usually due to a bloodborne infection with *staphylococci* derived from some other focus of infection such as a boil in the skin.

Perinephric abscess (perirenal abscess)—this is an abscess that forms in the fatty tissues around the kidney. It may be due to bloodborne infection or direct spread of infection from a lesion within the kidney.

Obliteration of the shadow of the psoas muscle on the side of the lesion is a common radiographic sign of a perinephric abscess.

Renal tuberculosis—tuberculosis infection of the kidney is due to bloodborne infection. The causative *tubercle bacilli* may be derived from an active or a reactivated primary tuberculous lesion in a site such as the lung, hilar or mesenteric lymph glands or less commonly, from the lesions of postprimary tuberculosis. Hence is classified as a form of metastatic tuberculosis.

Fortunately renal tuberculosis nowadays occurs less frequently than formerly. When it does develop, its highest incidence is in young adults.

The infection first causes inflammatory lesions in the cortices of the kidneys, which may heal or may progress so as to spread both in the solid part of the kidney and into the renal pelvis. *Tubercle bacilli* are discharged in the urine and foci of infection may as a result develop in the ureters and bladder. In males spread of disease to the reproductive organs may occur resulting in tuberculous infection in sites such as the prostate, seminal vesicles, epididymis and testis.

Among the clinical features of chronic renal tuberculosis are general ill-health, loss of weight, frequency of micturition, pyuria, haematuria and pain in the loin.

Radiological examination is of value in showing evidence of the disease. Pathological calcification is common in areas of tissue necrosis resulting from the inflammation, and is demonstrable on plain film. Destructive lesions which involve the pelvicalyceal system of the kidney produce changes demonstrable by intravenous urography.

The diagnosis is established by demonstration (using bacteriological methods) of the causative *tubercle bacilli* in the urine.

Associated bladder lesions may be demonstrated by cystoscopy.

Treatment is by antituberculous drugs and measures to improve the general condition of the patient. Surgery is necessary in certain types of kidney lesions and for some of the complications of the disease.

Glomerulonephritis (Nephritis)

Several diseases, most of which are of inflammatory origin and all of which are non-suppurative and affect glomeruli in both kidneys, fall in the group or disorders referred to as **glomerulonephritis** or, more shortly, as **nephritis**.

Houston *et al.* (3) indicate that many of these disorders have an immunological basis and further state 'there is no entirely satisfactory classification of glomerulonephritis'.

Accounts given by different authorities show that most cases of glomerulonephritis appear to be of four main types (or subtypes of these):

- **acute glomerulonephritis** (acute nephritis, acute diffuse glomerulonephritis, acute poststreptococcal glomerulonephritis);
- a type that produces the **nephrotic syndrome** (membraneous nephritis, nephrotic nephritis, subacute nephritis);
- **chronic glomerulonephritis** (chronic diffuse glomerulonephritis, chronic nephritis, chronic proliferative glomerulonephritis);
- **focal nephritis.**

Mixed types also occur.

The first of these types, frequently referred to briefly as **acute nephritis**, is widely thought often to be a manifestation of hypersensitivity to streptococcal infection. It follows a streptococcal tonsillitis and takes the form of an acute illness; among its characteristic features frequently are albuminuria, haematuria, oedema (often affecting the face as well as the dependent parts of the body), pleural effusions, ascites and high blood pressure. This disease may clear up completely or may undergo slow progression to a **chronic glomerulonephritis**, which ultimately leads to **chronic renal failure**, i.e. failure or normal kidney function.

In the **nephrotic syndrome** there is no acute phase, the condition being chronic from the outset and associated with the excretion of large amounts of protein in the urine, the presence of diminished amounts of protein in the blood, and the development of oedema.

Cases which fail to respond to treatment progress ultimately to chronic glomerulonephritis and eventual chronic renal failure.

Note: Certain forms of kidney disease in which there is damage to the renal tubules may develop features with a resemblance to the nephrotic syndrome and are called **nephroses**.

Focal nephritis differs from the types of nephritis described above in that its lesions are scattered instead of diffuse. It is not generally in itself a serious disease but may occur as a complication of severe diseases such as subacute bacterial endocarditis and certain connective tissue diseases.

Renal function tests are of great value in the diagnosis and assessment of progress in patients with various types of glomerulonephritis. Renal biopsy is used to establish the diagnosis in some cases.

Specific dietetic measures with special reference to the intake of fluids, protein and salt are of great importance in treatment. Diuretics, i.e. drugs that increase the secretion of urine, are often required in chronic cases with oedema. Cases of nephrotic syndrome may benefit considerably from steroid therapy. An increasing number of patients who develop chronic nephritis and subsequently severe renal failure are being treated by haemodialysis (see p 162), and some of these by subsequent renal transplantation.

Neoplasms

Neoplasms may arise in the solid part of the kidney and in the renal pelvis and ureter. The most important are given below.

Adenocarcinoma (hypernephroma)—a carcinomatous growth of the solid part of the kidney which occurs in adult life, most usually in middle age and is of fairly common incidence. It is frequently referred to as a **hypernephroma**, owing to a formerly held belief that it derived from misplaced adrenal tissue. (The adrenal glands lie above the kidneys—**hyper**—above; **nephr**—kidney; **-oma**—tumour.)

In some patients the growth may remain confined to the kidney for a considerable time. In others, early bloodborne metastases may occur in sites such as the lungs and bones.

Haematuria is often the first sign of the disease. Pain in the loin tends to be a fairly late feature, as does the development of a palpable mass due to the tumour. Occasionally a metastatic deposit may produce the first evidence of the disease in the form of a haemoptysis or a pathological fracture of bone. In such instances the primary tumour may be difficult to detect and be referred to as a **hidden primary tumour**.

Blood and occasionally malignant cells may be demonstrable in the urine.

Treatment is by surgery, usually combined with radiotherapy.

Radiological investigation with contrast urography, and sometimes renal angiography are important diagnostic measures. In the former, frequently demonstrable changes are displacement and distortion of the renal pelvis and calyces, the presence of a filling defect within these structures, and abnormality of renal outline. CT or radioactive isotopes may also be useful in demonstrating the presence of hypernephroma.

Some hypernephromas present appearances on urograms indistinguishable from those of solitary renal cysts (see later). Ultrasonic examination, followed when indicated by renal cyst puncture and cytological examination of aspirated fluid, is commonly used in differentiating between the two conditions.

Embryoma (Wilms' tumour, nephroblastoma, adenosarcoma)— this is a rare neoplasm of the solid part of the kidney, which occurs in infants and young children. It is believed to originate in remnants of embryonic tissue which persist in the kidney, and to be of sarcomatous type. In clinical practice it is usually known by its old name of **Wilms's tumour**, after M. Wilms, a German surgeon.

The neoplasm is usually unilateral, but cases have been reported in which tumours have been found in both kidneys.

Growth of a Wilms's tumour is usually rapid and produces a very large abdominal swelling. Haematuria, usually a common feature of renal neoplasms, is rare. Widespread early metastases are common, the lungs being one of the principal sites for their occurrence.

Plain radiographs, intravenous urography and sometimes renal angiography are of considerable help in diagnosis.

Surgical removal of the kidney, followed by radiotherapy, is the usual treatment if the disease is diagnosed before there is evidence of metastatic spread. Metastases are treated by radiotherapy.

Carcinoma of the renal pelvis—this tumour of the hollow part of the kidney may take the form of a **transitional cell carcinoma** or less commonly a **squamous cell carcinoma**. The former has a tendency to produce secondary 'seedling' growths in the lower part of the ureter and in the bladder. Haematuria is the cardinal symptom of both types. The growth may produce a filling defect in the renal pelvis, demonstrable by ascending or descending pyelography. Treatment is surgical in all suitable cases.

Cyst Formation

Renal cysts are not very common but when they do occur it is important to differentiate them from renal neoplasms.

The occurrence of multiple cysts in the disorder called **congenital polycystic kidneys** has already been mentioned. **Solitary cysts of the kidney** are usually thought to develop as a result of acquired abnormality.

Renal Calculus (Stone in the Kidney, Renal Lithiasis)

Chemical salts may be precipitated from the urine to form solid bodies known as **calculi**. Calculus formation in the kidney usually starts in a calyx. From this site the calculus may migrate into the renal pelvis. Here it may remain and may gradually increase in size, as a result of further precipitation of urinary constituents. Alternatively, it may migrate into the ureter and pass through the bladder and urethra, being ultimately voided in the urine. Sometimes a calculus which has entered the ureter may become lodged in this structure, when it is described as an **impacted ureteric calculus**.

Renal calculi usually consist of a mixture of chemical substances but are named according to their principal constituents, e.g. **phosphate calculi, calcium oxalate calculi, uric acid** and **urate calculi**.

A great many factors may operate in the production of calculi. Among these may be mentioned urinary stasis, resulting from congenital or acquired obstructive lesions within the urinary system; urinary infections; urinary stasis from prolonged lying in bed as a result of operation or illness; diseases in which there is marked loss of calcium in the blood and urine (e.g. hyperparathyroidism, see p 219); excessive sweating, such as occurs in hot countries and leads to the passage of unduly concentrated urine.

It should be noted that calculus formation in the urinary system is not confined to the kidney but may also occur in the bladder and occasionally in the urethra. In the male reproductive system calculi may form in the prostate gland.

Renal calculi may form in one or both kidneys, and may be single or multiple. They occur in childhood and adult life and are found in both sexes. In some cases they are symptomless, but in most cases they cause pain in the loin and not infrequently haematuria.

Passage of a stone down the ureter causes pain of a type called **renal colic**. These pains are felt in the abdomen and often radiate into the groin or external genital organs.

Most renal calculi contain sufficient calcium salts to render them visible on plain radiographs, but contrast radiography is generally necessary to differentiate them from other calcified opacities which can be found in the abdomen or cavity of the pelvis, e.g. opaque gall stones, calcified mesenteric glands, **phleboliths** (i.e. small calcified thrombi in pelvic veins).

A calculus may cause a partial obstruction of the pelviureteric segment resulting in the development of a hydronephrosis or a partial obstruction of a ureter, causing hydroureter and hydronephrosis (see later).

Urinary stasis due to obstruction, urinary infection and calculus formation are quite often found in association, and it may be difficult or impossible to determine which of these abnormal conditions was the first to develop.

Surgery is necessary in a high proportion of patients with renal calculus and may also be required in cases of impacted ureteric calculus, when the stone fails to pass onwards into the bladder after a reasonable period of observation.

Hydronephrosis and Hydroureter

The term **hydronephrosis** indicates a condition of dilatation of the renal pelvis and its calyces, and **hydroureter**, dilation of the ureter.

It is generally only a partial or intermittent obstruction that leads to any pronounced degree of hydronephrosis. Complete obstruction of a ureter generally leads to cessation of secretion of urine, i.e. **anuria**, from the kidney above it and, if the obstruction is not relieved, eventually to atrophy of the affected kidney.

Hydronephrosis may, or may not, be accompanied by hydroureter and may develop on one or both sides according to the site of the obstructing lesion, or lesions, e.g. bilateral hydronephrosis and hydroureters may occur as a result of obstructive lesions at the bladder neck or in the urethra, whereas a partial obstruction of the pelviureteric region on one side only will produce a unilateral hydronephrosis.

In many cases of hydronephrosis, no obvious mechanical cause for the condition can be discovered and the condition is therefore described as **idiopathic hydronephrosis**. Notley (4) has shown that in this disorder there is narrowing together with a considerable increase in fibrous tissue in the pelviureteric segment.

The same writer (5) in describing the clinical features of the condition indicates that infants may present with an abdominal mass or a history of failure to thrive and infected urine, and older children and adults with pain arising in the loin.

Idiopathic hydronephrosis may be treated by various forms of an operative procedure called **pyeloplasty**.

Unilateral hydronephrosis is most commonly of the idiopathic type referred to above. Among the many other causes of this condition are: (*a*) impaction of the calculus in the ureter or at the pelviureteric segment; (*b*) partial blockage of the pelviureteric segment by a renal neoplasm; (c) kinking of the upper end of the ureter by an **aberrant renal artery** (i.e. a renal artery which, as a result of developmental error, is abnormal in position); (d) pressure on the lower end of one ureter by a pelvic neoplasm (e.g. an advanced carcinoma of the uterine cervix); (e) an uncommon condition, called **periureteric fibrosis** or **retroperitoneal fibrosis**, where ureteric compression, by surrounding inflammatory fibrosis in the retroperitoneal tissues, leads to partial obstruction and medial displacement of the ureter on one or both sides. Treatment is surgical. In most cases it is not possible to determine the cause of development of the fibrous tissue.

Bilateral hydronephrosis may be due to congenital bladder neck obstruction. Among its other causes are: congenital strictures and valves in the urethra; obstruction of the urethra by an enlarged prostate gland; acquired urethral stricture; lesions that cause obstruction of both ureters, e.g. bilateral calculi, extensive pelvic neoplasms, periureteric fibrosis.

> Slight and moderate degrees of hydronephrosis can readily be demonstrated by intravenous urography and this examination may indicate the cause of the obstruction. With a large hydronephrosis, however, destruction of renal tissue may be of such a degree that no concentration of the dye occurs on the affected side. Retrograde pyelography is then necessary to demonstrate the condition.

Hydronephrosis in its early stages is often reversible and a return to normal may follow removal of its cause, when this is possible. **Nephrectomy** (surgical removal of the kidney) is frequently required in advanced degrees of unilateral hydronephrosis.

It is to be noted that during pregnancy some dilatation of the upper parts of both renal tracts, but more pronounced on the right side, develops as a normal physiological change and subsides normally after delivery over a period of about 3 months.

Renal Failure

This term describes a condition in which the kidneys are unable adequately to carry out their normal function. Accordingly, waste products accumulate in the blood, the normal water and electrolyte balances are upset, and alterations occur in the reaction of the blood.

Accumulation of acid waste products in the circulating blood results in a condition termed **acidosis**. Accumulation of waste products generally, including urea—a nitrogenous protein breakdown product—causes a clinical picture with features such as headache, drowsiness, mental confusion, convulsions, coma, and sometimes accompanying haemorrhages; signs and symptoms which are referred to as being due to **uraemia**. The term **azotaemia** is used to describe an excess of urea and other nitrogenous substances in the blood.

According to the factors responsible, renal failure may present in acute or chronic form. In the acute type excretion of urine is either scanty (**oliguria**) or stops altogether (**anuria, suppression of urine**) in the early phase of the disorder. In chronic renal failure, however, there is, characteristically, **polyuria**, i.e. the passage of excessive amounts of urine.

Long-standing chronic renal failure may result in overgrowth of the parathyroid glands and **secondary hyperparathyroidism**, and also abnormalities of vitamin D metabolism, both of which produce bone lesions. This condition is thus one of the causes of renal osteodystrophy (see p 254).

Appropriate chemical tests may show abnormalities in the blood and urine arising from renal failure, e.g. estimation of blood urea, plasma bicarbonate, plasma potassium and sodium, urea concentration tests, etc.

Three main types of renal failure are described.

Prerenal—in which there is a sustained diminution of blood flow through the kidneys from lowering blood pressure or a decreasing volume of blood circulating through them e.g. caused by haemorrhage, burns, severe vomiting and diarrhoea or obstruction of the renal artery or vein.

Renal—when there is extensive damage to kidney substance e.g. from chronic pyelonephritis, chronic glomerulonephritis, essential or malignant hypertension, eclampsia, diabetes (diabetic neuropathy), phenacetin and other analgesic drugs (analgesic nephropathy), transfusion of incompatible blood.

Postrenal—due to obstruction in the flow of urine through the urinary system by obstructive lesions of both ureters or of the lower urinary tract e.g. extensive pelvic neoplasms, prostatic enlargement. Renal failure resulting from obstruction is referred to as **obstructive uropathy**.

> Intravenous urography may be of considerable value in investigating the cause of chronic renal failure, provided the condition is not too severe. As the concentrating power of the kidneys is diminished, it is however necessary to administer a high dose of contrast medium by injection or infusion in order to obtain diagnostic films. Dehydration can be dangerous and should not be used as a preliminary to X-ray examination in this condition.

The treatment of renal failure is directed to treating its cause when practicable, correcting abnormalities of blood reaction and water and electrolyte balance, taking a suitable diet, and preventing the development of intercurrent infections.

When appropriate, the principles of osmosis are applied in a method of treatment called **intermittent haemodialysis**. This is designed to remove accumulated waste products by passing the whole of the circulating blood over a semipermeable membrane contained within a machine known as an **artificial kidney**.

In suitable patients intermittent haemodialysis may be followed by **renal transplantation**.

In some patients, notably those unsuitable for haemodialysis, **continuous ambulatory peritoneal dialysis** (CAPD) may be carried out through a tube introduced through the anterior abdominal wall into the lower part of the general peritoneal cavity.

Hypertension of Renal Origin

This term indicates high blood pressure caused by certain diseases of the kidney and of its arterial blood supply, e.g. chronic pyelonephritis, some types of glomerulonephritis, renal artery stenosis.

In **renal artery stenosis** there is a narrowing of the main trunk of one or both renal arteries, resulting in **renal ischaemia**, i.e. a diminution in the amount of blood circulating through affected kidneys. The condition is usually due to atheroma. It is demonstrable by renal angiography.

Some Other Terms Referring to Kidney Diseases

Referring to renal tubular defects (i.e. disorders in which the renal tubules are unable to carry out their normal functions with respect to the reabsorption of certain of the substances excreted by the glomeruli).

(i) **Renal tubular acidosis** (Lightwood-Albright syndrome)—a disorder in which acid substances are retained in the blood. The type described as **idiopathic renal acidosis of infancy** and also the type that occurs in older children and adults are both frequently associated with **nephrocalcinosis**, i.e. the deposition of calcium salts in the solid part of the kidney, and also with the development of rickets or osteomalacia.

(ii) **Fanconi syndrome**—a congenital disorder of the renal tubules often complicated by rickets or osteomalacia.

Referring to vascular disorders of the kidney (i.e. disorders in the renal blood supply).

(i) **Acute tubular necrosis**—a condition which may complicate the prerenal type of renal failure, and be due to diminished renal blood supply; or may result from certain severe infections and chemical poisonings.

(ii) **Atheroma of the renal arteries**—this arterial disease may lead to localised or diffuse renal ischaemia according to its distribution. Renal artery stenosis is usually due to atheroma.

Referring to other diseases which may produce kidney lesions. The following are among the other diseases which may produce kidney lesions, and are referred to in other parts of the book: essential hypertension, causing **hypertensive nephrosclerosis** (**nephrosclerosis** means hardening of the kidneys and indicates the hardening which occurs when damaged renal tissue is replaced by fibrous tissue); diabetes mellitus, causing **diabetic kidney** (diabetic nephropathy); primary hyperparathyroidism causing calculus formation and nephrocalcinosis; amyloid disease; myelomatosis causing **myeloma kidney** with which is associated the passage in the urine of an abnormal protein, referred to as **Bence-Jones protein**, eclampsia, gout, systemic lupus erythematosus and polyarteritis nodosa.

Renal Osteodystrophy

This term indicates defective bone formation occurring in association with renal disease. It is discussed further under Metabolic Bone Diseases.

Diseases of the Urinary Bladder

Congenital Abnormalities

Congenital bladder neck obstruction—this is a fairly common condition especially in males. The obstruction is due to hypertrophy of muscle fibres around the bladder neck (i.e. the region where the urethra leaves the bladder). It may produce obstructive symptoms in childhood but more often produces no symptoms until adult life is reached.

The symptoms in men resemble those of benign prostatic enlargement but develop at an earlier age.

Incomplete bladder emptying due to the obstruction and any resultant dilation of the ureters and pelvicalyceal systems, due to back-pressure effects, are readily demonstrable by intravenous urography.

The condition may be treated by transurethral resection of the bladder neck.

Ectopia vesicae (extrophy of the bladder, extroversion of the bladder)—a rare anomaly in which, as a result of developmental failure, the anterior wall of the bladder and part of the anterior abdominal wall are absent. The two pubic bones are widely separated at the symphysis pubis, and the posterior wall of the bladder and the urethral orifices lie on the anterior surface of the lower abdomen.

Patent urachus—this condition results from partial or complete failure of obliteration of the lumen of a structure called the *urachus*, which is connected with the bladder and normally patent only during certain stages of fetal life. Such failure results in a condition called **patent urachus** which may present as:

  (i) a **vesicoumbilical fistula**, i.e. a patent track connecting the bladder and umbilicus;

(ii) a type of cyst termed a **urachal cyst**; or

(iii) a congenital pouch arising from the superior surface of the bladder termed a **urachal diverticulum**.

Traumatic Conditions

The bladder may be torn as a result of injury and, according to the site of the tear in its wall, the injury is termed **intraperitoneal rupture** or **extraperitoneal rupture of the bladder**. The former condition results in leakage of urine into the peritoneal cavity and consequent peritonitis. In extraperitoneal rupture, urine is extravasated into the soft tissue behind and above the pubis. Both injuries are frequently associated with fractures of the pelvis.

Infective Diseases

Infection of the bladder wall results in a condition of inflammation termed **cystitis** which may develop in acute or chronic form. Such infection may be caused by pathogens reaching the organ via either the bloodstream, the ureter or the urethra. In the latter instance infection may ascend from the bladder to involve the kidney pelvis and solid part of the kidney, the organisms being carried up through the ureter as a result of vesicoureteric reflux (see p 154).

Cystitis is commoner in females than in males. In females, the shortness of the urethra predisposes to ascending infection from the perineum, while in males the disease often develops as a secondary result of some obstructive lesion (e.g. enlarged prostate, urethral stricture) in the lower urinary tract.

Among other conditions associated with cystitis are vesical calculi, diverticula of the bladder, carcinoma of the bladder, neuropathic bladder disorders and foreign body in the bladder.

In the tropics and semitropics, cystitis may be caused by parasitic worms in the disease called schistosomiasis (bilharziasis).

Passage of a catheter into the bladder always carries some risk of introducing infective organisms and thus causing cystitis; hence the need for strict asepsis during this procedure.

The causal pathogens of cystitis may be demonstrated in specimens of urine by bacteriological methods. The commonest infecting microorganism to be thus found is the *Escherichia coli*.

A small propotion of bladder infections are due to tuberculous infection and are secondary to tuberculous infection in the kidneys.

Sulphonamides, antibiotics, and certain other drugs are used to treat simple cystitis.

Neoplasms

Two types of neoplasm are fairly common in the bladder.

Papilloma of the bladder—the word **papilla** means a nipple and, strictly speaking, **papilloma** means a nipple-like tumour. The term is, however, used to describe a class of benign tumour of epithelium that is raised above normal surrounding epithelium but is of varying size and shape.

A bladder papilloma arises in the epithelial lining of the organ and gives rise to painless haematuria. In most cases it is single, but multiple growths sometimes occur. The diagnosis is usually made by cystoscopy and biopsy.

The tumour may be destroyed by **diathermy**, i.e. a method in which a high frequency current is used to generate heat in an area of body tissue. In surgical diathermy the heat is such as to cause death of tissues touched by the operating electrode. When dealing with bladder growths, the electrode is introduced into the interior of the organ through a cystoscope.

Malignant change may develop in a papilloma, the condition then developing into one of **papillary carcinoma**.

Carcinoma of the bladder—a carcinomatous growth arising in the epithelial lining of the bladder may be of the papillary type described above or take the form of a solid tumour.

A connection has been established between the use of certain chemicals in industrial processes and the development of bladder carcinoma. This neoplasm is also a not uncommon complication of schistosomiasis (see p 313).

The condition is more common in males than in females.

Haematuria and frequency of micturition are common early features of the disease and cystitis often develops as a complication.

Both lymphatic and bloodborne metastases may occur and the latter may be found in lungs and bone.

The diagnosis of bladder carcinoma is usually made at cystoscopy and confirmed by biopsy. Local complications of the disease include bladder neck obstruction; involvement of a ureteric orifice leading to hydroureter and hydronephrosis, or a non-functioning kidney; and spread to neighbouring organs with fistula formation, e.g. vesicocolic fistula.

Intravenous urography is valuable for investigating the complications of the disorder, and will usually also demonstrate the primary growth in the form of a filling defect in the shadow produced when the interior of the bladder is outlined by the contrast medium.

Localising cystograms are used when planning treatment by radiation.

Treatment is by surgery or radiotherapy, used singly or in combination.

Neuropathic (Neurogenic) Bladder Disorders

In this group of disorders there is interference with normal nervous control of the bladder. The disorders may be congenital in origin or result from various types of diseases and injuries of the spinal cord. They may cause bladder neck obstruction with retention of urine. Resulting from such retention, urine may overflow from the full bladder down the urethra, a state of affairs termed **retention with overflow** and giving rise to **overflow incontinence** (false incontinence).

In other neuropathic bladder disorders there may be no bladder neck obstruction and inability of the bladder to hold urine may result in a continual leakage of fluid into the urethra, producing what is known as **true incontinence**.

Other Bladder Disorders

Vesical calculus—calculi (stones) found in the urinary bladder may have formed there or migrated from the kidney. Small calculi may be voided through the urethra. Calculi which remain in the bladder frequently show a gradual increase in size owing to repeated deposition of urinary constituents on their external surfaces.

Vesical calculi may be single or multiple; the majority are radio-opaque. They are similar in composition to renal calculi and similar factors operate in their production (see p. 159). Urinary obstruction (e.g. due to an enlarged prostate or urethral stricture) is often a predisposing factor in their formation.

Painful and frequent micturition, often associated with haematuria, are the chief clinical features. Treatment is surgical.

Bladder diverticula—diverticula, or pouches, of the bladder may be congenital or acquired, and single or multiple. They consist of protrusions of mucosa through the muscular wall of the organ. The acquired variety tend to develop as a secondary result of some obstruction to the outflow of urine from the bladder (e.g. due to an enlarged prostate or urethral stricture).

Stasis of urine, with subsequent infection, is common in diverticula, and calculi and neoplasms may form within them. Diverticula are readily demonstrated by descending or ascending cystograms.

Vesical fistula—fistulae of the bladder may be congenital, or may form between the bladder and adjacent organs as a result of disease or injury, e.g. **vesicovaginal fistula**, **vesicocolic fistula**. Contrast radiography may be employed to demonstrate such fistulae.

Vesicocolic fistula may occur as a complication of diverticulitis of the colon, or a carcinoma of the colon. The condition results in cystitis and the passage of intestinal gas in the urine. This latter symptom is called **pneumaturia**.

Diseases of the Male Urethra

Congenital Abnormalities

These include the following diseases.

Congenital urethral stenosis (congenital stricture)—this malformation usually takes the form of a localised stenosis (narrowing) at some point during the course of the urethra. If it occurs at the external urinary meatus (external urethral orifice) it produces a condition referred to as **pinhole meatus**.

Congenital urethral stenosis is one of the causes of obstruction of the lower urinary system and may lead to bilateral hydroureter and hydronephrosis.

Congenital urethral valves—these are abnormal folds of mucous membrane which exert a valve-like action causing obstruction to the flow of urine through the urethra. They are found only in males and occur predominantly in the posterior urethra (i.e. the part of the urethra that includes its prostatic and membranous portions).

Hypospadias—a rare condition in which the external opening of the urethra lies on the undersurface of the penis, or in the perineum. The name of the anomaly means drawn beneath.

Epispadias—this is the opposite to hypospadias being a condition in which the external urethral orifice is situated on the dorsal surface of the penis. It is extremely rare.

Traumatic Conditions

Traumatic rupture of the urethra is a not uncommon injury in males, the membranous portion being especially liable to damage. It may be associated with fracture of the pelvis. Urethral stricture is a frequent sequel to urethral injury.

Foreign body in the urethra—various types of foreign body may be inserted into the urethra. X-ray investigation is often of value in suspected cases.

Inflammatory Conditions

Inflammation of the urethra is called **urethritis**. Taylor and Cotton (6) list as causes of this condition gonorrhoea, instrumentation of the urethra, non-specific causes and the presence of an indwelling catheter.

Urethral stricture is a not uncommon sequel of urethritis.

It has already been noted that urethritis is sometimes associated with arthritis and conjunctivitis in a condition called **Reiter's syndrome** (see p 59).

Urethral Stricture

A stricture (stenosis) of the urethra may be of congenital, traumatic, postoperative or inflammatory origin.

The cardinal symptom of this lesion is difficulty in passing urine, which may progress to a condition in which the patient can pass hardly any urine or no urine at all. This is referred to as a condition of **retention of urine**, or more simply spoken of as **retention**.

Urethral stricture may lead to back-pressure changes with distension of the bladder and bilateral hydronephrosis and hydroureter. Cystitis is also a common complication, and vesical calculi and diverticula may also form.

Valuable information regarding the site and severity of a stricture may be obtained by performing a urethrogram. The extent of any back-pressure changes can be shown by intravenous urography.

Treatment may be by dilatation of the stricture by instruments called **bougies** or by a surgical procedure called urethroplasty.

Urethral Calculus

A calculus which has been voided from the bladder may lodge in the urethra. It is then referred to as a urethral calculus. Calculi may also form in the urethra in patients who have some pre-existing abnormality in this structure, e.g. urethral stricture.

Neoplasms of the Urethra

These are very rare. **Carcinoma of the urethra** may be treated by surgery or by radiotherapy.

Diseases of the Female Urethra

The female urethra is very much less liable to disease or injury than that of the male. Among the disorders which may uncommonly affect this structure are injury to the urethra during childbirth or surgical operations, urethritis, carcinoma, urethral diverticulum and **urethral caruncle**—a small localised inflammatory swelling, presenting in the region of the external urethral orifice and often associated with trichomonas infection. Lesions in the female urethra may rarely cause urinary obstruction.

Urethral abnormalities in women are among the causes of a type of incontinence of urine called **stress incontinence**, a condition in which urine escapes from the bladder involuntarily when the patient coughs or strains.

The displacement of the urethra and bladder neck which may occur in genital prolapse (p 184) is an important cause of stress incontinence.

Diseases of the Penis

These diseases include the following.

Balanitis—inflammation of the glans penis and foreskin and **primary chancre**, the initial lesion of syphilitic infection.

Phimosis—constriction of the distal end of the foreskin preventing its normal retraction so as to completely uncover the glans penis. This condition is treated by the surgical operation of **circumcision**, i.e. excision of the *prepuce* (i.e. the foreskin).

Paraphimosis—a condition wherein the prepuce having been retracted cannot be replaced and causes a constriction at the distal part of the penis just below the glans with resultant marked swelling of the glans.

Priapism—a condition of persistent erection of the penis, usually the result of venous thrombosis within the organ.

Carcinoma of the penis—an uncommon type of neoplasm which is largely confined to uncircumcised men and occurs in the glans. Radiotherapy is the treatment of choice.

Diseases of the Prostate Gland

The prostate gland lies below the base of the bladder and the prostatic urethra runs through its substance.

Compression of the urethra, with resultant urinary obstruction, is a common secondary feature of diseases that cause prostatic enlargement. The most important of these are benign enlargement and carcinoma. Among the other conditions which may affect the gland are **prostatitis** (inflammation of the prostate), which is of infective origin and may be acute or chronic, and **prostatic calculi** which are usually symptomless but show as well-defined opacities on X-ray film.

Benign Enlargement of the Prostate Gland (Simple Prostatic Enlargement, Senile Hyperplasia of the Prostate, Adenoma of the Prostate)

This is a common disease because, in many men, some degree of enlargement of the prostate occurs as old age approaches. This frequently causes some degree of compression of the prostatic urethra and consequent interference with normal micturition. Hormonal imbalance is thought to be an important factor in causation.

Urinary symptoms may be slight and non-progressive. In other instances the disease may result in a degree of obstruction that prevents the bladder from achieving complete expulsion of its contents. This organ then always contains some residual urine after micturition. Cystitis is a common complication. Acute retention may supervene. Other complications which may develop as a consequence of the urinary obstruction are bilateral hydronephrosis and hydroureter; calculus and diverticulum formation in the bladder, and disordered renal function which may progress to renal failure.

In most instances the enlarged prostate gland can be felt at rectal examination. Renal function tests, including blood urea estimation, are important in assessing whether there is any secondary renal damage.

Radiological investigation by intravenous urography is a most important measure in assessing the patient's condition, as from it the following information may be derived: (a) it serves as a rough test of renal function by showing the extent to which the kidneys are capable of concentrating the dye; (b) it reveals the presence of complications such as hydronephrosis, hydroureter, vesical calculus, bladder diverticula; (c) the hypertrophied gland frequently produces a filling defect in the base of the bladder, thus in many instances indicating enlargement; (d) a post-micturition film gives an indication of the amount of residual urine; (e) evidence of unsuspected metastases may be seen in the spine, ribs, hip bones or femora, thus revealing that clinical features, initially thought to be of simple prostatic enlargement, are due in reality to prostatic carcinoma.

Surgery is frequently indicated for benign enlargement of the prostate, prostatectomy being performed. In patients with retention a period of catheter drainage of the bladder may be necessary as a preoperative measure.

Carcinoma of the Prostate Gland

Like benign enlargement of the prostate, prostatic carcinoma also occurs in elderly men but is much less common than the former condition.

The growth causes disturbances of micturition and leads to urethral compression which in turn results in complications such as cystitis and bilateral hydronephrosis and hydroureter.

Bony metastases are often an early feature in the disease and may cause pain in the back. Pulmonary metastases may occur as a late feature.

The growth may be palpable on rectal examination. Radiological investigation is valuable in showing changes produced in the urinary system and metastases in bones.

If the tumour has spread outside the gland blood examination may show increased amounts of an enzyme called *serum acid phosphatase* and, when bony metastases are present, another enzyme called *serum alkaline phosphatase* may also show increased blood concentrations. (This latter enzyme is raised in conditions in which there is increased activity of osteoblasts e.g. Paget's disease, sclerotic metastases.)

Radical surgery may be used in very early cases but, in the majority, palliative treatment is used and includes administration of female hormones (oestrogens). This is frequently successful in relieving pain and producing temporary regression of both the primary growth and any metastases present. The operation of subcapsular **orchidectomy** (removal of the testes) may sometimes be used as an alternative to hormone therapy.

Radiation may be employed in the treatment of bony metastases and sometimes in the treatment of the primary growth.

Diseases of the Testis, Epididymis, and Scrotum

Imperfect Descent of the Testis

The testes develop during fetal life in the retroperitoneal tissues in the region of the kidneys and descend into the scrotum shortly before birth. Upset of the normal processes of descent may result in the testis remaining in the abdomen, or being arrested at some point along its normal route of descent. This constitutes the condition known as **undescended testis**, Alternatively, such upset may result in the testis descending to some abnormal position when the condition is referred to as **ectopic testis**, the word **ectopic** meaning abnormally placed.

Undescended testis and ectopic testis may both occur as unilateral or bilateral abnormalities. When an undescended testis is retained in the abdomen or inguinal canal on one or both sides, the condition is termed unilateral or bilateral **cryptorchidism** the component **crypto-** meaning hidden.

Undescended testes may descend spontaneously into the scrotum, but if this does not occur in early childhood surgery is necessary.

Torsion of the Testis

A condition in which, as a result of imperfect fixation of the testis within the scrotum, the *spermatic cord* (i.e. the structure which suspends the testis within the scrotum and is formed by the distal part of the vas deferens and the blood vessels and nerves of the testis) becomes twisted, compressing the veins draining blood from the testis. As a result the testis becomes swollen and tender and there is severe pain. Unless the conditon is speedily relieved, permanent damage to the tissues of the testis will result.

An undescended testis is more liable to torsion than a normal testis.

Inflammatory Diseases

Acute inflammatory changes in the testis are practically always accompanied by similar changes in the epididymis, the condition being called **epididymo-orchitis**.

Acute epididymo-orchitis may occur as a complication of infections in the urethra and prostate gland and during the course of mumps.

Chronic inflammatory changes may often affect only the epididymis as is frequent in **tuberculous epididymitis**, or only the testis as is common in **syphilitic orchitis**.

Tuberculous epididymitis is usually secondary to renal tuberculosis and is often accompanied by **tuberculous vesiculitis** (i.e. inflammation of the seminal vesicles).

Neoplasms

Neoplasms of the testis are rare, but those that develop usually show a high degree of malignancy with early glandular spread and subsequent bloodborne metastases in the lungs. Lymphangiography (contrast radiography of the lymphatic system) is of great value in demonstrating metastases in the iliac and para-aortic lymph glands as is CT also.

Malignant tumours of the testis are of two main types.

(i) **Seminoma** (spermatocytoma)—a carcinomatous tumour, the name of which derives from its origin from epithelial cells lining the seminiferous tubules, i.e. the structures in which spermatozoa are produced from the *spermatocytes.*

(ii) **Teratoma**—thought to arise from embryonic cells which persist into adult life. A very rare type of teratoma is called a **chorioncarcinoma** or **chorionepithelioma of the testis**. This tumour is of considerable interest because, although in this instance arising in the male, it produces cells resembling those normally only found in chorionic epithelium formed within the uterus during pregnancy. (*Note:* the **chorion** is the outer of the fetal membranes.)

The usual treatment of testicular neoplasms is by **orchidectomy** (removal of the testis) followed by postoperative radiotherapy to the iliac and para-aortic lymph glands. Chemotherapy may be given to patients with widespread metastases.

Carcinoma of the scrotum—a malignant tumour arising from the skin of the scrotum. It is nowadays seldom seen but formerly was common in chimney sweeps.

Other Disorders

These include:

Hydrocele—used without qualification this term indicates a collection of fluid contained in a structure in the scrotum called the tunica vaginalis.

Hydro– means water or fluid, and **–cele** a tumour or swelling. This latter suffix is usually only applied to swellings other than those due to neoplasms.

A hydrocele of the tunica vaginalis may develop as a result of inflammatory or other diseases of the testis and epididymis, or be due to trauma or of unknown causation.

Haematocele—a collection of blood in the tunica vaginalis (see above) resulting from trauma or other cause.

Varicocele—a swelling produced by varicosity of the veins of the *pampiniform plexus*, i.e. a plexus of veins which lie in the spermatic cord anterior to the vas deferens.

Spermatocele—a cyst arising in the epididymis or in close relation to this structure.

> Soft tissue radiography of the testes, using a technique developed from mammography, has been described by Price and Loveday (7) as a useful diagnostic aid to differentiate between benign and malignant swellings.

Some Genitourinary Operations

Kidney and Ureter

Nephrectomy—removal of a kidney.

Nephrostomy—surgical drainage of the renal pelvis.

Nephroureterectomy—removal of a kidney and its ureter.

Pyeloplasty—this term describes a number of plastic operations on the renal pelvis which are used in certain cases of hydronephrosis to relieve obstruction at the pelviureteric junction. One of the best known is called the **Anderson-Hynes operation** and involves excising the pelviureteric segment and anastomosing (i.e. making a communication between) the residual part of the renal pelvis and the upper end of the ureter.

Renal transplantation—transplantation of a kidney from a living donor or from a cadaver to another individual. This operation is used in certain selected cases as a form of treatment for severe bilateral and irreversible kidney damage.

Ureteric reimplantation—an operation for correcting vesico-ureteric reflux.

Bladder and Urethra

Cystectomy—removal of the urinary bladder. This may take the form of partial or total removal of the organ.

When total cystectomy is performed, some operative procedure must also be carried out to effect satisfactory drainage of urine. This is termed **urinary diversion** and at the present time the most favoured method is by the construction of an **ileal conduit**. This involves transplanting the lower ends of the ureters into a segment of ileum which is isolated from the rest of the small bowel, and made to open on to the anterior abdominal wall, the operation being termed **ileoureterostomy**.

Another method is called **ureterocolostomy** and includes transplantation of the lower ends of the ureters into the colon.

Cystotomy—opening the bladder by a surgical incision.

Lithotomy—this term means the opening of an organ to remove a calculus. Used without qualification, it denotes surgical opening of the bladder to remove a vesical calculus.

Suprapubic cystostomy—surgical drainage of the bladder through an incision made through the anterior part of the lower abdominal wall just above the pubis.

Urethroplasty—a plastic operation for relief of a urethral stricture.

Prostate

Prostatectomy—removal of the prostate gland.

According to the route employed to gain access to the gland the operation may be referred to as a **suprapubic** or **retropubic prostatectomy** or **transurethral resection of the prostate** (TUR).

(Another form of prostatectomy is a recently developed method called **cryosurgery** in which tissues are destroyed by the action of severe cold.)

Testis and Epididymis

Epididymo-orchidectomy—removal of the testis and epididymis.

Orchidectomy—removal of the testis.

Orchiopexy—an operation to fix the testis in the scrotum, employed in certain cases of undescended testis.

Vasectomy—division of the vasa deferentia. This operation may be performed in association with prostatectomy to prevent spread of infection from the prostatic bed along the vasa to the epididymes. It may also be carried out with the specific object of producing sterility.

REFERENCES

(1) Sherwood, T. (1975). *Recent Advances in Radiology* (Lodge, T., Steiner, R. E., eds.) Edinburgh: Churchill Livingstone.

(2) Hodson, C. J., Edwards, D. (1960). Chronic pyelonephritis and vesicoureteric reflux. *Clinical Radiology*; **4**: 219.

(3) Houston, J. C., Joiner, C. L., Trounce, J. R., (1982). *A Short*

Textbook of Medicine, 7th Edn. p 464. London: Hodder and Stoughton.

(4) Notley, R. G. (1971). The structural basis of normal and abnormal ureteric motility. *Annals of the Royal College of Surgeons of England*; **49**.

(5) Notley, R. G. (1976). *Urology*. (Blandy, J., ed.) Oxford: Blackwell.

(6) Taylor, S., Cotton, L. (1982). *A Short Textbook of Surgery*, 5th Edn. p 409. London: Hodder and Stoughton.

(7) Price, J. L., Loveday, B. J. (1975). Preliminary Communication: Soft tissue radiography of the testicles. *British Journal of Radiology*; **44**: 179–80.

FEMALE REPRODUCTIVE SYSTEM

Some Anatomical and Physiological Considerations

The **female reproductive system** includes (*a*) the *internal genital organs*, namely the two *ovaries*, the *uterus* and the two *uterine (Fallopian) tubes* and the *vagina*, (*b*) the *external genital organs*, which collectively constitute the *vulva*.

The female *breasts* are accessory organs of this system but terminology related to diseases of the breast is later dealt with more conveniently in a separate section.

The ovaries are the reproductive glands of the female and produce the female germ cells which are called *ova* (singular: *ovum*). The discharge of a mature ovum into the peritoneal cavity is called **ovulation**.

The ovaries also, acting under the influence of the anterior lobe of the pituitary gland, secrete the female sex hormones *oestrogen* and *progesterone*.

The processes of reproduction begin after **coitus** (sexual intercourse) when an ovum is fertilised by a spermatozoon, a process described as **conception**. **Pregnancy** is a condition which exists from the time of conception until the end of labour (childbirth) and has an average duration of 40 weeks as reckoned from the first day of the last menstrual period.

The active phase of reproductive life in both sexes starts with a period referred to as **puberty**. In the female this period is marked by the onset of menstruation, enlargement of the breasts and other changes.

The end of reproductive activity in the female is characterised by cessation of menstruation and is called the **menopause**. It is sometimes also termed the **climacteric**.

The prefixes **utero-** and **hystero-** both refer to the uterus, while **salpingo-** refers to the uterine tubes, and both **vagino-** and **colpo-** refer to the vagina.

The prefix **metro-** also means pertaining to the uterus, e.g. **metritis** means inflammation of the uterus.

Some General Aspects

Diseases of the female reproductive system may be congenital, traumatic, inflammatory, neoplastic or due to other causes.

The branch of medicine concerned with diseases of the female reproductive organs is called **gynaecology** and is closely allied with the specialty of **obstetrics** which deals with the management of pregnancy, labour and the puerperium. Terms relating more specifically to the practice of obstetrics will be discussed in the next section.

Among the principal signs and symptoms of gynaecological disorders are disorders of menstruation; vaginal discharge, which may take the form of a blood-stained discharge, or a discharge without blood known as **leucorrhoea**; abnormal bleeding from the vagina; pain in the pelvis, lower abdomen and back; **dyspareunia**, i.e. difficulty or pain on sexual intercourse; and **sterility** (see p 183).

Special Methods of Investigation

These include (i) microscopic examination of **curettings** from the uterus, i.e. specimens of the lining mucosa of the uterus obtained during a procedure called **dilatation and curettage** (D & C), wherein the cervix of the uterus is dilated and the mucosa of the cavity of the uterus is scraped with an instrument called a uterine **curette**; (ii) demonstration of the interior of the uterus and uterine tubes by a form of contrast radiography called **hysterosalpingography**; (iii) demonstration of the ovaries by another form of contrast radiography called **pelvic pneumography**; (iv) **Ultrasonic investigation** and **CT scanning**; (v) biopsy of suspected neoplasms; (vi) **cervical cytology**—see p 182; (vii) **laparoscopy**, whereby the pelvic organs and other intra-abdominal organs can be inspected visually by an instrument inserted into the peritoneal cavity through the anterior abdominal wall; (viii) **Colposcopy**—visual inspection of the interior of the vagina with an instrument called a colposcope.

When using ionising radiation for diagnostic or therapeutic purposes in females below or of reproductive age care must be taken to limit as far as practicable the dose of radiation to the ovaries and thus minimise not only somatic but also genetic hazards (see p 316). Special care, moreover, must be taken when using such radiation during pregnancy on account of the fact that fetal tissues are more sensitive to the effects of radiation than adult tissues.

Congenital Abnormalities

There are various congenital abnormalities of the female reproductive system but none of them are common. The names of a few of them are as follows: **ovarian dysgenesis** (defective development of the ovaries), seen in a genetic disorder called Turner's syndrome; **hypoplasia of the uterus** (underdevelopment of the uterus); **double uterus** (the body of the uterus consists of two portions. The neck of the uterus is often also double and the vagina is **septate**, i.e. divided by a partition of tissue called a **septum**); **bicornuate uterus** (the uterus is incompletely divided so its upper part consists of two structures resembling horns); **atresia of the vagina** (failure of the development of the normal lumen of the vagina, usually in its lower part)—a condition which may lead after puberty to retention of menstrual blood in the vagina and uterus—conditions called respectively **haematocolpos** and **haematometra**.

It is to be noted that certain congenital abnormalities of female and male reproductive organs may be associated with a condition termed **hermaphroditism**. A true **hermaphrodite** is an individual possessing tissue of the sex glands of both sexes (i.e. ovaries and testes).

An individual who possesses external genitalia and secondary sexual characteristics resembling those of one sex and gonads (sex glands) of the other sex is termed a **pseudohermaphrodite**.

As stated by Clayton and Newton (1) 'the ill-defined term of **intersex** is applied to patients in whom the diagnosis of sex is difficult'.

Inflammatory Diseases

Salpingitis—this term means inflammation of the uterine tubes. Such inflammation is frequently accompanied by inflammation of the ovaries, when the condition is more correctly called **salpingo-oophoritis**.

Salpingitis may be acute or chronic. Infection may reach the tubes via the uterus or bloodstream, or as a result of direct spread from an infective process in the peritoneal cavity. Among the causes of infection are streptococcal or other infection after childbirth or abortion, gonorrhoea, possibly chlamydial infection, and chronic infection due to tuberculosis. Acute salpingitis may result in a development of a **pyosalpix** (a tube distended with pus) or an abscess involving both tube and ovary and termed a **tubo-ovarian abscess**. Chronic salpingitis may result in a tube becoming distended with clear fluid; a condition termed a **hydrosalpinx**.

In either type of salpingitis, infection may spread from the tubes to the connective tissues of the pelvis causing **pelvic cellulitis** also referred to as **parametritis**, a term indicating inflammation of connective tissues around the uterus.

Salpingitis, salpingo-oophoritis, and pelvic cellulitis and other infections in the region of the pelvis (e.g. acute appendicitis), when due to pyogenic organisms, may result in the formation of a **pelvic abscess**. Such an abscess may burst and drain into the rectum or vagina or be drained surgically through the posterior fornix of the vagina, but should it burst into the general peritoneal cavity it will cause a generalised infection termed **general peritonitis**.

Endometritis—a condition of inflammation of the **endometium** i.e. the mucous membrane lining the interior of the uterus. In its acute form it may occur as a result of infection following on childbirth or abortion, or of gonococcal infection. Spread of infection readily occurs from the endometrium to the uterine tubes and ovaries. Endometritis occurs also in chronic form and may then be due to tuberculosis.

Cervicitis—a term used to denote inflammation of the cervix or neck of the uterus. The causes of acute cervicitis include those described above as being causes of acute endometritis and also genital herpes.

An important type of chronic inflammation of the cervix occurs in the benign condition termed **cervical erosion**. (An **erosion** is a localised area which has lost its normal epithelial covering and thus appears raw; it tends to bleed easily.)

Erosions of the cervix may be congenital or acquired as a result of trauma during childbirth, or infection. Both types cause vaginal discharge and sometimes bleeding.

Most cervical erosions are treated by cauterisation, using a high frequency electric current or sometimes laser beams.

Vaginitis—inflammation of the vagina, which may result from a variety of infections including infection with a protozoan organism called *Trichomonas vaginalis*: infection with a fungus called *Candida albicans* or *Monilia albicans*; and gonococcal infection. Trichomonas vaginitis is a fairly common disease and is frequently transmitted by sexual intercourse. Irritant douches may also cause vaginitis.

Inflammatory changes in the vagina are often accompanied by similar changes in the vulva and the condition is then described as **vulvovaginitis**.

Puerperal infections—(see Puerperal Sepsis p 193).

Neoplasms

Ovarian Neoplasms and Cysts

A large variety of cystic and solid tumours may arise in the ovaries, and some of them may be of sufficient size to produce a soft-tissue swelling demonstrable by plain radiography. The type known as a **cystadenoma** may attain a tremendous size and occupy a considerable portion of the pelvis and abdomen, causing marked displacement of other viscera and elevation of the diaphragm.

Calcification may sometimes be shown radiologically in ovarian tumours. Of particular interest is the **ovarian dermoid cyst**, as it may contain imperfectly formed teeth which may be shown on radiographs.

In so-called **Meigs's syndrome** the presence of a benign ovarian tumour is associated with the presence of bilateral pleural effusions and ascites.

Endocrine disturbances are found in some uncommon types of ovarian tumour.

The ovaries may be the site of metastases from carcinoma of other organs. The so-called **Krukenberg tumours** are metastic growths from primary carincomas of the stomach, breast or colon.

The following is a list of some of the main types of primary ovarian neoplasms and cysts.

Benign—pseudomucinous cystadenoma, papillary cystadenoma, fibroma, dermoid cyst, endometrioma, follicular cyst, luteal cyst, serous cyst, granulosa cell tumour (sometimes locally malignant), arrhenoblastoma (produces endocrine changes, occasionally malignant), Brenner tumour, dysgerminoma (sometimes malignant), simple teratoma.

Malignant—carcinoma, papillary adenocarcinoma, malignant teratoma.

Speaking generally, the commonest form of spread of malignant ovarian neoplasms is by direct extension into the peritoneum, with resultant ascites. Bloodborne metastases are also common but lymphatic spread occurs infrequently.

Benign ovarian tumours and cysts are treated surgically. Radiotherapy is extensively used in treating malignant ovarian neoplasms either singly or in combination with surgery. Chemotherapy may also be employed.

Uterine Neoplasms

Those most frequently encountered are given below.

Leiomyoma (fibromyoma)—this benign tumour consists of a mixture of fibrous and muscle tissue, as indicated by its name. In clinical practice it is more usually referred to as a **fibroid**. Fibroids are usually multiple. They are common tumours which develop in women of childbearing age. They are generally of slow growth, and usually undergo some degree of atrophy after the menopause. Degenerative changes are also common after the menopause and subsequent pathological calcification within the lesions may then be readily demonstrable on radiographs.

In many cases, fibroids are symptomless, but in others may cause ill-effects through pressure on adjacent organs, e.g. bladder or pelvic colon, or as a result of changes in the tumours themselves (e.g. degeneration). The presence of fibroids may also be associated with certain forms of menstrual disorder, e.g. menorrhagia and dysmenorrhoea. Malignant change may occur in a fibroid but this is extremely rare. Among other conditions which may also be attributed to fibroids are certain cases of sterility and abortion. Large fibroids may also obstruct the birth canal in cases when pregnancy has otherwise proceeded normally. Their presence may then necessitate caesarean section. Fibroids which are causing symptoms usually require surgical removal. Removal of one or more tumour masses is called **myomectomy**. In some cases this operation will suffice. In others hysterectomy (removal of the uterus) must be performed.

Polyp—a benign tumour with a stem-like process termed a pedicle. Uterine polyps may be single or multiple and may arise in the cervical canal (**cervical polyps**), or in the cavity of the uterus (**endometrial polyps**).

Carcinoma of the body of the uterus—(carcinoma corpus uteri, endometrial carcinoma)—a fairly common form of carcinoma arising from the endometrium lining the cavity of the uterus and occuring more frequently in women who have never borne children. It usually arises after the menopause.

The chief clinical features are postmenopausal bleeding from the uterus, offensive vaginal discharge and later pain in the pelvis.

Diagnosis is made by microscopic examination of curettings obtained from the uterine mucosa.

Spread of growth outside the uterus is relatively slow in some cases but in others lymphatic metastases may occur relatively early in the disease. Bloodborne metastases are usually a late feature and are found most commonly in the lungs.

Suitable cases are treated by a combination of surgery, radiotherapy and hormones; advanced cases by radiotherapy alone.

Carcinoma of the cervix uteri (cervical carcinoma)—a common type of carcinoma arising from the mucuous membrane on the vaginal surface of the cervix uteri or within the cervical canal. It is usually referred to more shortly as **carcinoma of the cervix** or **cervical carcinoma**.

In contradistinction to carcinoma of the body of the uterus, carcinoma of the cervix occurs more frequently in women who have borne children.

The cardinal symptoms caused by the neoplasm are irregular vaginal bleeding and bloodstained vaginal discharge.

While the growth is confined to the epithelium of the cervix, it is termed a **preinvasive carcinoma** or **carcinoma-in-situ** (often denoted by the letters CIN, meaning cervical intraepithelial neoplasia) and when it starts to spread outside this epithelium it is described as **invasive carcinoma of the cervix**. Direct spread of the growth may occur in any direction. It is generally slow but may eventually lead to involvement of the rectum, vagina, bladder or lower ends of one or both ureters.

Spread to the rectum may cause the formation of a fistula between that organ and the vagina, i.e. a **rectovaginal fistula**, whereas bladder involvement may result in a **vesicovaginal fistula**. Pressure on a ureter may cause some degree of urinary obstruction on the affected side with resultant hydroureter and hydronephrosis.

Lymphatic spread may be a fairly early feature but bloodborne metastases are uncommon until a very late stage of the disease.

Lymphangiography is used to investigate spread by lymphatic vessels and intravenous urography to investigate ureteric involvement. Complicating fistula formation may be demonstrable by contrast radiology.

X-ray films are also taken to show the position of radium or caesium sources in the uterus and vagina when these are used to treat the neoplasm.

As in carcinoma of the breast, the extent of the growth as assessed by clinical examination may be indicated by a type of classification called **clinical staging**, stages 0, 1, 2, 3 and 4 being described. Carcinoma-in-situ (preinvasive carcinoma) is classified as stage 0. A growth which has distant metastases or has involved the rectum or bladder falls into stage 4.

Early diagnosis of cervical carcinoma in its preinvasive stages has been greatly facilitated by the extended use of **cervical cytology**, an investigation where smears taken from the uterine cervix are examined microscopically for malignant exfoliated cells. (*Note:* **Cytology** is a branch of science concerned with the study of cells.) In cases which give positive findings by this method, and in other clinically suspected cases, the diagnosis may be confirmed by microscopic examination of curettings from the cervix or by a type of biopsy called **cone biopsy**.

The treatment of the disease may be by surgery, radiotherapy or by a combination of these methods; or in carcinoma-in-situ by laser beam therapy.

Other Neoplasms

These include chorion carcinoma of the uterus (see p 193), carcinomas of the uterine tubes, vagina and vulva, all of which are uncommon.

Disorders of Menstruation

The following terms are among those used in the description of menstrual disorders.

Amenorrhoea—a term indicating absence of menstruation.

Amenorrhoea is a normal condition before puberty, during and shortly after pregnancy, and also after the menopause. In all other circumstances it is abnormal and may be due to one or other of a variety of causes. These include disorders of the pituitary, adrenal and thyroid glands, abnormal conditions of the ovaries and uterus, chronic pulmonary tuberculosis and other debilitating diseases, and sometimes after taking oral contraceptives. In other instances the condition may result from pyschological causes.

Cryptomenorrhoea—a term meaning hidden menstruation and referring to a rare condition in which menstruation occurs but blood is retained within the vagina (**haematocolpos**) and sometimes also within the uterus (**haematometra**) as a result of conditions such as imperforate hymen or atresia of the vagina.

Dysmenorrhoea—painful menstruation.

Menorrhagia—excessive loss of blood during menstruation.

Metrorrhagia—bleeding from the uterus other than that due to menstruation.

Dysfunctional uterine bleeding—this name indicates abnormal bleeding which occurs in the absence of any evidence of organic cause (e.g. trauma, infection, neoplasm, etc.), and is thus ascribed to disordered function.

One common type of dysfunctional bleeding is associated with changes in the endometrium described as being due to **metropathia haemorrhagica**. This condition is due to endocrine disorder.

Dysfunctional bleeding from the uterus occurs most frequently at or near the time of the menopause.

Polymenorrhoea—menstruation occurring more frequently than normal.

Sterility (infertility)

Barnes (2) states that 'infertility or sterility may be said to occur when pregnancy does not occur after one year during which coitus takes place at regular intervals'.

Failure of conception may result from factors affecting either or both the male and female partner.

Female sterility may result from absence of **ovulation** (i.e. the process of shedding an ovum by the ovary) or from other causes, local or general. Among the former are various congenital and acquired disorders of the reproductive system, e.g. congenital malformations such as atresia of the vagina, double uterus; inflammatory diseases of the reproductive system such as salpingitis; uterine tumours; acquired displacements of the uterus such as **retroversion** (i.e. a condition in which the uterus is tilted backwards).

General causes include various debilitating and systemic diseases and endocrine disorders, including hyperprolactinaemia (see p 216).

The investigation of sterility includes taking histories and clinical examination of both wife and husband. Special investigations are often required, e.g. uterotubal insufflation and hysterosalpinography in the female spouse; analysis of the seminal fluid in the male spouse.

Hysterosalpingography is of value in demonstrating blockage of the uterine tubes, hydrosalpinx, tuberculous salpingitis, congenital uterine abnormalities and may also on delayed film show evidence of peritoneal adhesions in the regions of the abdominal openings of the uterine tubes.

Prolapse

In gynaecology, this means a protrusion of one or more pelvic organs into the vagina or through the pelvic floor. Prolapse is most commonly due to injury to the pelvic floor during childbirth. It is an important cause of stress incontinence (see p 169).

A prolapse of the bladder is called a **cystocele** and a prolapse of the rectum, a **rectocele**.

Prolapse may be treated surgically by one of the operations known collectively as **repair operations**. Alternatively, when surgery is not deemed advisable it may be treated by a supporting instrument, called a **pessary**, which is inserted into the vagina.

Endometriosis

Endometrium is the name given to the mucous membrane lining the uterine cavity. The presence of endometrial tissue in other sites constitutes a disorder termed **endometriosis**. This disorder may occur in the form of **uterine endometriosis**, also called **uterine adenomyosis**, when endometrial deposits are found in the muscular wall of the uterus, and **external endometriosis**, when deposits occur in other sites such as the ovaries, uterine tubes, intestine, peritoneum and umbilicus.

Endometrial deposits undergo premenstrual changes and bleed at the time of the menstrual periods. They thus cause pain which begins with a menstrual period and reaches its peak on the second or third day of the period.

Uterine endometriosis is associated with menorrhagia. Ovarian endometriosis produces blood-containing cysts which may be of a type termed **chocolate cysts**.

Surgery or laser beam treatment is often required in the treatment of endometriosis but some patients respond to treatment with hormones.

Other Disorders

Pruritus vulvae—the word **pruritus** means itching. Pruritus vulvae may be due to one of a great many different causes. Among these are certain skin diseases, infective conditions of the vulva and vagina, glycosuria, external irritants and psychogenic causes.

Leucoplakia vulvae—a condition of unknown origin in which there is thickening of the skin of the vulva associated with the development of the white patches which give the disease its name. Malignant changes may supervene.

Kraurosis vulvae—a degenerative postmenopausal condition in which there is atrophy of the tissues of the vulva.

Vaginismus—a term describing a condition of spasm of the muscles of the pelvic floor.

Diseases of Bartholin's glands—*Bartholin's glands* (greater vestibular glands) lie one on either side of the opening of the vagina. They may sometimes be the site of infection and abscess formation, cyst formation, and very rarely of a carcinoma. Inflammation of these glands is called **bartholinitis**.

Stein–Leventhal syndrome—an ovarian disorder in which **hirsutism** (hairiness) and amenorrhoea develop in association with a cystic condition affecting both ovaries.

Contraception

The prevention of conception may be achieved by sterilisation (e.g., by tubal ligation or hysterectomy in the woman, vasectomy in the man) or by methods designed to prevent impregnation and termed **contraceptive methods**. These include taking oral contraceptives (the pill method), the insertion of an intrauterine contraceptive device (IUCD), the use of the safe period, the wearing of a condom (sheath) by the male partner, the insertion of a diaphragm and spermicide (a substance that destroys spermatozoa), and coitus interruptus (withdrawal method).

Nowadays, as pointed out by Clayton and Newton (3), advice on family planning is an important part of gynaecological practice.

Some Gynaecological Operations

Colpoplasty—a plastic operation on the vagina.

Dilatation of the cervix and uterine curettage. (D & C). (See p 177.)

Hysterectomy—removal of the uterus. In **total hysterectomy** the whole of the uterus is removed. In **subtotal hysterectomy** the cervix uteri is left in situ, the remainder of the organ being removed.

Pan-hysterectomy is total removal of the uterus together with the uterine tubes and ovaries. **Wertheim's hysterectomy** is removal of the whole of the uterus together with the tubes, ovaries, pelvic cellular tissues, pelvic lymph glands and upper part of the vagina.

Myomectomy—removal of a leiomyoma (fibroid).

Oophorectomy—removal of an ovary.

Salpingectomy—removal of a uterine tube. The operation of bilateral partial salpingectomy may be employed as a method of **sterilisation**, i.e. rendering the subject incapable of reproduction.

Salpingostomy—making a new opening from a uterine tube into either the peritoneal cavity or the cavity of the uterus. This operation is undertaken in certain cases of sterility caused by tubal occlusion.

Repair operations—a group of operations undertaken for genital prolapse. The group includes the operations of anterior colporrhaphy, posterior colpoperineorrhaphy, and the Manchester operation for prolapse.

Vulvectomy—excision of the vulva.

Artificial insemination—used in the treatment of infertility and involving injection of seminal fluid, obtained from the patient's husband (**AIH**) or from a donor (**AID**), into the cervical canal of the uterus.

Fertilisation-in-vitro—involves removing one or more ova from the patient, fertilisation of these in a laboratory and reimplantation within the uterus. This is the method by which so-called 'test-tube' babies are produced. (*Note:* in-vitro means literally in glass.)

REFERENCES

(1) and (3) Clayton, S. G., Newton, S. R. (1983). *A Pocket Gynaecology*, 10th Edn. Edinburgh: Churchill Livingstone.
(2) Barnes, J. (1983). *Lecture Notes on Gynaecology*, 5th Edn. Oxford: Blackwell.

OBSTETRIC CONDITIONS (NORMAL AND ABNORMAL)

The branch of medicine concerned with the management of pregnancy, labour and the puerperium is termed **obstetrics** or **midwifery**.

Pregnancy is a condition which exists from the time of **conception** (fertilisation of an ovum by a spermatozoon) until the end of labour. The normal duration of pregnancy is 40 weeks. A woman in her first pregnancy is called a **primipara**, and in a second and any subsequent pregnancies a **multipara**. (*Note:* **parous** means bearing or having borne offspring.)

The processes which result in the expulsion of the fetus and subsequently the **afterbirth** (i.e. the placenta and fetal membranes) from the uterus constitute **labour** and may also be referred to as **childbirth** or **parturition**. The birth of a child is often referred to as a **delivery**, the mother being set free of, i.e. delivered of the child.

The period immediately following labour, during which the uterus returns gradually to its non-pregnant size and **lactation** (secretion of milk by the breasts) begins, is termed the **puerperium**. This period lasts about six weeks and the early part is sometimes also referred to as the **lying-in period**.

Fertilisation of an ovum occurs normally in one of the Fallopian tubes. Subsequently the fertilised ovum makes its way into the uterus and embeds itself in the uterine wall forming an **embryo** which as it develops is referred to as **fetus**. The meaning of the word fetus is an offspring.

Developed with the growing fetus are the placenta to which the fetus is connected by the *umbilical cord* and fetal membranes.

The *placenta* is a vascular structure which is firmly attached to the uterine wall during pregnancy but after the birth of the child becomes separated and is then, together with the membranes, expelled from the uterus. The *fetal membranes* are structures which develop within the uterus so as to enclose the fetus. There are two, the outer being called the *chorion* and the inner, the *amnion*. The amnion bounds the *amnoitic cavity* in which the fetus lies surrounded by the *amniotic fluid* (liquor amnii). This fluid permits movement of the fetus during pregnancy and also serves as a protection against external injury.

Signs and symptoms of pregnancy—these include the symptom of: amenorrhoea, nausea, morning sickness, feeling of fetal movements (18th–20th weeks) and abdominal swelling (16th–18th weeks); signs are palpable uterine enlargement, swelling of the breasts, audible fetal heart sounds (24th week onwards).

Pregnancy tests—these depend on the fact that a pregnant woman, from an early stage of her pregnancy, excretes increased amounts of a particular hormone (called chorionic gonadotrophin) in her urine. Such increased amounts may be demonstrated in various ways, e.g. by immunological tests which show a reaction between the urine and certain specially prepared types of antibody and will diagnose pregnancy at about 6 weeks.

Early pregnancy can also be demonstrated by ultrasonography at about 6–7 weeks.

Diagnostic imaging in pregnancy—this may include ultrasonic or X-ray investigations (or, rarely, radionuclide imaging). As far as is known no harmful effects arise from the use of ultrasound. In contradistinction the use of X-rays carries certain radiation hazards (p 316) and radiological methods should only be used when they provide information not obtainable by ultrasonography (e.g. in the diagnosis of disproportion).

Ultrasonic diagnosis is valuable to the obstetrician in managing both normal and abnormal pregnancy. Some examples of its use are: the diagnosis of early pregnancy, multiple pregnancy and certain types of fetal abnormality; estimation of fetal maturity; demonstration of fetal heart movements; demonstration of the site of the placenta.

Note that with X-ray examinations generally, it is most important in radiological practice to avoid irradiation of a pregnancy in its earliest stages. Hence all non-urgent examinations of females of childbearing age which include irradiation of the lower abdomen or pelvis should be carried out between the onset of a menstrual period and the presumed date of ovulation—i.e., as recommended in the *Code of Practice for the Protection of Persons against Ionising Radiations arising from Medical and Dental Use* (HMSO, 1972) within the ten days immediately following the first day of the last menstrual period. This official recommendation is popularly known as the **10-day rule**. Note that modification of this rule has more recently been advocated, in accordance with advice given by the National Radiation Protection Board: ASP8 (March, 1985) HMSO.

Some important terms related to the practice of obstetrics are given below.

Viability and Maturity

The normal duration of pregnancy is 40 weeks—but at the 28th week the fetus is considered to have reached a state of development which renders it capable of survival, should premature labour take place. During and after the 28th week of uterine life, therefore, the fetus is said to be **viable**. A 40-week-old fetus is described as being **mature** or **at term**.

A living baby born before the 40th week of pregnancy is said to be **immature**, and if it weighs less than 5½ pounds it is described as **premature**.

A dead baby born after the 28th week of pregnancy is called a **stillbirth**.

Expulsion of the uterine contents before the 28th week of pregnancy is known as **abortion** or **miscarriage**.

A baby born after the 40th week of pregnancy is described as being **postmature**.

Ultrasound is of value in estimating fetal maturity as the biparietal diameter of the fetal skull may readily be measured by A-scan techniques.

Ectopic Pregnancy (Ectopic Gestation, Extra-Uterine Pregnancy)

This term indicates that the fertilised ovum has become embedded in some site other than the cavity of the uterus. The term **ectopic** means abnormally placed or displaced.

The commonest form of ectopic pregnancy is **tubal pregnancy** (i.e. the ovum becomes embedded in the wall of one of the Fallopian tubes). This condition usually terminates with rupture of the affected tube, accompanied by severe haemorrhage into the peritoneal cavity and pronounced shock.

Multiple Pregnancy

This term indicates the presence of more than one fetus, e.g. twins, triplets, etc.

Fetal Presentation

The part of the fetus which lies in the lowermost portion of the body of the uterus is termed the **presenting part**. A **normal presentation** is one in whch the vertex of the fetal skull forms the presenting part because in normal labour the fetus enters the birth canal head first.

Any form of presentation other than a vertex presentation constitutes a **malpresentation**. The commonest form of malpresentation is a **breech presentation**, when the buttocks form the presenting part.

Fetal Abnormality

This term is used to describe abnormalities that may affect the fetus as a result of developmental errors, or due to disease acquired during intrauterine life.

A large variety of developmental errors may occur during fetal life. In many, the causes are unknown but, in some, hereditary factors are known to play a part. As noted when discussing diseases of the heart an association has been shown in some cases between the occurrence of rubella in the mother during early pregnancy and the birth of child with abnormalities such as congenital heart disease, congenital deafness and congenital cataract.

Serious congenital malformations also developed in the offspring of mothers who had taken a drug called thalidomide in early pregnancy, e.g. amelia and phocomelia (see p 244).

Certain types of severe fetal abnormality may be demonstrated on antenatal X-ray films. Among these are the following.

Anencephaly—a rare developmental abnormality, the name of which means absence of the brain. The brain fails to develop and as a result there is associated failure of development of the bones of the vault of the fetal skull and deformity of the bones of the skull base.

Anencephaly is associated with the presence of increased amounts of *alphafetoprotein* in the amniotic fluid, as are another group of fetal abnormalities in which **neural tube defect** is associated with a spinal abnormality called **spina bifida** (see p 241).

Hydrocephalus—a condition of excessive accumulation of cerebrospinal fluid within the cranium which may occur as a result of developmental error in fetal life or be due to acquired disease in postnatal life. The former type is called **fetal hydrocephalus** and leads to enlargement of the skull. Such enlargement may be marked and render normal delivery of the fetus impossible.

Fetal death in utero (FDIU)—this is often referred to as **intrauterine death** and referred to by the initials **IUD**. (*Note:* this abbreviation is, however, confusing as it is also applied to certain contraceptive appliances which are collectively known as intrauterine devices, e.g. Lippes loop. Such appliances are better designated by the letters **IUCD**.)

Hydrops fetalis (see under Erythroblastosis fetalis—haemolytic disease of the newborn, see p 191).

Anencephaly, hydrocephalus and hydrops fetalis all produce abnormal radiographic appearances.

Fetal death also produces X-ray changes but these latter are slow to appear. One sign of particular value is the appearance, before the onset of labour, of overlapping of the bones of the fetal cranial vault. This radiographic abnormality is referred to as **Spalding's sign**.

Placental Insufficiency

This is a condition in which placental function is inadequate for transfer from the maternal bloodstream to the fetus of nutrient substances in amounts necessary for normal fetal growth. Such growth is therefore retarded as may be shown by measuring the biparietal diameter of the fetal skull by ultrasound at prescribed intervals. Diminished hormonal secretion by the placenta may also be shown by measuring the amounts of *oestriol* present in maternal serum or excreted in the maternal urine.

Placental insufficiency may develop in association with postmaturity, or as a result of pre-eclampsia and other diseases. Often, however, its cause is unknown. It is sometimes responsible for fetal death in utero.

Erythroblastosis Fetalis—Haemolytic Disease of the Newborn

These terms are both used to indicate a group of diseases which are characterised by anaemia developing in intrauterine life as a result of **haemolysis** (destruction of red blood cells with setting free of their haemoglobin in the bloodstream). The term **erythroblastosis** indicates another feature of the disease—the presence of primitive red blood cells called **erythroblasts** in the circulation. Unlike mature red blood cells, i.e. **erythrocytes**, erythroblasts possess nuclei.

Red blood cells may, in late pregnancy and labour, cross the placenta in limited numbers, passing from the fetal to the maternal bloodstream and in the reverse direction.

In races of Caucasian origin, 85% of individuals possess blood of a type called **Rh+ve** (Rhesus positive) and their red blood cells all contain an antigen known as **Rh+ve** antigen. The other 15% of individuals have **Rh−ve blood**.

If an Rh−ve mother produces an Rh+ve fetus, Rh+ve antigen may be carried across the placenta. If entering the maternal bloodstream in sufficient amounts it may provoke the production of maternal anti-Rh+ve antibodies.

These latter may then cross the placenta in the reverse direction and cause an antibody–antigen reaction in the fetal circulation.

This reaction is rarely of any marked degree in a first pregnancy as it takes time for antibodies to form, but produces effects of varying seriousness in subsequent pregnancies with haemolysis of fetal blood cells and resultant anaemia. (*Note:* an Rh-negative female may also develop antibodies against Rh-positive blood cells, as a result of receiving a blood transfusion of Rh-positive blood. In this case the fetus produced in a first pregnancy may develop erythroblastosis fetalis.) If the reaction is not too severe, a living infant with a **haemolytic anaemia** may be born. A more marked reaction may result in a condition termed **icterus gravis neonatorum** and meaning severe jaundice of newborn. Babies with severe jaundice may develop cerebral damage associated with a pathological condition affecting the brain called **kernicterus**.

More serious forms of the disease, which are uncommon, result in a disorder called **hydrops fetalis**, in which together with pronounced anaemia there is oedema of fetal tissues and ascites; or in death and maceration of the fetus and resultant stillbirth.

The blood of an infant born with haemolytic disease of the newborn will give a positive result to a test called a **direct Coombs' test**. Such an infant may need a type of blood transfusion called an **exchange transfusion**, further untoward reactions being prevented by replacing most of its Rh-positive blood by Rh-negative blood from a donor with a compatible blood group.

A recent advance in the treatment of this disease is the development of a technique of **intra-uterine fetal blood transfusion**.

The determination of the rhesus factors and ABO (see p 205) blood groups is nowadays an important procedure in antenatal care.

An Rh-negative mother who gives birth to an Rh-positive child may be prevented from producing antibodies to the rhesus +ve antigen by injection of anti-D immunoglobulin, immediately after the birth of the first such child and, thereafter, immediately after the birth of any subsequent Rh-positive children.

Asphyxia Neonatorum

A condition in which **asphyxia**, i.e. a failure of normal respiratory function occurs immediately after birth.

A **neonate** is a newly born infant.

Disproportion

This term refers to a condition in which the relative sizes of the fetus and the maternal pelvis are such as to render passage of the former through the birth canal difficult or impossible. It may arise from the presence of a large fetus or abnormality of shape or size of the pelvis, or a combination of these factors.

In suspected disproportion valuable information regarding the internal measurements of the bony pelvis and the shape of this structure may be obtained from a radiological investigation termed **X-ray pelvimetry**.

Disproportion may necessitate forceps delivery of the child or, in severe cases, Caesarean section.

Hydramnios

A condition in which an excessive amount of amniotic fluid forms. It is frequently associated with uniovular twin pregnancy; with some fetal disorder in which there is difficulty in swallowing e.g. oesophageal atresia; anencephaly; erythroblastosis fetalis; or maternal diabetes. (*Note:* the opposite condition to hydramnios in which there is deficiency of amniotic fluid is called **oligohydramnios**.)

Antepartum Haemorrhage

Antepartum means before the birth of the child. **Antepartum haemorrhage** is the name given to bleeding from the genital tract after the 28th week of pregnancy and before delivery. The two commonest types of antepartum haemorrhage are as follows.

Accidental haemorrhage—in this condition the placenta is normally situated in the upper uterine segment but becomes partially or completely separated from the uterine wall before delivery.

Unavoidable haemorrhage—in this condition either the whole or part of the placenta is attached to the wall of the lower segment of the uterus. A placenta with such an abnormal site of attachment is termed a **placenta praevia**.

Antepartum haemorrhage is a serious condition, and it is of prime importance to the obstetrician to determine whether it is of the accidental or unavoidable variety because the treatment of the two types and the subsequent management of labour follows different lines.

Location of the placental site by ultrasound is therefore of considerable importance when such haemorrhage occurs.

Hydatidiform Mole

This is a benign tumour of chorionic tissue and is sometimes referred to as a **chorion adenoma** (the chorion is the outer of the fetal membranes and is derived from the developing ovum).

The term **mole** means mass, and this tumour consists of masses of small cysts which have been likened to the cysts which can occur as a result of hydatid infection.

Hydatidiform mole is an uncommon complication of pregnancy and results in enlargement of the uterus, uterine haemorrhage, and usually failure of development of the fetus. It is occasionally associated with severe preeclampsia.

If a pregnancy ends with the formation of a hydatidiform mole another rare complication of pregnancy may ensue. This is the development of a chorionepithelioma in the uterus.

Chorionepithelioma (Chorion Carcinoma)

This malignant tumour of chorionic tissue may develop either after: (*a*) a pregnancy which has ended with the formation of a hydatidiform mole; (*b*) a pregnancy which has ended in abortion; or (*c*) more uncommonly after the conclusion of a normal pregnancy. This neoplasm is usually highly malignant and early metastases in the lungs are frequent.

The curious fact that a chorionepithelioma may in rare instances develop in the male testis has already been noted (see p 173).

Modern treatment of both primary growth and metastases is by cytotoxic drugs. After the conclusion of treatment, follow-up examinations are carried out with regular estimations of β-human chorionic gonadotrophin (β-HCG) in the blood or urine.

Puerperal Sepsis

Puerperal sepsis was defined by Gibberd (1) as 'an infection which has entered the birth canal during or after labour or abortion'. Such infection may be due to streptococci, staphylococci, or various other pathogenic bacteria. Fever together with increased pulse rate are important clinical features, and signs and symptoms due to the localised effects of the infection in the birth canal may be present. The infection may sometimes spread to the uterine tubes causing salpingitis, and the connective tissues in the pelvis resulting in pelvic cellulitis (parametritis).

Puerperal sepsis is only one of a number of conditions which may be responsible for **puerperal pyrexia** which, as stated by Clayton and Newton (2), 'has been defined as a fever of 38°C or more arising from *any cause* within 14 days of labour or miscarriage'.

Toxaemias of Pregnancy

A group of common diseases of completely unknown causation are commonly referred to as toxaemias of pregnancy. (*Note:* **toxaemia** means the presence of poisonous substances, i.e. **toxins**, in the blood.)

Included in this group are the following.

Hyperemesis gravidarum—a condition of excessive vomiting occurring during pregnancy.

Pre-eclamptic toxaemia (albuminuria of pregnancy)—a condition in which there is raised blood pressure, oedema and protein albumen is passed in the urine, and in which rarely eclampsia may develop.

Eclampsia—a condition in which a raised blood pressure, oedema and albuminuria are accompanied by convulsions referred to as **eclamptic fits**.

This disease is associated with lesions in the kidneys and liver, which usually seem to resolve completely after the conclusion of the pregnancy, although occasionally the liver lesions may lead to permanent liver damage and eventual hepatic failure (p 138). Intrauterine death of the fetus is common in the more severe types of eclampsia. Induction of labour is frequently necessary to avoid this complication of the disease.

Postpartum Haemorrhage

This term indicates excessive bleeding from the uterus during the process of separation of the placenta during the last stage of labour, or shortly after the conclusion of labour.

Some Obstetric Procedures and Operations

Version (i.e. turning)—a manipulative procedure to remedy an unfavourable fetal presentation.

Altering a malpresentation into a normal vertex presentation is called **cephalic version**, whereas turning some other type of malpresentation into a breech presentation (the type of malpresentation least unfavourable to delivery of the fetus per vaginam) is termed **podalic version**. According to the method employed version may be described as **external** or **internal version**.

Forceps delivery—delivery of the fetus per vaginam by traction on its skull with instruments called **obstetric forceps**. This procedure is employed in certain cases when labour has failed to progress normally as a result of the more minor degrees if disproportion, in certain cases of malpresentation, and in **uterine inertia** (i.e. a condition in which the uterine contractions are inadequate to expel the fetus), etc.

Induction of labour—the employment of various procedures, medical or surgical, with the object of starting the processes of labour.

Medical induction may be achieved by administration of syntocinon, a synthetic preparation whose action is similar to that of the posterior pituitary hormone oxytocin, or by synthetic preparations of substances called prostaglandins. (*Note:* **prostaglandins**—are naturally occurring unsaturated fatty acids, with a wide range of physiological activities, including the ability to cause contraction of smooth muscle and their main clinical use is in the induction of labour or abortion.) The name **oxytocin** is derived from oxytocia a word of Greek derivation meaning quick labour.

Surgical induction involves the forcible **rupture of the membranes**, a procedure also referred to as **amniotomy**.

Caesarean section—the delivery of the fetus through a surgical incision made through the abdominal wall and the wall of the uterus. This operation is employed in patients with marked disproportion, and in some cases of malpresentation, placenta praevia etc.

Episiotomy (perineotomy)—the making of an incision in the perineum when it is unduly rigid and interferes with the normal passage of the fetus through the vulva to the exterior. This operation thus prevents severe perineal tearing during childbirth.

Vacuum extraction—a method used in certain circumstances to assist delivery of the fetus by applying suction to the fetal skull with an instrument termed a vacuum extractor.

Induction of abortion—this may in certain circumstances be necessary for medical reasons and the law on this subject is set out in the Abortion Act of 1967.

Amniocentesis—the obtaining, by a percutaneous puncture of the anterior abdominal wall and wall of the uterus, of a sample of amniotic fluid. This may then be subjected to chemical or cytological examination.

Special studies can be made on desquamated fetal skin cells in the amniotic fluid enabling the sex of the fetus to be determined as early as the 14th or 15th week of pregnancy, these investigations being termed **antenatal sexing**.

Studies of the amniotic fluid may also be employed in the antenatal diagnosis of certain genetic disorders e.g. Down's syndrome, anencephaly.

REFERENCES

(1) Gibberd, C. F. (1965). *A Short Textbook of Midwifery*. London: Churchill.
(2) Clayton, S. G., Newton, J. R. (1983). *A Pocket Obstetrics*, 10th Edn. p 125. Edinburgh: Churchill Livingstone.

THE BREAST

In females the two *breasts* or *mammae* (mammary glands) are accessory organs of the reproductive system. They undergo considerable changes at puberty and further development occurs during pregnancy in preparation for *lactation* (milk secretion) subsequent to childbirth. Later, at the time of the menopause, they are the subject of certain atrophic changes referred to as being due to **involution** of breast tissue.

Contained in the female breast are glandular structures called *alveoli* which are composed of epithelium. Clusters of *alveoli* are grouped together to form *lobules* and these communicate with a system of ducts called *lactiferous (milk-carrying)* ducts. The main ducts open to the exterior on the surface of each *nipple*.

In the male, the breasts are rudimentary in nature.

The breast may be the site of congenital abnormality, traumatic disorder, infection, neoplasm, cyst formation, or be affected by endocrine disorder or idiopathic disease.

Some of the diseases that occur in the female breast can also occur in the rudimentary breast tissue of the male. Abnormal endocrine influences or the administration of oestrogens (e.g. in the hormone treatment of prostatic carcinoma) may sometimes result in enlargement of the breasts in men. This disorder is called **gynaecomastia**.

Among the signs of breast disease are **mastodynia**, i.e. pain in the breast; enlargement of the breast; tenderness in the breast; the presence of a palpable tumour; discharge from the nipple; and nipple retraction.

Special methods of investigation of breast disease include a form of soft tissue radiography called **mammography**; **ultrasound** which is particularly useful in distinguishing between solid and cystic swellings and as indicated by Bloomberg *et al.* (1) enables cysts, even when impalpable, to be located and subjected to fine needle aspiration biopsy; and **thermography**, an investigation in which recordings of emission of infrared rays are made at different points over the surface of the breast. Radionuclide scanning is widely used to detect early metastases from breast carcinoma in bone.

In addition to conventional mammography using X-ray film and chemical processing, a process called **xeroradiography** may be employed in obtaining mammograms. In this system the X-ray image is recorded on a charged selenium-coated plate, and then rendered visible by blowing a charged powder over the plate. The development process is thus completely dry. If desired the X-ray image can be transferred from the plate to special xeroradiographic paper thus providing a permanent record of the examination.

The prefixes **mammo-** and **masto-** both mean referring to the breast. The prefix **mazo-** is also sometimes used with reference to the breast, especially in American publications.

Congenital Abnormalities

Congenital abnormalities of the breast are not common. They include the development of **supernumerary nipples**.

Inflammatory Diseases

Inflammation of the breast is termed **mastitis**. **Acute mastitis** of infective origin may result in the formation of a **breast abscess** (mammary abscess), a not uncommon condition during lactation.

Neoplasms

Neoplasms of the breast are common and may be benign or malignant.
The most important are given below.
Benign neoplasms

(i) **Fibroadenoma**—a common tumour in young women and composed of glandular epithelium and fibrous tissue.
(ii) **Duct papilloma**—an epithelial tumour usually arising in a main lactiferous duct. This tumour frequently causes bleeding from the nipple.

Malignant neoplasms

Carcinoma of the breast (mammary carcinoma)

This condition is the most common form of malignant disease in the female sex and shows its highest incidence in middle age.

The tumour may arise either in the epithelium of the alveoli or of the lactiferous ducts and may be of slow or rapid growth. Metastatic spread of disease, by the lymphatics or bloodstream, may be either an early or late feature of the disease but lymphatic spread is usually earlier than spread by the bloodstream.

Lymphatic metastases may be found in glands in the axilla and supraclavicular region, and later in the mediastinum and opposite breast. The principal sites for bloodborne metastases are the lungs, pleural membranes, bones and liver.

Rarely, carcinoma of the breast may occur in pregnancy or during lactation and it may then show rapid progression. It may rarely develop in the male sex, when it usually also shows a high degree of malignancy.

Another uncommon form of breast carcinoma occurs in association with an eczematous condition of the nipple called **Paget's disease of the nipple**.

Breast carcinomas may, according to their pathological type, be referred to as **scirrhous carcinomas**, **adenocarcinomas**, **encephaloid carcinomas**, **anaplastic carcinomas**, **intraduct carcinomas**, **acute carcinomas of pregnancy** or **lactation**, etc., the commonest type being the scirrhous carcinomas. (*Note:* **scirrhous** means hard and **scirrhous carcinomas** are hard as a result of their forming much dense connective tissue; **adeno-** means pertaining to glands and **adenocarcinomas** arise from glandular tissue; **encephaloid** means resembling brain tissue and **encephaloid carcinomas**, also called **medullary carcinomas** are soft growths containing much epithelial tissue and little connective tissue; the term **anaplasia** indicates an absence of development and anaplastic carcinomas contain large numbers of primitive cells and are often highly malignant.

In any individual patient, the extent of the disease, may be indicated by a procedure termed **clinical staging**. This is now carried out using a system known as the **TNM system** and also referred to as the **UICC classification**. The letter T refers to tumour size and the letters N and M indicate the presence or absence of lymph node involvement and of distant metastases, e.g. $T_1N_0M_0$ indicates a tumour of less than 2 cm diameter without associated palpable lymph nodes and without evidence of distant metastases.

The cardinal clinical sign of breast carcinoma is the presence of a palpable lump in the breast. It is, however, to be noted that a lump in the breast can be due to other causes, e.g. inflammation, benign neoplasm, cyst formation, fibroadenosis. Mammography is often helpful in differentiating between these conditions and, in cases which come to operation, immediate microscopic examination of a **frozen section** of tissue taken from the tumour is frequently of the highest value in deciding the correct line of operative treatment.

Among the signs of breast carcinoma which may be shown by mammography are the demonstration of a mass, usually with spiculated or irregular margins; fine pathological calcification of a type described as microcalcification; and changes in normal trabecular pattern seen in the breast. To show such abnormalities it is esential to obtain good contrast and fine detail. The former is obtained by a low kilovoltage technique and the latter by the use of fine grain film. It is also important to limit radiation as far as is consistent with the production of satisfactory results.

Price and Butler (2), in 1970 described a technique to secure a low radiation dosage. Subsequently, using this technique with a rare earth screen-film combination Price and Nathan (3) showed skin doses in mammographic examinations as low as 0.15 to 0.3 rads (1.5 to 3.0 mGy) per exposure could be obtained.

Mammographic localisation of breast lesions is now widely used as an aid to fine-needle aspiration biopsy.

In some cases the assessment of small mammographic abnormalities may be facilitated by the additional technique of magnification mammography (macromammography).

The following methods of treatment may be used for carcinoma of the breast, and two or more of them are often employed in combination.

Surgical—mastectomy, i.e. removal of the breast. This may be described as radical or simple (conservative), according to the amount of tissue removed. (*Note:* when the operative procedure is confined to localised excision only of a tumour or other breast swelling the operation may be described as a **tilectomy**.)

Radiotherapy—treatment with ionising radiation.

Hormone therapy—certain malignant neoplasms are referred to as being hormone dependent and progress of growth in both the primary tumour and metastases may be temporarily controlled by giving appropriate hormones (e.g. testosterone) by mouth or, in other cases, by diminishing the secretion of hormones (e.g. oestrogens) by surgical operations such as bilateral **oophorectomy** (removal of the ovaries), bilateral **adrenalectomy** (removal of the adrenal glands) and **hypophysectomy** (removal of the pituitary gland).

As an alternative to adrenalectomy the activities of adrenal cortex can be suppressed by the suprarenal hormone cortisone. It is also possible to abolish pituitary function by implantation of radioactive yttrium, a radioactive isotope, into the pituitary gland.

Treatment with cytotoxic drugs, e.g. methotrexate, cyclophosphamide, 5-fluorouracil. Since 1979 The Department of Health and Social Security has been conducting trials at centres in the UK to try to determine the efficacy of screening for breast cancer in reducing mortality from this disease. One of the screening programmes in these trials, involving both clinical examination and mammography, is described by Pearce (4) together with details of the mammographic technique employed.

Cysts of the Breast

These are of several varieties. They may be found in connection with simple or malignant tumours but are most commonly seen as a feature of fibroadenosis (see below).

One type of cyst which occurs during lactation is known as a **galactocele** or **milk cyst**, and is due to blockage of a main lactiferous duct.

Other Diseases

Included among these are the following.

Dysplasia of the breast (mammary dysplasia)—this is a most important condition on account of the difficulty that frequently arises in differentiating its clinical manifestations from those that can be caused by carcinoma of the breast.

Dysplasia of the breast is a term which includes the disorders referred to as **fibroadenosis**, **cystic hyperplasia of the breast**, and **fibrocystic disease of the breast**. These conditions used to be referred to collectively as **chronic mastitis**, as a result of a former belief that they were conditions of inflammatory origin. Now, however, it is widely thought that some abnormality of the hormones acting on breast tissue is likely to be responsible for their development.

The principal pathological features of breast dysplasia are overgrowth of fibrous tissue (fibrosis), overgrowth of epithelium (epithetial hyperplasia), and cyst formation of varying degree in one or both breasts. Such changes may be diffuse and affect both breasts, or be localised to a relatively small area in one breast.

Taylor and Cotton (5), describe two types of **epithelial hyperplasia**, namely **adenosis** (formation of new glandular acini) and **epitheliosis** (proliferation of the duct lining).

The condition called **sclerosing adenosis** is a variant of adenosis.

Hormonal treatment may sometimes be given in the diffuse form of the disease. In the localised form surgery is often advocated as the disease often results in a lump undistinguishable clinically from a carcinoma.

As has been indicated when discussing breast carcinoma, mammography is often of considerable value in investigating mammary dysplasias and assisting in their differentiation from malignant disorders.

Traumatic fat necrosis—in this condition a hard lump develops in the breast as a result of injury. Marked pathological calcification frequently occurs within the lump.

REFERENCES

(1) Bloomberg, T. J., Chivers, R. C., Price, J. L. (1984). Real-time ultrasound characteristics of the breast. *Clinical Radiology*; **35**: 21–7.
(2) Price, J. L., Butler, P. D. (1970). The reduction of radiation and exposure time in mammography. *British Journal of Radiology*; **43**: 251–5.
(3) Nathan, B. E., Price, J. L. (1976). Radiology now screening for breast cancer. *British Journal of Radiology*; **49**: 817–19.
(4) Pearce, P. (1982). The Guildford breast screening project. *Radiography*; **48**: 39–43.
(5) Taylor, S., Cotton, L. (1982). *A Short Textbook of Surgery*, 5th Edn. p 198. London: Hodder and Stoughton.

LYMPHATIC AND MONONUCLEAR PHAGOCYTIC SYSTEMS

General Considerations

The **lymphatic system** consists of *lymph vessels* and *lymphoid tissue*. The latter consists of small aggregations of such tissue widely dispersed throughout the body, and larger aggregations concentrated in the *lymph glands* (lymph nodes) spleen, tonsils, adenoids, submucosa of the gastrointestinal tract, bone marrow and thymus.

The fluid which circulates through the system is called *lymph*. It is drained from tissue spaces throughout the body, filtered in the lymph nodes and ultimately reaches the bloodstream via the *thoracic duct* and *right lymph duct*.

Note: the tissue spaces contain tissue fluid which is formed from the circulating blood by diffusion through the walls of the capillaries and carries nourishment to the tissue cells.

The **mononuclear phagocyte system** (phagocytic cell system) is, as indicated by Thomson and Cotton (1), a term which replaces the earlier designations of this system as the *reticuloendothelial system* or *lymphoreticular system*. This system is composed of (i) mobile phagocytic cells found in the tissue spaces where they are called *macrophages* or *histiocytes*, and in the circulating blood where they are known as *monocytes*; and (ii) static (fixed) phagocytic cells, also called *macrophages* which like lymphoid aggregations are widely distributed in the body, but are most plentiful within the sinuses of the lymph nodes and in the spleen and liver. (In this latter organ they line the liver sinusoids and are known as *Kupffer cells*.)

It is also to be noted that *osteoclasts* found in bone and *microglial cells* of the neuroglia, the specialised supporting tissue of the central nervous system, have phagocytic properties and also belong to the mononuclear phagocyte system; as indicated by Govan et al (2).

The lymphatic and phagocytic cell systems have close anatomical and functional relationships. Consequently although usage of the term differs, it seems that the designation of **lymphoreticular tissues** may be taken as referring jointly to the tissues of both systems.

Phagocytes are concerned with the removal and disposal of pathogenic micro-organisms and other 'foreign' material and products of cell breakdown, from the blood, tissue fluids and lymph; and in the lymph nodes act in concert with lymphoid tissue which filters off particulate material of these types from the lymph. Thus the two systems together play an important role in the internal defence mechanisms of the body against infection.

Other functions include the manufacture of lymphocytes by *stem cells* of lymphoid tissue contained in the bone marrow, destruction of worn-out red cells, and liberation of their haemoglobin by phagocytic cells, and storage by these latter cells of fatty substances called lipids.

The role of B-lymphocytes, plasma cells and T-lymphocytes in immunity has been briefly noted when discussing immunity (p 35).

General Aspects of Diseases of the Lymphatic and Mononuclear Phagocyte Systems

Among the diseases that may affect these systems are: (i) infective disorders, generalised or localised resulting in inflammation of lymph glands, referred to as **lymphadenitis** (or often more simply as **adenitis**), and sometimes inflammation of lymphatic vessels, called **lymphangitis**; (ii) neoplastic disorders—primary neoplasms of lymphoreticular tissue called **lymphomas**, carcinomatous metastases in lymph glands, and rarely tumours of lymph vessels called **lymphangiomas**; (iii) **lipid storage diseases** (lipoidoses); and (iv) sarcoidosis.

Any disease of lymph glands may be termed **lymphadenopathy**.

The former classification, in which certain disorders of the lymphoreticular tissue were classified as benign or malignant **reticuloses**, is gradually being replaced.

Common features of diseases of the lymphoreticular tissues include enlargement of the lymph glands, spleen (splenomegaly) and liver (hepatomegaly).

Lymph node biopsy is often an important procedure in the investigation of lymphadenopathy.

Ultrasound, CT, and contrast radiology in the form of **lymphangiography** may be used to demonstrate glandular masses in the abdomen and plain film, tomography and CT those within the mediastinum and hilar regions. Enlarged submucous lymphoid aggregations in the alimentary tract may be demonstrated by barium studies.

Glandular Fever (Infectious Mononucleosis)

This infection is probably due to the *Epstein-Barr* virus. It is characterised by fever, pharyngitis, enlargement of cervical lymph glands and often other lymph glands; and also numbers of large abnormal mononuclear leucocytes in the circulating blood. These features explain the two alternative names of the disease.

Other clinical features may include splenomegaly and the development of a rubella-like rash.

A blood test called the **Paul-Bunnell test** is positive in most cases at some stage of the disease.

There is no specific treatment but spontaneous recovery occurs— usually over a period of a few weeks.

Lymphomas

The lymphomas are generally regarded as primary neoplasms of lymphoreticular tissue, although their exact nature has not yet been established.

They are now classified as being of two principal types: Hodgkin's disease and non-Hodgkin's lymphomas.

Hodgkin's disease—this condition was named after Thomas Hodgkin a 19th century British physician. Its basic pathological feature is infiltration of lymphoid tissue by so-called Hodgkin's tissue, containing giant cells called **Reed-Sternberg cells** and presenting in one of four histological types.

The infiltration primarily affects lymph glands, causing them to enlarge. It may be confined to a single gland or group of glands or may be widespread involving superficial and deep glands and, in advanced cases, lymphoid tissues in the spleen, liver, bone marrow and elsewhere. Extralymphatic deposits (i.e. deposits outside the lymphatic system) may sometimes develop.

A widely applied system of staging recognises four different clinical stages of the disease, stage IV being the most advanced.

Plain radiographs are of value in demonstrating enlarged mediastinal and hilar glands, lung deposits, pleural effusions and bone lesions. Lymphography is used to show deposits in the iliac and para-aortic lymph glands.

As the disease advances, fever, wasting and anaemia develop, together with symptoms caused by pressure of enlarged glands on various internal structures, e.g. jaundice owing to pressure of glands on the bile ducts in the porta hepatis.

Treatment is usually by a combination of radiotherapy and cytotoxic drugs. Surgical excision is sometimes combined with radiotherapy when the disease is localised to a single group of glands.

Non-Hodgkin's lymphomas—this, at present rather ill-defined group of neoplasms, is generally taken to include various types of **follicular lymphomas** and **diffuse lymphomas**, derived from lymphoid tissue; and **histocytic lymphomas**, derived from the mononuclear phagocyte system.

All these diseases are uncommon. Some, while having a different histology from Hodgkin's disease, present a similar clinical picture (e.g. glandular enlargement, splenomegaly, anaemia).

Some authorities classify myelomas (plasma cell tumours—p 252) as lymphomas. Leukaemia, arising in lymphoid tissue (pp 212 and 213) may also be regarded as a lymphoma, or more commonly as a condition closely related to non-Hodgkin lymphoma.

Radiotherapy and chemotherapy are both used to treat these diseases.

Note: the disorder formerly known as **lymphosarcoma** is now widely regarded as a form of diffuse lymphoma; and, that termed **reticulum cell sarcoma** may now be described as an undifferentiated non-Hodgkin's lymphoma.

Lipid Storage Diseases (Lipoidoses)

These disorders are characterised by the accumulation of lipid substances in cells of the mononuclear phagocyte system, and resultant lipid deposits in sites such as the spleen, liver, bone marrow and lymph glands.

Lipid storage diseases are rare. The one seen most commonly in the UK is called **Hand-Schüller-Christian disease** (xanthomatosis) and is a form of a group of disorders known as histiocytosis X; other members of which are **eosinophil granuloma** and **Letterer-Siwe disease**.

Gaucher's disease and **Niemann-Pick disease** are other types of lipid storage diseases.

REFERENCES

(1) Thomson, A. D. and Cotton, R. E. (1938). *Lecture Notes on Pathology*, Oxford: Blackwell.
(2) Govan, A.T.D., Macfarlane, P. S., Callander, R. (1981). *Pathology Illustrated*. Edinburgh: Churchill Livingstone.

THE BLOOD

Some Anatomical and Physiological Considerations

Blood is composed of a fluid called *plasma* in which are suspended *red corpuscles*, *white cells* and *platelets*.

Red corpuscles, or **erythrocytes**—are formed in red bone marrow, which in childhood is found in all bones, but in the adult is limited mainly to the skull, vertebrae, sternum, ribs, pelvic bones, and the upper-end of the femora and humeri. The red corpuscles contain haemoglobin (an iron-containing substance which combines readily with oxygen), and their function is the carriage of oxygen to the tissues.

White cells, or **leucocytes**—are the two main types:

(*a*) **granulocytes** (neutrocytes) which have a granular cytoplasm and are divided into: *polymorphonuclear leucocytes*—often referred to more simply as **polymorphs**, and also called neutrophils; *eosinophil leucocytes*; *basophil leucocytes* (known as mast cells when they migrate into the tissues).

(*b*) **Hyalines** which have a clear cytoplasm and are divided into *lymphocytes* and *monocytes* (large mononuclears, known as macrophages or histiocytes when they migrate into the tissues).

The granulocytes are formed in red bone marrow. It is generally believed that the hyalines are formed in lymphoid tissue.

Polymorphs, eosinophils and monocytes possess the property of **phagocytosis**, i.e. the ability to take up foreign matter (e.g. infective bacteria, fragments of dead tissue) into their cytoplasm.

The important role of the polymorphs in inflammatory reactions was noted on p 37. In many types of acute infection there is an increase in the numbers of polymorphs in the circulating blood. An increase in the circulating white cells is called a **leucocytosis**, and, according to the type of increase, may take the form of a **polymorphonuclear (neutrophil) leucocytosis**, a **monocytosis**, a **lymphocytosis**, or an **eosinophilia**.

A deficiency of white cells in the circulation is called **leucopaenia**. When such deficiency is due to a diminution in the numbers of granulocytes it is called **granulopaenia**, and when due to a diminution in the lymphocytes, **lymphocytopaenia**.

Lymphocytes play an important part in immunity (see page 35). *B-lymphocytes* develop into *plasma cells*, produce antibodies, and are concerned in humoral immunity. *T-lymphocytes* are subject to the influence of the thymus gland and are concerned with cell-mediated immunity.

Basophil leucocytes carry both histamine and heparin in their cytoplasm.

Platelets, or **thrombocytes**—play an important part in the process of clotting of the blood. An increase above the normal of the numbers of platelets in the circulating blood is called **thrombocytosis**, and a deficiency of platelets is known as **thrombocytopaenia**.

All human blood belongs to one of four main types known as **blood groups**, and these, under what is termed the A B O blood group system, are described as A, B, AB, and O. Most individuals possess an antigen in their red blood corpuscles termed the **rhesus factor**, on account of the same factor being present in the red cells of rhesus monkeys. Such individuals are said to be **Rhesus positive** (Rh+ve), while those lacking this factor (i.e. about 15% of people) are said to be **Rhesus negative** (Rh−ve).

The blood contains circulating substances which, when shed, cause it to **coagulate**, i.e. to form a clot. The platelets are involved in this process of blood coagulation together with a soluble protein called *fibrinogen* and other substances. The actual clot consists of blood cells and platelets entangled in a mesh of *fibrin* which is an insoluble form of *fibrinogen*. Also circulating in the blood are substances such as *heparin*, which prevent clot formation and are termed **anticoagulants**.

The fluid part of a quantity of blood in which clot formation has occurred is called *blood serum*.

The prefix **haem-** means referring to the blood and the branch of medicine concerned with the study of the blood and its diseases is called **haematology**.

The process of formation of red blood corpuscles is termed **erythropoiesis** and of white blood cells, **leucopoiesis**.

Haematopoiesis (haemopoiesis) is a word used either to indicate the formation of both red and white blood cells, or with particular reference to red cell formation.

Some General Aspects of Diseases of the Blood

Blood diseases may be associated with either excessive or deficient production of various cells of the blood and the blood platelets; deficiency of factors essential for the production of red cells (e.g. iron); abnormal destruction of red cells; hereditary factors; defects in coagulation; structural defects in the blood capillaries, etc.

Some important diseases of the blood are: anaemias, haemophilia, polycythaemia vera, agranulocytosis, leukaemias, thrombocytopaenic purpura, and reactions due to transfusion of incompatible blood.

Special Methods of Investigation

Blood examinations

These consist of various laboratory investigations of specimens of circulating blood taken from the patient. Among these are the following.

Haemoglobin estimation—the haemoglobin content being expressed as a percentage of the normal, or in grammes of haemoglobin per 100 millilitres of blood; expressed as g/dl.

Blood counts—i.e. the counting of the numbers of red cells, white cells and platelets per litre (l) of blood. In addition to the counting of the total numbers of white cells, the numbers of each type of white cell (e.g. polymorphs, lymphocytes) may be counted; a procedure known as a **differential white cell count**.

Investigations such as estimations of the **PCV** (packed cell volume—also known as the **haematocrit value**); **MCV** (mean corpusular volume); **MCD** (mean cell diameter); **MCH** (mean corpuscular haemoglobin); serum iron, etc.

Estimation of bleeding time and **clotting time**.

Estimation of the serum bilirubin—to indicate degree of blood destruction (haemoglobin liberated by destruction of red cells is converted into bilirubin).

Bone marrow biopsy

This is microscopic examination of a small quantity of bone marrow obtained by instrumental puncture of some superficial bone such as the sternum.

Blood Grouping

Examination of a specimen of blood to determine its A B O and Rhesus groups.

Blood Transfusion

Blood transfusion, a procedure that transfers blood from one individual (the donor) to another (the recipient), is frequently employed for patients suffering from anaemia due to loss of blood or other causes.

It is to be noted that, when blood is transfused it must first be ensured that the blood of the donor and of the recipient belong to compatible blood groups. It must then be further ascertained, in each separate transfusion, that no incompatibility exists between the cells of the donor and the serum of the intended individual recipient. This is done by carrying out a procedure called **cross-matching** before the transfusion.

Giving a transfusion of incompatible blood will provoke an immune response in the recipient which may lead to a severe reaction, with destruction of transfused red cells, lowered blood pressure and shock. Subsequently jaundice appears and in some cases there may be anuria and renal failure.

Anaemias

The anaemias are a group of diseases in which the blood is lacking in either, or both, a normal content of haemoglobin in its red corpuscles or normal numbers of red cells.

Anaemias may be due to haemorrhage, due to interference with red cell production, or due to excessive destruction of red cells within the circulation (see later).

The presence of anaemia is usually determined initially by performing a haemoglobin estimation on a specimen of blood.

Some forms of anaemia are characterised by the red cells generally being of greater or lesser size than normal. In the former instance, the cells are termed **macrocytes** (i.e. large cells) and the anaemia is called a **macrocytic anaemia**. Red cells which are smaller than normal are called **microcytes**, and those of normal size **normocytes**.

Red corpuscles, whose haemoglobin content is less than normal stain more faintly than normal in a blood film. They are thus described as being **hypochromic** (i.e. deficient in colour). Hypochromic cells are frequently below normal size, i.e. they are microcytes.

In all types of anaemia the oxygen-carrying capacity of the blood is diminished.

Common clinical features of anaemia are tiredness, shortness of breath on exertion, and a characteristic pallor of the mucous membranes and skin. If the condition is of marked degree, the heart rate may also be increased and dilation of heart may occur in severe cases. Splenic enlargement occurs in many types of anaemia and enlargment of the liver may also occur.

There are many different forms of anaemia and descriptions by different authorities frequently show a differing use of nomenclature. It will be possible here to indicate the names and nature of only a limited number of these disorders, most of which, as was stated by Dible (1) many years ago, fall into three main groups which he described as being due to loss of blood, due to defective blood formation, and due to excessive intravascular destruction of blood.

Posthaemorrhagic Anaemias

This term indicates anaemias resulting from loss of blood due to either injuries to blood vessels or diseases which cause bleeding, e.g. bleeding peptic ulcer, bleeding haemorrhoids, menorrhagia, bleeding due to the group of diseases called the **haemorrhagic diseases**, e.g. **haemophilia** and **Christmas disease** (see p 211), **thrombocytopaenic purpura** (see p 213).

Anaemias Due to the Defective Production of Red Blood Cells

A large number of factors may interfere with normal production, by the bone marrow, of mature red blood corpuscles. Among these may be mentioned deficiency of essential factors in the diet (e.g. iron, vitamin B12, folic acid, vitamin C), and failure of absorption of such factors from the food into the body (e.g. in malabsorption syndromes); deficiency of intrinsic factor (see below), replacement of red-cell producing bone marrow tissue by neoplastic tissue (e.g. secondary carcinomatous deposits, leukaemic deposits, multiple myelomata); depression of the activity of red bone marrow by serious diseases in other organs and tissues (e.g. chronic suppurative infections, malignant neoplasms, nephritis); damage to the red marrow by toxic agents (e.g. cytotoxic drugs and certain other drugs) and ionising radiation.

Factors which interfere with normal red cell production may also cause depression of the activity of cells that produce white blood cells of the granulocyte variety and, also cells that make blood platelets. Thus leucopaenia and thrombocytopaenia are also features of some of these anaemias.

Among the anaemias of this type are the following.

Iron deficiency anaemias—due either to a deficiency of iron in the diet or to inadequate absorption of iron from the food.

Iron-deficiency anaemias are treated by giving iron by mouth or parenteral administration. (*Note:* the term **parenteral** means external to the intestine and thus implies some form of injection. Certain preparations of iron are suitable for intravenous or intramuscular injection.)

Female patients with certain types of iron-deficiency anaemia may suffer from **Plummer-Vinson syndrome** (also known as **Paterson-Brown-Kelly syndrome**), i.e. a combination of dysphagia (difficulty in swallowing), glossitis (inflammation of the tongue) and anaemia.

Pernicious anaemia—also called **Addison's anaemia**, after Thomas Addison, a nineteenth century English physician. (*Note:* Addison's disease of the adrenal medulla was also so-called after this physician.)

Pernicious anaemia is due to deficient absorption of vitamin B12 (cyanocobalamin), a substance essential for normal red cell and also white cell production. Such deficient absorption results from changes in the lining mucosa of the stomach, which cause a failure of production by this organ of **Castle's intrinsic factor**, a substance whose presence is essential for the assimilation of vitamin B12 from the food into the body.

The disease has its maximum incidence in middle age. In addition to the general clinical features of severe anaemia, there is often soreness of the tongue and gastric disorder. Neurological symptoms, due to a complicating disease of the spinal cord called **combined subacute degeneration of the cord**, develop in about 10% of cases.

Pernicious anaemia is a macrocytic type of anaemia, the average size of the erythrocytes being greater than normal in this condition. The bone marrow in this disease shows an abnormally high percentage of primitive forms of red cells known as **megaloblasts** and of other forms of immature red cells. It is thus also referred to as a **megaloblastic anaemia**. In addition to the interference with normal red cell production, the deficiency of vitamin B12 also has the effect of interfering with the production of white cells of the granulocyte type, and also of blood platelets. There is thus accompanying leucopaenia and thrombocytopaenia.

Treatment was formerly by injection of specially prepared extracts of liver, this organ being a rich source of vitamin B12. Nowadays, however, its treatment is by preparations of vitamin B12 administered by intramuscular injection. (*Note:* in addition to pernicious anaemia there are a number of other forms of megaloblastic anaemia. These may develop as a result of deficiency of vitamin B12 or of *folate*, the active form of *folic acid*, a vitamin belonging to the vitamin B complex, e.g. certain anaemias associated with **malabsorption syndromes**, the anaemia of **tropical sprue** and **macrocytic anaemia of pregnancy**.)

Aplastic and hypoplastic anaemias—anaemias in which red cell production is brought to a stop or depressed as a result of a varying degree of disappearance of red-cell-forming tissue from the bone marrow; or absence or depression of the normal functional activity of such tissue. These anaemias may be due to unknown causes, or result from damage to the bone marrow from certain drugs, infections, damage from ionising radiations, etc.

The formation of granulocytic white cells and platelets may also be depressed in these disorders.

Leucoerythroblastic anaemia—this type of anaemia is due to the replacement of blood-forming bone marrow tissue as a result of certain disease processes (e.g. multiple carcinomatous metastases in bone, multiple myelomata, fibrous tissue formation accompanied by increased bone formation in a rare disorder called **myelosclerosis**).

Anaemias Due to Excessive Destruction of Red Cells

These are known collectively as **haemolytic anaemias**.

Haemolysis means destruction of red cells and in haemolytic anaemias an excessive premature destruction of these cells takes place, either within phagocytic cells of the lymphoreticular tissues, or within the circulating blood, the rate of destruction being such that the red cells cannot be replaced by the production of new red cells by the bone marrow.

Note: At the end of their usual life span, which is about four months, red cells are normally destroyed by the action of macrophages of the mononuclear phagocyte system; the site of such destruction being mainly in the liver and spleen.

Although haemolytic anaemias are uncommon, they are of various types and various different factors operate in their production; e.g. rhesus incompatibility (see erythroblastosis fetalis); inherited fragility of red cells (see acholuric jaundice); inherited defects in the manufacture of haemoglobin (see later); transfusion with blood of incompatible types; malarial infection; blackwater fever; certain severe bacterial and viral infections; extensive burns; certain chemical substances; sensitivity to certain drugs; and autoimmunity.

Excessive destruction of red corpuscles leads to raised amounts of *bilirubin* (an iron-free breakdown product of haemoglobin) in the blood and, if the disorder is severe, clinical jaundice may develop as well as anaemia (see p 140). When such destruction occurs in the circulating blood, however, haemoglobin is set free in the plasma and **haemog-lobinaemia** is then said to be present. This condition results in **haemoglobinuria**, i.e. passage of haemoglobin in the urine.

Inherited defects in the manufacture of haemoglobin, referred to above and occurring principally in natives of countries with warm climates, are found in a group of disorders called **haemo-globinopathies**, and also in a form of anaemia called **thalassaemia** (also known as Cooley's anaemia or Mediterranean anaemia).

Sickle-cell anaemia is one form of haemoglobinopathy and its name derives from an appearance of sickling of the red cells which can be demonstrated on examination of blood films taken from patients with this disease.

> In children with severe thalassaemia skeletal changes secondary to pronounced overgrowth of bone marrow tissue may be seen on radiographs. These include cortical thinning and destruction of cancellous bone with consequent bone expansion, often most apparent in the tubular bones of the hands and feet.
>
> In sickle-cell anaemia osteosclerosis and evidence of bone infarction, i.e. localised necrosis of bone tissue are not uncommon X-ray findings.

An interesting type of haemolytic anaemia occurs in the hereditary disease called **acholuric jaundice (hereditary spherocytosis)**, in which excessive breakdown of red cells develops in childhood as a result of inherited abnormal fragility of the red corpuscles. Increased amounts of bilirubin are present in the blood leading to jaundice. Splenic enlargement is a common feature of the disease and the development of gall stones, composed of bile pigment, is a common complication.

Important blood examinations in the diagnosis of haemolytic anaemias include **estimation of the serum bilirubin**—('direct' or 'indirect'), and **Coombs test** (a test for antibodies associated with destruction of red cells).

Haemophilia

This rare hereditary disease belongs to the group of blood disorders called haemorrhagic diseases and is due to a defect in the coagulability of the blood. It normally only affects males but can be transmitted by females in affected families.

The condition is characterised by severe attacks of bleeding which may occur without apparent cause or result from minor injuries, tooth extraction, etc. Common sites in which haemorrhage occurs include the skin and subcutaneous tissues, the nose, the joints, and the urinary tract.

Christmas disease and **Von Willebrand's disease** are other examples of inherited disorders due to coagulation deficiency. Both are rare.

Vitamin K deficiency may also be responsible for defective clotting of the blood. The condition called **haemorrhagic disease of the newborn** (not to be confused with haemolytic disease of the newborn, p 190) is one manifestation of such deficiency.

Polycythaemia

The prefix **poly-** means many and the term **polycythaemia** is used to indicate that the circulating blood contains many more red blood cells than normal.

Increased numbers of red cells may be produced as a physiological response to residence at high altitudes in order to increase the oxygen-carrying capacity of the blood, and thus offset the effects of lowered atmospheric pressure. This is referred to as **physiological polycythaemia**.

Secondary polycythaemia may develop as a compensatory mechanism in certain diseases of the heart and lungs which cause interference with the oxygenation of the blood.

Primary polycythaemia occurs as a result of a primary disease of the bone marrow in which there is overgrowth of tissue producing red cells, accompanied also by proliferation of tissue producing white cells and platelets. This disorder is more commonly termed **polycythaemia rubra vera** but may also be referred to as **erythraemia** or **Vaquez–Osler disease**. It is predominantly a disorder of middle age, characterised by headaches, thrombus (clot) formation in blood vessels, and bleeding from sites such as the nose, alimentary and urinary tracts. Thrombi may form in the vessels of the limbs, heart or brain. In some cases there is associated renal disease, sometimes in the form of a hypernephroma (adenocarcinoma of the kidney).

Treatment with radioactive phosphorus is often of considerable benefit in polycythaemia vera and chemotherapy e.g. using busulphan, is also employed as an alternative form of treatment.

Granulocytopaenia and Agranulocytosis

A deficiency in the total number of white blood cells is termed **leucopaenia**. The leucopaenia may be due to **lymphocytopaenia**—deficiency of lymphocytes, or to **granulocytopaenia**—deficiency of granulocytes. In most instances of the latter condition the deficiency affects principally the polymorphonuclear leucocytes and, as these cells may also be described as neutrophil granulocytes, the condition may be termed **neutropaenia**.

Deficiency of granulocytes may be due to various infections, certain drugs (e.g. gold salts, cytotoxic drugs), ionising radiation, etc., or may be of unknown causation. Granulocytes, like red cells, are formed in red bone marrow. Many of the causes which produce a deficiency of granulocytes in the blood may also depress red cell formation and thus granulocytopaenia is often seen as a concomitant of anaemia.

A marked degree of granulocytopaenia is referred to as **agranulocytosis** and may result in clinical features such as fever and infective lesions in the mouth and throat, which may proceed to severe ulceration.

Leukaemias

The literal meaning of the name **leukaemia** is white blood.

The leukaemias are diseases in which there is an overgrowth of tissue responsible for producing white blood cells. This overgrowth, moreover, does not remain confined to sites of normal leucocyte production, but is found in the form of widely scattered deposits in various internal organs and sometimes also in the skin. Such deposits are termed **leukaemic infiltrations**. They may occur in the lungs, bones and hilar and mediastinal lymph glands, and then be demonstrable on X-ray films.

In the vast majority of cases the presence of leukaemia is associated with a considerable increase in the numbers of leucocytes in the circulating blood. In most cases the diagnosis may be readily established by performing a white blood cell count. Sometimes, however, marrow puncture is necessary to determine the nature of the condition.

Anaemia is an invariable accompaniment of leukaemia owing to interference with red corpuscle formation. Haemorrhages are also common owing to reduced production of blood platelets.

Leukaemias may develop in either acute or chronic form. In any single case there is overproduction of only one type of leucocyte or its parent cells. Thus, according to whether granulocytes, lymphocytes, or monocytes, or their parent cells are involved the principal types of leukaemia as designated as: **acute myeloblastic, chronic myeloid, acute lymphoblastic, chronic lymphocytic**, and **monocytic leukaemia**.

Myeloblasts are immature cells found in bone marrow and ancestral cells of granulocytic leucocytes. Myeloid means pertaining to bone marrow. *Lymphoblasts* are parent cells of lymphocytes and like monocytes are found in the lymphoreticular tissues.

Splenic enlargement is a common feature in the leukaemias, being especially marked in chronic myeloid leukaemia. Generalised enlargement of lymph glands and lymphoid tissue is seen in lymphatic leukaemia.

The cause of leukaemia is unknown. There is, however, evidence to suggest exposure to high doses of ionising radiation has played a part in the genesis of some cases.

Accompanying anaemia is combated by blood transfusion. Leukaemias are treated principally by chemotherapy; radiotherapy sometimes being used as an adjunct in chronic leukaemia. Bone marrow transplantation may be used as a form of therapy in some cases of acute leukaemia.

Essential Thromboctyopaenia

This is a rare disease which, as indicated by the term thrombocytopaenia, has as its basic pathological feature a deficiency of blood platelets (thrombocytes). The cause of this deficiency is unknown and, as the disease is characterised by **purpura**, i.e. spontaneous haemorrhage into the skin and subcutaneous tissues, it is often referred to as **idiopathic thrombocytopaenic purpura**.

In addition to the skin haemorrhages, bleeding occurs from mucous membranes and may cause haematemesis, melaena or haematuria.

Note: Purpura may also occur in other diseases in which there is a deficiency of platelets due to disease of the bone marrow, e.g. leukaemias, some anaemias; certain infections; as a reaction to certain drugs, and also in diseases in which there is some abnormality of the capillary blood vessels, e.g. scurvy. It may also be seen as a manifestation of hypersensitivity to various agents as in the condition called **Henoch-Schönlein purpura** or **anaphylactoid purpura**.

The Spleen

The spleen acts as a reservoir for blood, manufactures red and white blood cells during fetal life and white cells of the lymphocyte variety during adult life. It contains much lymphoreticular tissue and its phagocytic cells destroy worn out red blood cells and infective micro-organisms.

Splenomegaly, i.e. enlargement of the spleen is a common feature in many diseases of the blood and of the lymphoreticular tissues. It also occurs frequently in several infective disorders (e.g. malaria, typhoid fever, glandular fever). Among its other causes are chronic right-sided heart failure and portal hypertension.

Primary disorders of the spleen are uncommon and malignant neoplasms other than lymphomas hardly ever develop in this organ.

Traumatic rupture of the spleen is a not uncommon abdominal injury and often results in severe haemorrhage.

Spontaneous rupture of the spleen is a condition which occasionally occurs in some disorders associated with enlargement of this organ, e.g. glandular fever.

REFERENCE

(1) Dible, J. H., (1950). *Dible and Davie's Pathology*. London: J. and A. Churchill.

ENDOCRINE SYSTEM

The endocrine system consists of a number of ductless glands, i.e. the *pituitary*, *pineal*, *thyroid*, *parathyroid*, *thymus*, *adrenal glands*, and also certain cells within the *pancreas*, *ovaries* and *testes*. All its components possess the common property of elaborating secretions called *hormones*. These latter pass from the endocrine cells into the bloodstream and produce effects of various kinds in other organs and tissues.

The anterior lobe of the pituitary gland exercises a general control over many of the activities of the other components of the endocrine system and in its turn is subject to control by the hypothalamus.

The *hypothalamus* is a part of the forebrain, which lies above the pituitary gland and is connected to it by the pituitary (infundibular) stalk, containing blood vessels and nerves which supply the gland. The secretion of various hormones by the anterior lobe of the pituitary is either stimulated or inhibited by what are termed releasing and inhibiting factors, produced in the hypothalamus. This structure is also the site of production of the hormones stored and secreted into the blood by the posterior lobe of the pituitary (see later).

The branch of medicine which deals specifically with diseases of the endocrine system is called **endocrinology**. There are a great many disorders resulting from **hyperfunction** (overactivity) or **hypofunction** (underactivity) of endocrine organs. These range from minor disorders to severe and disabling diseases.

Certain complex relationships exist between a number of the endocrine glands and, accordingly, some of the diseases of this system are highly complex in nature. In general, it is only proposed here to refer to terms which describe some of the more clearly defined endocrine diseases.

The Pituitary Gland

The *pituitary gland*, or *hypophysis*, lies in the pituitary fossa (sella turcica) of the sphenoid bone, being connected to the base of the brain by the *pituitary stalk*. It consists of two lobes which differ in origin, structure and function. Both these lobes are however, as noted, subject to the control of the *hypothalamus*. As a consequence conditions, in which there is overactivity or overactivity of the pituitary gland, may, as in the description by Harrison (1), be referred to as disorders of the *pituitary—hypothalamic system*.

The **anterior pituitary lobe** *(adenohypophysis)* develops from the buccal (mouth) cavity of the embryo and secretes hormones connected with growth and lactation, and other hormones which affect the activity of the thyroid gland and adrenal cortex, and also the activities of endocrine cells in the ovaries and testes, i.e. *growth hormone (GH), prolactin (PRL), thyroid stimulating hormone (TSH), adrenocorticotrophic hormone (ACTH)*, and the *gonadotrophic hormones* called *follicle stimulating hormone (FSH)* and *luteinising hormone (LH)*, whose two names do not give any indication that, in the male sex, the former stimulates spermatogenesis and the latter production of testosterone by the testes.

It also secretes a hormone which increases skin pigmentation and is called *melanocyte-stimulating hormone (MSH)*.

Overactivity of the anterior lobe is called **hyperpituitarism** and underactivity **hypopituitarism**.

Tumours of glandular tissue, called **pituitary adenomas** may develop in the anterior pituitary. These are of three types called **eosinophil**, **basophil** and **chromophobe adenomas**, so-called according to the staining properties with certain dyes of the cells which compose the tumours (e.g. the cells of an eosinophil adenoma have an affinity for an acid dye called **eosin**).

Eosinophil adenoma is associated with overproduction of growth hormone and if it develops before growth of the skeleton is complete leads to **pituitary gigantism**. After growth has ceased, however, such a tumour causes a condition called **acromegaly**, the name of which means large extremities. Sufferers from acromegaly show overgrowth of certain bony structures and generalised overgrowth of soft tissues. They have large hands and feet and prominent lower jaws. Enlargement of the pituitary fossa also occurs and can be shown on X-ray film of the skull. Severe headaches are common and, if the tumour extends outside the pituitary fossa, it frequently causes disturbances of vision, ultimately resulting in blindness.

Basophil adenoma is very rare. It is usually small and thus does not enlarge the pituitary fossa. It may be associated with a disorder of the adrenal glands called **Cushing's syndrome** (see 'adrenal glands').

Chromophobe adenoma is the most frequently occurring type of pituitary tumour. It often attains a large size resulting in enlargement of the pituitary fossa and destruction of its bony walls, changes demonstrable by skull radiography. It causes headaches, vomiting and blindness. In addition there is often amenorrhoea in women and **impotence** (i.e. inability to perform the sexual act) in men, as a result of deficient hormone secretion.

Pituitary adenomas sometimes cause increase of secretion of the hormone prolactin, and are therefore one cause of **hyperprolactinaemia**, i.e. high levels of prolactin in the blood. This condition may result in menstrual disorder and infertility in women, impotence in men, and **galactorrhoea**, i.e. excessive or abnormal secretion of milk.

Other disorders of the anterior lobe of the pituitary gland include the following conditions which develop as a result of factors causing hypopituitarism.

(i) **Pituitary dwarfism**, the main types of which are called **Lorain dwarfism** (pituitary infantilism) and **Frohlich's syndrome** (dystrophia adiposo-genitalis).

(ii) **Simmonds's disease** (panhypopituitarism) a condition of severe hypopituitarism seen most frequently in women, in whom it occurs as a result of destruction of the anterior lobe after childbirth. It is associated with amenorrhoea, wasting and premature senility.

The **posterior pituitary lobe** (*neurohypophysis*) develops as a downgrowth from the brain and consists of nervous tissue. The hormones, referred to as *posterior lobe hormones* are actually manufactured in the hypothalamus in the base of the brain, but are stored in the posterior lobe of the pituitary, and are released from this structure into the blood stream. These hormones can raise the blood pressure, stimulate contraction of the muscles of the uterus during and after labour, and exercise what is termed an **antidiuretic effect** on the kidneys, i.e. prevent secretion of greater than normal amounts of urine. *Note:* **diuresis** means excretion of greater than normal amounts of urine.

It secretes two hormones: *oxytocin*, which stimulates contraction of the muscles of the uterus during labour; and *antidiuretic hormone* (ADH), also known as *vasopressin*, which prevents the excretion by the kidneys of excessive amounts of urine.

As a result of disease affecting the posterior lobe of the pituitary gland, pituitary stalk or certain structures in the base of the brain, secretion of the antidiuretic hormone may be impaired causing **diabetes insipidus**, a disease characterised by severe thirst and **polyuria**, i.e. the passage of excessive amounts of urine.

Surgical removal of the pituitary gland is termed **hypophysectomy**.

Pituitary function can also be abolished by implantation of radio-active yttrium into the gland.

The Thyroid Gland

The thyroid gland lies in the lower part of the neck. It consists of two lateral lobes, joined by an isthmus which lies in front of the upper part of the trachea. Its activities are subject to the control of thyroid-stimulating hormone (TSH) secreted by the anterior lobe of the pituitary gland. It secretes iodine-containing hormones called *thyroxine* (T4) and *triiodo-thyronine* (T3) which exert a considerable influence on the metabolism of tissues throughout the body. (**Metabolism** is a term used to describe the processes whereby absorbed foodstuffs are modified for tissue building and repair, and whereby waste products are broken down into forms which can be excreted from the body.)

Warwick (2) states that 'too much or too little thyroxine in circulation results in a metabolic rate which is incorrectly balanced to the needs of the body'.

Methods to measure the activity of the thyroid gland include: measurement by a method called radioimmunoassay of the concentrations in the blood of the thyroid hormones T4 and T3, and of the anterior pituitary hormone TSH (see above); and measurement of the uptake by the thyroid gland of radioactive iodine.

In addition to secreting thyroxine and triiodo-thyronine, the thyroid gland also secretes a hormone called *calcitonin*, which has the property of lowering the serum calcium.

Overactivity of thyroid secretion is known as **hyperthyroidism**, and underactivity as **hypothyroidism**.

Enlargement of thyroid gland, diffuse or localised, is a feature of many thyroid diseases and any enlargement of thyroid tissue is termed a **goitre**.

Goitres may exert pressure effects on the trachea causing dyspnoea (difficulty in breathing) and on the oesophagus causing dysphagia (difficulty in swallowing).

Enlarged thyroid tissue may sometimes extend behind the sternum into the upper thorax. Such an extension is termed a **retrosternal goitre** and may be demonstrable on chest X-ray films.

Types of goitre—some important types of goitre are given below.

(i) **Simple goitre** (non-toxic goitre)—this condition is not associated with any abnormality of endocrine secretions. One type is thought to result from a deficient intake of iodine. In another type, known as **non-toxic adenomatous goitre**, single or multiple nodular overgrowths of glandular tissue called **thyroid adenomas** develop in the gland.

(ii) **Toxic goitre**—a name used to describe any goitre associated with hyperthyroidism (i.e. overactivity of the thyroid gland) resulting from oversecretion of the thyroid hormone, thyroxine.

The presence of abnormally high amounts of this hormone leads to a general increase of cellular metabolic processes throughout the body. This is evidenced clinically by signs and symptoms such as rapid pulse, excessive sweating, loss of weight, restlessness, nervousness and tremor of the hands, i.e. the so-called toxic features of the disorder which lead to it also being referred to as **thyrotoxicosis**.

In one form of toxic goitre, known as **exophthalmic goitre**, or **Graves's disease**, in addition to evidence of hyperthyroidism there develops also **exophthalmos**, i.e. a condition of pretrusion of the eyeballs.

In another type of toxic goitre, thyrotoxic features may develop in a patient who has had a non-toxic adenomatous goitre for many years. This type is sometimes called a **toxic adenoma**.

Toxic goitres in middle-aged and elderly subjects may be complicated by the development of a form of heart disease known as **thyrotoxic heart disease**. Atrial fibrillation is common in this condition.

The treatment of toxic goitres may be surgery, antithyroid drugs (e.g. carbimazole) or radioactive iodine.

(iii) **Malignant goitre**—this disorder is also termed **carcinoma of the thyroid gland** and is not usually associated with overactivity of the gland but it often produces metastases at an early stage of its growth. These develop most frequently in lymph glands in the neck and in the lungs and bones.

Surgery, radiotherapy or radioactive iodine may be used to treat the primary growth. Radiotherapy, radioactive iodine or hormone therapy may be used in the treatment of metastases.

Hypothyroidism—a condition of underactivity of the thyroid gland associated with defective secretion of thyroxine and consequent diminution of metabolic activities of cells throughout the body.

In certain cases of hypothyroidism occurring in adults, there is a characteristic thickening of the subcutaneous tissues which simulates swelling of the tissues due to oedema. This type of hypothyroidism is called **myxoedema** and among its other features are an abnormally slow pulse rate, obesity, lethargy, slowing of mental processes, loss of hair, and enlargement of the heart. Treatment is by administration of thyroxine.

Cretinism (infantile hypothyroidism) is another type of hypothyroidism. It may occur as a congenital condition due to absence or underdevelopment of the thyroid gland. It can also develop in early childhood, when it appears to result from iodine deficiency and may be associated with a goitre.

Among the clinical features of cretinism are lethargy and retarded mental and skeletal development. The tongue is enlarged and protruding, and the infant is potbellied. Treatment is by thyroxine. Hypothyroidism may be detected or excluded by estimation of the plasma thyroid-stimulating hormone (TSH) and this investigation is now widely used as a screening procedure in neonates during the first few days of life.

Other diseases—other diseases of the thyroid gland include several uncommon inflammatory disorders, e.g. **acute thyroiditis, Hashimoto's thyroiditis** (an autoimmune disorder), **Riedel's thyroiditis**.

The Parathyroid Glands

The parathyroid glands are normally situated on the posterior aspect of the thyroid gland. They vary in number, four usually being present. Rarely, ectopic (abnormally placed) parathyroid glands may be sited in the superior mediastinum.

The parathyroids secrete a hormone called *parathormone* which is concerned with the maintenance of a normal level of calcium in the blood plasma and a normal balance between the amounts of calcium and phosphorous in the blood.

Hyperparathyroidism—in this uncommon condition there is overactivity of parathyroid tissue resulting in oversecretion of parathormone, and increased amounts of calcium are found in the blood. This latter feature is termed **hypercalcaemia**.

Primary hyperparathyroidism may result from the presence of a benign tumour called a **parathyroid adenoma** or from hyperplasia (overgrowth) of the parathyroids. **Secondary hyperparathyroidism** may develop as a secondary effect of certain kidney diseases and malabsorption syndromes, of a type which result initially in low levels of serum calcium, and thus stimulate overactivity of the parathyroid glands.

In both types of hyperparathyroidism there is increased absorption of calcium from the bones. The bones become osteoporotic and may develop a condition termed **generalised osteitis fibrosa**. Renal stones are also common as a result of the increased blood calcium leading to increased excretion of calcium in the urine; a condition is called **hypercalciuria**.

In the early stages of hyperparathyroidism radiographs may show evidence of general osteoporosis (see p 238) and also typical changes in the phalanges of the hands referred to as **subperiosteal erosions**.

Lateral views of the skull may show a characteristic mottled appearance due to numerous small translucencies resulting from the osteoporosis.

As the disease progresses cystic areas and deformities may be apparent in skeletal films and the presence of renal calculi may be demonstrated by urography.

Hypoparathyroidism—is a rare condition, resulting from deficiency of parathormone, and is usually seen as a result of accidental removal of the parathyroid glands duing thyroidectomy (surgical removal of the thyroid gland).

In this disorder the blood calcium is below normal, resulting in an undue excitability of nervous and muscular tissue. This excitability may lead to the development of **tetany**, a condition characterised by painful muscle spasms. (*Note:* tetany occurs in other disorders in which blood calcium levels are below normal and in diseases in which the blood has a more alkaline reaction than normal, i.e. in various forms of **alkalosis**.)

The Adrenal Glands

There are two *adrenal (suprarenal) glands* and each lies in close apposition to the upper pole of the corresponding kidney, in the posterior part of the abdomen.

Each gland consists of an outer part called the *cortex* and an inner part called the *medulla*. These structures are of different developmental origin and thus differ from each other in structure and function (cf the anterior and posterior lobes of the pituitary gland).

The adrenal cortex—produces a large number of endocrine secretions and its principal functions are concerned with the metabolism of carbohydrates, minerals and water. It also produces *sex hormones* of both male and female type. These latter play some part in the development of secondary sexual characteristics and the functioning of the sex glands; but the production of sex hormones by the adrenals is small in relation to production of these substances by the gonads (i.e. the testes and ovaries). It is interesting to note that small quantities of *androgens* (male sex hormones) are secreted normally by the adrenals in females, and small quantities of *oestrogens* (female sex hormones) are secreted in males both by the adrenals and by endocrine cells in the testes.

The secretion of hormones concerned with carbohydrate metabolism by the adrenal cortex is stimulated by the anterior pituitary hormone called *corticotrophin* or ACTH (adrenocorticotrophic hormone).

The prefixes **adrenocortico-** and **cortico-** are both used with reference to the suprarenal cortex.

Adrenocortical hormones may thus be classified into three main groups: (i) *glucocorticoids*—which affect carbohydrate metabolism, e.g. cortisol and corticosterone; (ii) *mineralocorticoids*—which affect mineral metabolism, and in particular are concerned with the retention of sodium and water in the body and the excretion of potassium, e.g. aldosterone, deoxycorticosterone; (iii) *sex hormones*, i.e. *androgens* (e.g. testosterone) and *oestrogens* (e.g. oestriol, progesterone). (See also *Note:* corticosteroid therapy p 222).

Diseases of the adrenal cortex are not common. Overactivity of the adrenal cortex is referred to as **adrenocortical hyperfunction** and may be associated with hyperplasia (overgrowth) of adrenocortical tissue on both sides, the presence of one or more benign tumours called **cortical adenomas** or, in rare instances, **carcinoma of the adrenal cortex**. The principal diseases which occur as a result of adrenocortical hyperfunction are:

(i) **Cushing's syndrome**—a condition usually associated with bilateral hyperplasia of the suprarenals, but sometimes with a cortical adenoma or with cortisone therapy. Other causes include oversecretion of ACTH by a basophil adenoma of the pituitary gland and, rarely, secretion of ACTH by neoplasms arising in structures other than the pituitary or adrenal glands, e.g. bronchial carcinoma. It is characterised by overproduction of carbohydrate-regulating hormones (glucocorticoids).

Among the clinical features of Cushing's syndrome are obesity of the face (producing the characteristic moonface appearance), obesity of the trunk with accompanying wasting of the limbs, hypertension and glycosuria, osteoporosis, impotence in men and amenorrhoea and virilisation in women (**virilisation** means the development, in female subjects, of male secondary sexual characteristics, e.g. deepening of the voice, growth of a beard.)

Biochemical investigation into a suspected case may include measurement of the plasma cortisol and its diurnal variation, measurement of urinary free cortisol and performance of a dexamethasone suppression test.

Treatment of the condition may be surgical, a cortical adenoma being dealt with by excision of the tumour and bilateral suprarenal hyperplasia by bilateral adrenalectomy together with hormone replacement therapy for the rest of the patient's life. Irradiation of the pituitary gland may be employed when a pituitary tumour is the cause.

(ii) **Conn's disease**—a rare condition, due usually to an uncommon type of cortical adenoma but sometimes due to cortical hyperplasia, and associated with overproduction of the mineralocorticoid called *aldosterone* and thus also known as **primary hyperaldosteronism**.

It is characterised by **hypokalaemia** (deficiency of blood potassium) and resultant muscular weakness, and by retention of sodium and water which may result in oedema. Hypertension develops in some cases.

(iii) **Adrenogenital syndrome**—an uncommon disorder associated with overproduction of male sex hormones and resulting in virilisation (see under Cushing's syndrome) in females and sexual precocity in boys. This disorder may be associated with either an adrenocortical adenoma, or a congenital enzyme deficiency and accompanying hyperplasia of the adrenal cortex.

Underactivity of the adrenal cortex is termed **adrenocortical hypofunction** and may present in acute form as a result of rapidly developing necrosis or of haemorrhage into the gland. The causes include shock and severe infections.

Such hypofunction also occurs in chronic form when its causes include atrophy of glandular tissue due to autoimmune disease, tuberculous infection and carcinomatous metastases in the adrenals.

Chronic adrenocortical hypofunction is seen clinically in the condition called Addison's disease. Sometimes, however, this disease is complicated by attacks of acute hypofunction with very marked lowering of blood pressure, coma in some cases and general intensification of symptoms. Such attacks are known as **Addisonian crises**.

Addison's disease (adrenal insufficiency) was named after Thomas Addison, an English physician after whom Addisonian anaemia was also named. It most commonly develops in middle-aged patients and is associated with a deficiency of cortical hormones concerned with both carbohydrate metabolism (glucocorticoids), and with metabolism of minerals (mineralocorticoids). Among its clinical features are severe general weakness, mental apathy, low blood pressure, brownish pigmentation of the skin and gastrointestinal disturbances. Treatment is by corticosteroids.

When the disorder results from tuberculosis infection, pathological calcification in the suprarenal glands may be demonstrable on abdominal radiographs.

Note: **corticosteroid therapy**—the word **steroid** literally means fat-like and describes a class of substances which includes the **corticosteroids**, i.e. steroid hormones produced by the suprarenal cortex, e.g. cortisol (hydrocortisone), corticosterone, aldosterone; and also includes certain non-hormone compounds such as cholesterol and ergosterol.

The treatment of diseases by corticosteroid hormones and certain synthetic substances with similar properties (e.g. cortisone, prednisone, prednisolone) is called **corticosteroid therapy**, or alternatively **steroid therapy**.

Naturally occurring and synthetic corticosteroids are widely employed in the treatment of a variety of different conditions, e.g. rheumatoid arthritis, ulcerative colitis, sarcoidosis, following bilateral adrenalectomy, in the emergency treatment of hypersensitivity reactions, in Hodgkin's disease and for vomiting resulting from courses of radiotherapy.

Some patients receiving corticosteroid therapy may develop undesirable side effects as a result of treatment, e.g. signs and symptoms similar to those of Cushing's syndrome, peptic ulceration, osteoporosis leading to vertebral collapse.

Disorders of this nature which are the direct result of remedies prescribed in treatment of the primary condition are often referred to as **iatrogenic diseases** meaning literally diseases caused by physicians. (Other examples of iatrogenic diseases include insulin coma and reactions to treatment with ionising radiation.)

Sudden cessation of corticosteroid therapy is dangerous as it may produce so-called **withdrawal symptoms** among which may be generalised muscular weakness and sometimes circulatory collapse. Patients on routine treatment with steroids may be given a steroid card to carry on their persons giving particulars regarding such treatment.

The adrenal medulla is derived from nervous tissue and secretes two hormones, *adrenaline* and *noradrenaline*, both of which belong to a class of substances called *catecholamines* and both of which stimulate *receptors* at sympathetic nerve terminals (*sympathetic* or *adrenergic receptors*—see p 28).

Adrenaline stimulates both α- and β- receptors. It raises the blood pressure and increases the output of blood by the heart, and the blood supply of the skeletal muscles during times of stress, while relaxing smooth muscle generally, and diminishing the circulation in the skin and gastrointestinal tract. As stated by McNaught (3) in a concise account of the endocrine system, 'adrenaline reinforces the action of the sympathetic nervous system in preparing the various systems of the body to meet all sorts of emergencies'.

Noradrenaline acts on α-receptors and has the property of raising the blood pressure.

Several rare types of tumour may develop in the adrenal medulla.

(i) **Phaeochromocytoma**—a rare tumour, of cells called phaeochromocytes, which may be benign or malignant. It secretes the adrenal medullary hormones, adrenaline and noradrenaline, and consequently produces hypertension (high blood pressure).

The hypertension may be persistent or, as is more common, occur in intermittent attacks. In this latter event it is referred to as **paroxysmal hypertension**.

(ii) **Neuroblastoma**—a rare but highly malignant tumour which is composed of nerve cells of primitive type called neuroblasts. It occurs in childhood and frequently produces metastases at an early stage in sites such as the lungs, liver and bones.

(iii) **Ganglioneuroma**—a very rare benign tumour of nerve cells.

Radiological studies are often of great value in the diagnosis of tumours of both the adrenal cortex and medulla. They may include plain films, intravenous urography, tomography, CT, ultrasound, also certain forms of angiography to show the arteries and veins supplying the adrenal glands.

The Gonads

Diseases of the ovaries and diseases of the testes are referred to earlier in Part IV (see pp 174 and 176).

The Pancreas Islets

The cells of the pancreas, which belong to the endocrine system, are arranged in collections known as the *pancreas islets* or *islets of Langerhans*. The islet cells are of three types A, B and G and rarely give rise to tumours (see p 144). The B cells, the most numerous type, secrete the hormone *insulin*, which plays an important role in carbohydrate metabolism. Deficient production or defective action of this hormone gives rise to the common and important disorder called diabetes mellitus.

Diabetes Mellitus

This is due to defective action of insulin and among the factors which may be responsible for this are: (i) deficient secretion of this hormone by the islet cells of the pancreas; (ii) oversecretion of *insulin antagonists*, i.e. other hormones in the body which render the action of insulin less effective than normal (the adrenocortical hormone cortisol and anterior pituitary growth hormone are examples of insulin antagonists); (iii) increased requirements of the body for insulin due to the development of obesity (when such requirements are in excess of what the pancreas can meet).

Diabetes may develop as a primary condition, the basic cause of which is unknown or may be secondary to other disease.

Two clinical types of primary diabetes are described: **type I diabetes**, also known as **early onset** or **insulin-dependent diabetes**, which occurs in young subjects, and in which hereditary factors and autoimmunity often play a part; and **type II diabetes** which occurs in middle-aged and elderly subjects and is termed **late onset** or **non-insulin-dependent diabetes**.

Certain endocrine disorders, prolonged corticosteroid therapy and diseases of the pancreas may give rise to secondary diabetes.

Defective action of insulin interferes with the normal utilisation of glucose by tissue cells and also with the production of glycogen and its storage. (*Note:* carbohydrates are converted into glucose during digestion and absorbed into the blood in this form. The absorbed glucose is then either utilised by tissue cells, or converted into a starch called glycogen and stored in the liver and muscles.) Such defective hormone action leads to **hyperglycaemia** (excessive amounts of glucose in the blood) and consequent **glycosuria** (passage of glucose in the urine).

Common symptoms of diabetes are excessive thirst (**polydipsia**), the passage of excessive amounts of dilute urine (**polyuria**), and loss of weight. A variety of other symptoms and signs may occur as a result of the disease and its many complications. The milder type of case may, however, be completely symptomless.

The passage of large amounts of urine, which contains glucose, gives the disorder its name—**diabetes** meaning to go through and **mellitus** meaning honey.

(*Note:* used without qualification the term diabetes indicates diabetes mellitus and not the uncommon pituitary disorder called diabetes insipidus.)

In the severer forms of diabetes, secondary disorders may also develop in the metabolism of fats and proteins. The former may result in accumulation of substances called **ketone bodies** in the blood, i.e. **ketosis** (ketoacidosis) and the presence of such substances in the urine, i.e. **ketonuria**. Diabetic ketosis is a serious development and may lead to a state of unconsciousness termed **diabetic coma** (hyperglycaemic coma).

Important diagnostic investigations in suspected diabetic subjects include the testing of the urine for sugar and ketone bodies, **blood glucose estimation**, and tests termed **glucose tolerance tests**.

Diabetes is a disease with many complications. Among these are **diabetic cataract** (opacity of the lens of the eye), **diabetic retinopathy** (also called diabetic retinitis—see p 293), **diabetic gangrene, diabetic neuropathy** (a disease of the nervous system) which may lead to the development of **Charcot joints** (see p 261). Diabetics are especially prone to septic infections, certain forms of renal disease, such as pyelonephritis, pulmonary tuberculosis, and the degenerative arterial disease called atheroma.

According to its type and severity the treatment of diabetes may consist of: dietetic measures combined with the injection of either short-acting or long-acting insulin preparations (e.g. early onset diabetes); dietetic measures alone (e.g. late onset diabetes); dietetic measures together with oral hypoglycaemic drugs such as tolbutamide and other sulphonylureas, or biguanides (e.g. late onset diabetes that cannot be controlled by dietetic measures alone).

It is to be noted that overdosage with insulin may lower the blood sugar to such an extent that a type of coma termed an **insulin coma** (hypoglycaemic coma) may develop.

The Thymus Gland

The thymus gland is situated in the superior mediastinum, secretes a hormone called *thymosin*, and contains much lymphoid tissue. As already noted it plays an important role in immunity because it influences or modifies the T-lymphocytes, which are responsible for cell-mediated immunity (see p 35).

It may be the site of lymphoid hyperplasia, or of cyst or tumour formation. Thymic tumours are called **thymomas**, and one variety of these may occur in association with myasthenia gravis (see p 265).

REFERENCES

(1) Harrison, R. J. (1980). *Textbook of Medicine*, 2nd Edn. London: Hodder and Stoughton.
(2) Warwick, R. (1961). *Whillis's Elementary Anatomy and Physiology*. London: Churchill.
(3) McNaught, A. (1983). *Companion to Illustrated Physiology*. Edinburgh: Churchill Livingstone.

SKIN AND SUBCUTANEOUS TISSUES

Some Anatomical and Physiological Considerations

The **skin** consists of an outer layer called the *epidermis* and an inner layer called the *dermis*.

The epidermis consists of epithelial cells among which are cells containing the pigment *melanin* and called *melanocytes*. It does not contain any blood vessels but receives its nourishment from the blood capillaries of the dermis. The deepest cells of the epidermis are known as *basal cells*. The most superficial layer of the epidermis is called the *horny layer*.

The dermis is richly supplied with blood vessels, lymphatic vessels and nerves. It also contains *hair follicles*, *sebaceous glands*, and *sweat glands*, and these structures together with the hair and the nails are sometimes referred to as the **appendages of the skin**.

The skin provides a waterproof protective covering for the body and the pigmentation in the epidermis protects the delicate underlying dermis from excessive ultraviolet radiation. It has functions concerned with the regulation of body temperature and is to some extent concerned with the excretion of water and salts. It is also able to absorb certain oily substances.

The prefix **derm-** and the adjective **cutaneous** mean pertaining to the skin.

The skin is separated from the deeper tissues of the body by the **subcutaneous tissues** composed of connective tissue and containing some of the main fat deposits of the body.

Some General Aspects of Skin Diseases

The branch of medicine concerned with diseases of the skin is known as **dermatology**.

Skin diseases produce effects which in most instances are readily discernible on visual inspection but bacteriological examination is an important procedure in some infective conditions, and biopsy is frequently required in certain cutaneous disorders.

Among the signs and symptoms of skin disorders are: **pruritus** (itching); **erythema** (redness of the skin); **rashes** (eruptions) composed of lesions, referred to as **macules**, **papules**, **vesicles**, or **petechiae** (see under Infectious fevers p 48), **urticaria** (nettle rash); **purpura** (see p 213); ulceration of the skin: crust formation, fissure formation, scarring; areas of skin thickening (such areas are termed **hyperkeratoses** when the thickening is due to overgrowth of the horny layer of the skin); areas of atrophy of the skin; shedding of upper layers of skin epithelium in scales or layers, referred to as **desquamation** or **exfoliation**; localised or diffuse areas of swelling in the skin and subcutaneous tissues; small localised swellings in the skin termed **nodules**; and tumour formation.

There are many primary disorders of the skin and a large variety of diseases of other systems of the body may produce secondary lesions within the skin. It will be possible here to indicate medical terms referring to only a selected number of common or otherwise important skin diseases.

Among the methods of treatment in dermatology are the external application of ointments, creams, lotions, paints, pastes and powders, to the skin; the internal administration of drugs, the giving of injections, the use of medicated baths; surgical procedures including plastic surgery and diathermy; graduated exposures of ultraviolet rays; and radiotherapy.

Radiotherapy is most frequently used in the form of superficial X-rays. It is used in skin carcinomas and, as indicated by Barnes and Rees (1), may be of considerable value in the following benign skin conditions: eczema, contact dermatitis, lichen planus, keloid scars, plantar warts and haemangioma.

Congenital Abnormalities

As a result of errors in development, in rare cases the opening of a congenital sinus or fistula may be present in the skin at birth. Such a condition results from persistence of structures which normally disappear during intrauterine life. Examples are **branchial sinus** and **branchial fistula** in the neck; and **urachal fistula** leading from the urinary bladder to the umbilicus.

Misplaced skin cells may in the course of development result in the formation of cysts in sites such as the neck (**branchial cyst**) or in the region of the outer *canthus* (i.e. the fissure between the eyelids). Such cysts are forms of **dermoid cyst**, the term **dermoid** being applied generally to a cyst lined with squamous epithelium.

Note: an acquired cyst which forms as a result of a fragment of squamous skin epithelium being pushed below the skin by a pentrating injury is called an **implantation dermoid**.

Traumatic Disorders

These include damage to the skin and subcutaneous tissues caused by violence, mechanical irritation, external physical agents and external chemical agents.

A breach in the continuity of the skin caused by violence is termed a **wound**.

Mechanical irritation or pressure as a result of long periods of lying in bed may produce open sores (i.e. breaches in the skin surface, skin ulcers) called **bedsores** or **pressure sores**. Pressure sores may also result from ill–fitting plaster splints and other appliances.

Intermittent pressure over the toes, or less commonly in other sites, may cause a localised thickening in the horny layer of the skin called a **corn**.

Damage to the skin from excessive heat, electric currents, certain chemical agents (e.g. strong acids and alkalies, phosphorous) produces injuries called **burns**. These may be classified as **superficial** (partial skin thickness) and **deep** (full skin thickness) **burns**. In these latter, there may·also be damage to underlying structures such as muscle and bone. Such damage may produce areas of dead tissue, which when they begin to separate off from surrounding tissue are referred to as **sloughs** or **eschars**. The more extensive type of burn is accompanied by considerable loss of blood plasma from damaged capillaries in the burnt area and resultant shock.

A burn caused by steam or hot liquid is called a **scald**.

Infections

These are of considerable variety and include inflammatory disease due to infection with bacteria, viruses, and fungi. Some examples are given below.

Pyogenic infections—as indicated in Part III infection with pus-producing bacteria may cause the following types of infection in the skin and subcutaneous tissues:

  (i) due to staphylococci—**furuncle** (boil), **carbuncle**, **paronychia** (whitlow), **pulp infection** of a finger, **wound infection**;
  (ii) due to streptococci—**cellulitis**, **erysipelas**.

In addition to the above, either staphylococcal or streptococcal infection may cause a contagious infection of the skin called **impetigo contagiosa**. The lesions of this disorder occur most frequently in the skin of the face and scalp in the form of small blisters known as **vesicles** and larger blisters termed **bullae**. These rupture and their contents form thick yellow crusts on the skin surface.

Tuberculosis of the skin—this may occur in the form of (i) **primary tuberculosis of the skin**, which is very rare, (ii) **lupus vulgaris**—an uncommon type of postprimary tuberculosis infection which produces small reddish brown nodules in the skin. These are seen most commonly on the face and neck and tend to heal, producing much scarring. Carcinoma may sometimes develop in an area of lupus. (*Note:* the conditions known as **tuberculides** are not due to actual infection of the skin with tubercle bacilli, but occur as allergic skin reactions to tuberculous infection elsewhere in the body.)

Syphilis—syphilitic infection of the skin may occur in the primary, secondary, or tertiary stages of the disease, and in congenital syphilis. The initial lesion of the disease known as the **primary sore** or **chancre** develops in the skin or a mucous membrane. In most cases it occurs in the external genital organ or in the anal region.

Syphilitic rashes are common in secondary syphilis and in early congenital syphilis. In tertiary syphilis the characteristic lesions known as **gummas** may develop within the skin and cause ulceration.

Gas gangrene—a disorder caused by putrefactive bacteria and usually seen as a result of a wound infection. The infecting organisms cause putrefaction and accompanying gas formation in skin, subcutaneous and muscle tissue. The condition is treated with penicillin or other antibiotics.

Anthrax—an uncommon bacterial disease in which infection is derived from infected animals such as cattle and pigs, or infected animal products such as wool, hides and bristle used in the manufacture of imported shaving brushes.

The word **anthrax** means a carbuncle (see p 54). Infection of the skin with the *bacillus anthracis* causes a lesion resembling a carbuncle and known as a **malignant pustule**, or less commonly a spreading type of infection affecting the skin and subcutaneous tissues and called **anthrax oedema**.

Another type of anthrax infection may affect either the lungs or gastrointestinal tract and is termed **wool sorter's disease**.

Leprosy and **yaws**, see Part V.

Herpes simplex—a virus infection which causes red skin and the formation of vesicles in affected areas. It develops most commonly on the lips (labial herpes) and surrounding skin. It may also occur elsewhere on the skin, and rarely may affect the central nervous system.

(*Note:* **Herpes zoster**, another condition characterised by a vesicular skin eruption, is primarily a disorder of the nervous system and will be referred to later. **Genital herpes** has already been referred to when discussing sexually transmitted diseases.)

Verruca vulgaris (common wart)—**verrucae**, or **warts** of this type are common and are localised overgrowths of epithelium due to a virus infection. They are sometimes classified as benign tumours of the skin. They have a roughened surface and occur chiefly on the hands, forearms, and soles of the feet (**plantar warts**). They are often resistant to treatment but sometimes disappear spontaneously.

Molluscum contagiosum—is a term used to describe another form of wart due to virus infection. In this condition the epithelial overgrowths have a smooth surface.

Ringworm (tinea)—is a term used to describe a group of diseases due to infection of the skin by a number of related fungi called **ringworm fungi**. The commonest members of the group are (i) **tinea capitis** (ringworm of the scalp), (ii) **tinea pedis** (ringworm of the foot)—also known as **epidermophytosis**, or **athlete's foot**, (iii) **tinea cruris** (ringworm of the leg)—also known as **dhobi itch**. (*Note:* dhobi is the Hindu name for a washerman.) This condition usually starts on the inner side of the upper part of the thigh and may spread from there to the skin of the groin, abdomen and genital organs.

Skin eruptions due to infectious fevers—these have been referred to in Part III.

Infestations

These disorders are due to animal parasites that provoke an inflammatory reaction in the skin. They include the following.

Scabies—due to infestation with a form of parasite called a **mite**. The mite which causes this highly contagious disease is called *Sarcoptes scabiei* and its presence in the skin causes severe itching and a rash composed of papules and small vesicles. The name of the disease is derived from a Latin word meaning to scratch.

Pediculosis—pediculus is the Latin word for a louse and this term describes three disorders resulting from infestation with lice. As denoted by their individual names, **pediculosis capititis**, **pediculosis corporis**, and **pediculosis pubis**, the infestation in these disorders affects respectively the head (scalp), body and pubic region.

Benign Neoplasms

Papilloma—a localised overgrowth of skin which consists of an outer covering of epithelium and an inner portion of connective tissue. In external appearance it may resemble a verruca.

Simple melanoma (pigmented mole)—a tumour of cells which produce pigment. A simple melanoma may be present at birth or first appear in adult life. It may, in some instances, undergo malignant change into a **malignant melanoma**.

Lipoma—a tumour which develops from fat cells in the subcutaneous tissue.

Haemangioma (angioma)—a tumour of vascular tissue of which there are several different forms. (*Note:* some authorities classify haemangiomas as benign neoplasms; others regard them as congenital malformations.) The **spider naevus** and the **capillary angioma** are both due to overgrowth of capillaries. The latter is popularly called a birthmark or port-wine stain.

Haemangiomas may also occur in muscles, bones and in the liver and brain. In the uncommon disorder called **Sturge-Weber syndrome** a haemangioma of the face occurs in association with a haemangioma of the brain and meninges of the same side.

Clotting of blood may take place within the vessel walls of haemangiomas. Subsequently calcium salts may be deposited in the clots, producing opacities in radiographs.

Certain types of haemangioma are treated by radiotherapy.

Lymphangioma—a rare tumour of the lymphatic system, which may be found in the skin or subcutaneous tissues or elsewhere. A type which grows in the deep tissues of the neck is called a **cystic hygroma**.

Malignant Neoplasms

Epithelioma (squamous carcinoma)—this is a carcinomatous new growth arising from cells of the epidermis. It may be seen on any part of the skin, but is commonest on the face and lips. It may present as an overgrowth of skin, or as an ulcer.

It is rarely seen before middle age. Chronic irritation is a factor in its causation in many cases, e.g. through exposure to certain types of oil used in industry, and exposure to excessive doses of ionising radiation. It may also develop in any area of extensive scarring, such as may follow old burns, or infection with lupus vulgaris.

The tumour usually grows slowly, but has a tendency to spread to involve deeper structures such as bone. Bone involvement may be demonstrated on radiographs. Spread by lymphatics may be an early or late feature of this disease, but bloodborne metastases are usually seen only in its later stages.

Treatment may be by surgical excision or by radiotherapy.

Rodent ulcer (basal-cell carcinoma)—this condition is also a carcinoma arising in cells of the epidermis. However, whereas an epithelioma originates from cells called *Malphigian cells*, a rodent ulcer is usually a growth of the *basal cells* of the epidermis.

Rodent ulcer is also rare before middle age. It is of slow growth and does not produce metastases. If not successfully treated, however, in the course of time it causes widespread destruction of the skin and deeper tissues. The face is by far the commonest site for its occurrence.

Treatment may be by surgical excision or radiotherapy.

Malignant melanoma—varies greatly in its degree of malignancy. It is a tumour of the pigment-producing cells of the skin or their ancestral cells. It may arise as a result of malignant change in pigmented mole, or alternatively, in an apparently normal area of skin. It may also originate within the eye.

Lymphatic and bloodborne metastases are sometimes early features of a malignant melanoma. Such metastases are commonly seen in lymph glands, lungs and liver, and not infrequently in bone.

Metastases—metastatic growths from primary carcinomas of other organs (e.g. breast) are sometimes found in the skin.

Kaposi's sarcoma—an uncommon neoplasm, believed to arise from blood vessels, and sometimes occurring in association with acquired immune deficiency syndrome (AIDS).

Urticaria (Nettle rash)

This term describes a type of inflammatory reaction which occurs in skin as a manifestation of allergy (hypersensitivity) to various agents. The reaction may be localised or generalised and is evidenced by the presence in the skin of areas of erythema, which cause itching and which often develop into wheals.

The name **urticaria** derives from the Latin word for a nettle and the condition may result from nettle stings, insect bites, eating certain protein foods and drugs, and the administration of iodine-containing radiographic contrast media, etc.

A type of urticaria of unknown causation, called **papular urticaria** is of common occurrence in childhood and is popularly referred to as heat spots. It is usually provoked by insect bites.

Eczema and Dermatitis

The term eczema is used to indicate a number of skin diseases which exhibit a special type of cutaneous inflammation called the **eczema reaction**. In most cases this reaction appears to be a manifestation of skin allergy.

In allergic or otherwise predisposed subjects, the eczema reaction may result from agents which reach the skin (i) from the exterior, e.g. the external application of certain drugs such as penicillin, and chemicals, certain chemical dyes and detergents and photographic chemicals, contact with certain plants (e.g. primulas), exposure to sunlight, (ii) via the bloodstream, e.g. ingested proteins.

Terms referring to different forms of eczema include the following: **contact eczema**, **infective eczema**, **infantile eczema**.

Eczema may present in acute or chronic form and among the clinical features produced by the eczema reaction are erythema, itching, the formation of vesicles and sometimes bullae, weeping (i.e. exudation of fluid from the skin lesions), crust formation and the development of areas of skin thickening.

Some authorities have classified eczema as a form of dermatitis. The term **dermatitis** when used in its widest sense may be employed to indicate any form of inflammation of the skin. Other authorities have used the term in a more restricted sense and differentiated between eczema and conditions which may be described as forms of dermatitis.

Some individual disorders described as dermatitis are **dermatitis herpetiformis**, **radiation dermatitis** (produced by ionising radiation), **contact dermatitis** (due to direct contact of irritant substances with the skin) and **neurodermatitis** (an eczematous condition in which psychological factors are thought to play a role), **light dermatitis, traumatic dermatitis**.

The description of **industrial dermatitis** is applied to certain non-infective types of cutaneous inflammation arising as a result of the patient's occupation.

The term **generalised exfoliative dermatitis** describes a condition in which there is shedding of the superficial layers of the skin over large areas of the body (shedding of the superficial layers of the skin is known as **exfoliation** or **desquamation**). It may develop as during the course of other skin disorders when these occur in generalised form (e.g. psoriasis, eczema, drug eruptions); as a complication of Hodgkin's disease or leukaemia; or may arise from unknown causes.

Some Other Skin Diseases

Psoriasis—the name of this inflammatory disorder means itching. It is a common disease of unknown origin and chronic course. The characteristic lesions consist of red papules covered by white scales. They may occur in any part of the skin, but are commonest over the knees and elbows and in the scalp. In older patients there is not infrequently an accompanying arthritis (inflammation of joints) referred to as **psoriatic arthritis**.

Chilblains (erythema pernio)—these are inflammatory lesions and represent an abnormal response to cold in affected areas of skin. They are due to the action of cold on the capillaries in sites such as the fingers and toes, heels, lobes of the ears, and tip of the nose.

Cutaneous sarcoidosis—sarcoidosis is a chronic inflammatory disease of unknown origin. Its lesions bear a similarity to those seen as a result of chronic tuberculosis. They occur most frequently in sites such as the skin, lungs, hilar glands and other lymph glands, bone, the eye and the parotid gland. In many instances they resolve without causing serious cellular damage; in others, however, they result in extensive fibrosis.

In bone, sarcoid lesions occur most commonly in the phalanges producing a condition known as **osteitis multiplex cystoides**. A combination of eye lesions and lesions in the parotid glands constitutes the condition called **uveoparotitis**. (*Note:* the *uveal tract* includes the iris diaphragm, ciliary body and choroid coat of the eye.)

In the skin, sarcoidosis may produce a nodular condition called **Boeck's sarcoid** or more rarely a condition called **lupus pernio** which affects the cheeks and nose.

Erythema nodosum (see below) may also develop in patients with sarcoidosis.

Drug eruptions (drug rashes)—this term is used to indicate skin rashes which develop as a result of the internal administration of certain drugs. It does not include eczema or dermatitis caused by the external application of drugs to the skin.

Percival (2) states that drug eruptions are examples of allergy but that 'the allergic processes involved in urticaria, eczema and drug rashes, differ basically from one another'.

Among the drugs which may cause eruptions are penicillin, sulphonamides, bromides and iodides.

Erythema Nodosum—a condition in which, as indicated by its name, tender reddish rounded areas of thickening appear in the skin, usually on the shins but sometimes on the forearms. There are usually only a few lesions.

In many cases this disease appears to be an allergic response to primary tuberculous infection or streptococcal infection elsewhere in the body. Erythema nodosum may also follow the taking of certain drugs and is quite often seen in patients with sarcoidosis.

Pemphigus—this word means a blister and is used to denote a group of uncommon diseases, of unknown origin, which are characterised by rashes in which the essential feature is the formation of bullae (i.e. fluid-containing blisters, larger than vesicles). The condition called **pemphigus vulgaris** is the least uncommon member of this group.

Angioneurotic oedema—is a rare condition which can affect both the skin and mucous membranes. It is of rapid onset and produces marked oedematous swelling of affected tissues, as a result of excessive leakage of fluid from the blood capillaries therein. It occurs most commonly in the region of the mouth and face. It can affect the throat and larynx and in severe cases the swelling may cause a degree of respiratory obstruction that necessitates tracheostomy.

Angioneurotic oedema is a disorder of unknown causation but can occur very rarely as a manifestation of sensitivity to iodine-containing radiographic contrast media.

Ichthyosis—a condition of abnormal dryness of the skin. Areas of the skin surface may present an appearance resembling those of fish scales and the name of the disease derives from the Greek word meaning a fish.

Dupuytren's contracture—a disorder in which thickened bands of fibrous tissue develop in the subcutaneous tissues of the palm and produce flexion deformities of fingers; usually the middle and ring fingers.

Pityriasis rosea—a self limiting conditon, of unknown origin, in which a maculopapular irritant rash develops over the trunk and upper parts of the extremities.

Lichen planus—lichen is a form of moss, and the word is also used as a name for several skin diseases, characterised by small firm papular eruptions. Lichen planus is one such disease in which the papules have a violet tinge and are irritant. Lesions may also develop in the mouth. The cause is unknown.

Some Disorders of the Skin Appendages

Acne vulgaris—is a common disorder in adolescents of both sexes but occurs more frequently in males. It is associated with **seborrhoea**, i.e. increased secretion of *sebum*, the oily secretion of the sebaceous glands which lubricates the skin and the hairs. (Seborrhoea is associated with other disorders besides acne, e.g. dandruff of the scalp, seborrhoeic dermatitis.)

Endocrine factors appear to play some part in the causation of acne and it seems to be aggravated in some individuals by certain foodstuffs.

In acne, lesions called **blackheads** or **comedones** form in the openings of the hair follicles, blocking these latter structures and causing a surrounding inflammatory reaction which results in the formation of red papules. Secondary infection of the follicles with staphylococci occurs and causes many of the papules to develop into pustules.

The lesions of acne occur mainly in the skin of the face, neck and upper part of the back. They tend to disappear spontaneously during early adult life.

Frequent skin cleaning; local applications, often containing sulphur; ultra-violet radiation; dietary measures; and oral antibiotics are measures commonly employed in treatment. Oestrogens are sometimes used to treat female patients.

Alopecia—this term means baldness, i.e. absence of hair from the scalp.

Diffuse baldness may be associated with seborrhoea or may follow severe infection, injuries or operations.

Localised areas of baldness may develop as a result of disease or injuries to the scalp or treatment with X-rays. They may also occur in a condition of unknown origin called **alopecia areata**.

Prickly heat (miliaria)—is a disorder in which blockage of sweat glands results in the development of an irritating skin rash. It is predominantly a disease of hot climates.

Acne rosacea—a conditon in which hyperaemia of the forehead and face is associated with overactivity and hypertrophy of sebaceous glands. Capillary dilatation results in marked reddening of the skin in affected sites.

REFERENCES

(1) Barnes, P. A., Rees, D. J. (1972). *A Concise Textbook of Radiotherapy*. London: Faber and Faber.
(2) Percival, G. H. (1967). *An Introduction to Dermatology*. Edinburgh: Churchill Livingstone.

LOCOMOTOR SYSTEM

The *bones* and *joints* together with the *skeletal muscles* and their *tendons* and *aponeuroses* constitute the **locomotor system**. As indicated by its name this system is concerned with movement (i.e. **locomotion** means movement from one place to another).

The bones are sometimes referred to as constituting the **skeletal system** and the joints as constituting the **articulatory system**.

Also connected with the locomotor system are certain of the structures called *bursae* (see later).

Some Anatomical and Physiological Considerations
Osteoporosis and Osteomalacia

Bones are structures composed of specialised connective tissue and are of four principal types: *flat bones* (e.g. skull vault), *irregular bones* (e.g. vertebrae), *long bones* (e.g. femora) and *short bones* (e.g. phalanges).

Individual bones when fully developed possess the following.
  (i) An investing membrane—the *periosteum*. This surrounds the bone except in such areas where bony surfaces entering into the formation of joints have a protective covering of *articular cartilage*.
     The periosteum consists of an outer layer of fibrous tissue and an inner layer, containing cells called *osteoblasts*, which readily lay down new bone if it is injured or affected by certain disease processes (e.g. infection; neoplastic disease).
 (ii) A complete outer shell of bone tissue of the type called compact or cortical bone—the *cortex*.
(iii) An inner portion composed of bone tissue of the type called cancellous or spongy bone—the *medulla*.

In long bones there is a hollow space in the middle of the medulla. This is called the *medullary cavity* and is lined by a fibrous membrane called the *endosteum*.

Compact bone consists of tightly packed layers of bony tissue within which are spaces containing blood vessels and nerves. Cancellous bone contains numerous plates of bony tissue, which are called *bone trabeculae* and are arranged in such a manner as to produce a sponge-like appearance. Between the trabeculae are spaces called *marrow spaces* which contain soft tissue known as *bone marrow*.

Bone marrow is of two types (i) *yellow marrow*, which consists mainly of fat; and (ii) *red marrow* which is very vascular and contains cells which form red blood corpuscles, granulocytic leucocytes and blood platelets.

It also contains a certain amount of lymphoreticular tissue and produces the white blood cells called monocytes, which are members of the mononuclear phagocyte system, and migrate into the tissues where they are termed macrophages or histiocytes.

In childhood red marrow is found in all bones, but in the adult it is limited chiefly to the vertebrae, sternum, ribs, skull and pelvic bones, and upper ends of the humeri and femora.

During fetal life bones are preformed in either *cartilage* (another type of specialised connective tissue, referred to in lay language as gristle), or a type of fibrous connective tissue called *membrane*. The processes of bone formation are referred to collectively as **ossification** or **osteogenesis**, and according to the type of tissue in which it originates, bone formation may take the form of **ossification-in-cartilage** (e.g. as in bones of the limbs) or **ossification-in-membrane** (e.g. as in the bones of the skull vault and clavicle).

Ossification in the great majority of bones begins in fetal life but in some (e.g. the carpal bones and some of the tarsal bones), it starts in childhood. The site, or sites, at which bone form commences within a developing bone are called *primary centres of ossification*. Some bones during their period of growth also develop *secondary centres of ossification*. These are generally all referred to as *epiphyses*, although certain of them (i.e. those which do not enter into the formation of joints) are more strictly termed *apophyses*.

During the formation of bone tissue, cells called *osteoblasts* lay down *osteoid tissue* which possesses an abundant intercellular substance called *matrix* (**osteoid** means bone-like and **matrix** a mould). This latter contains large amounts of a protein substance called *collagen*, which is an important constituent of all forms of connective tissue.

Osteoid tissue is converted into *bone tissue* proper by the deposition in the matrix of calcium salts from the bloodstream (mainly in the form of calcium phosphate) and matrix is then often referred to as *calcified matrix*. It is this process of calcification that gives bone tissue its characteristic rigidity.

The cells of fully formed bone are known as *osteocytes*. During the processes of bone formation, other cells called *osteoclasts*, which belong to the phagocytic system and have the ability to remove bone, model the newly formed bone tissue to its required shape. (*Note:* the removal of tissue or secreted substances by normal physiological processes, and also by pathological processes, is termed **resorption**.)

Osteogenesis does not cease when growth of the bony skeleton is complete. *The activities of osteoblasts and osteoclasts continue throughout life and all bone tissue is subject to a continual process of absorption of old bone and its replacement by newly formed bone.*

In early adult life and middle age the processes of bone production and bone replacement are exactly counterbalanced but with the onset of old age, the formation of new bone tissue decreases.

An upset in the processes of normal ossification may lead to two developments.

(i) **Osteoporosis**—a condition in which affected bones contain less bone tissue than do normal bones, and consequently less calcium than normal. They are thus more brittle, fracture more easily, and show a diminished density on X-ray films.

Osteoporosis may be either generalised or localised, and its development may result from either diminished bone formation or increased bone resorption.

Factors which operate in the causation of generalised osteoporosis include: normal ageing—**age osteoporosis** (senile osteoporosis, idiopathic osteoporosis); diminished ovarian activity—**postmenopausal osteoporosis**; other endocrine disorders (e.g. hyperparathyroidism) and hormone therapy (e.g. steroid therapy); protein deficiency, vitamin C deficiency (e.g. scurvy).

Localised osteoporosis may result from diminished mobility of a part of the body—**disuse osteoporosis**; certain infections (notably tuberculosis of bones and joints); and in association with neoplasms affecting bone.

Changes due to osteoporosis and osteomalacia may coexist in the same patient.

(ii) **Osteomalacia** (adult rickets)—a generalised disorder of ossification the name of which means softening of bone, and similar in nature and cause to the disorder of infancy and childhood called **rickets**.

As stated by Govan *et al* (1) the essential defect in both osteomalacia and rickets is 'failure of calcification of newly formed osteoid tissue, caused by vitamin D deficiency'.

Vitamin D controls the absorption of calcium and phosphorus from the small intestine and the utilisation of these substances by the body, and is also concerned with excretion of phosphates by the kidneys.

Deficiency of vitamin D is usually due to an inadequate diet, but lack of exposure of the skin to sunlight, malabsorption of the vitamin from the small intestine, and certain renal disorders (e.g. chronic renal failure) may also be factors in such deficiency.

The deficient calcification of osteomalacic and rachitic bones makes them less rigid than normal and may therefore result in the development of marked skeletal deformities, particularly in weight-bearing bones.

Osteomalacia and rickets will also be referred to further when discussing metabolic diseases of bone.

Joints (articulations) are formed whenever two or more bones come into contact. The opposing bone ends may be connected by fibrous tissue (e.g. sutural joints of skull), or cartilage (e.g. symphysis pubis). In most joints of the body, however, the bone ends are covered in *articular cartilage* and separated from each other by a joint cavity containing *synovial fluid*. This fluid is formed by the *synovial membrane* that lines the *joint capsule* surrounding the joint. The joint capsule is strengthened by *supporting ligaments* composed of connective tissue. Joints of this type are called *synovial joints* (e.g. shoulder, hip).

The skeletal muscles are all composed of muscle tissue of the type called *voluntary* (*striated*) *muscle*. (*Note:* the other two types of muscle tissue found in the body are known as *involuntary*, *smooth* or *non-striated muscle*, and *cardiac muscle*.)

These muscles are attached to bones by bands of dense white fibrous tissue called *tendons*, or sometimes by sheets of white fibrous tissue called *aponeuroses*. The fleshy part of a muscle is referred to as its *belly*. Tendons in certain sites possess *synovial sheaths* which contain *synovial fluid* between their inner and outer layers.

The skeletal muscles are all surrounded by coverings of fibrous connective tissue called *deep fascia*, and lie beneath the *superficial fascia*, a layer of fibrous tissue which is found immediately below the skin.

All forms of muscle tissue possess powers of contraction, which are subject to the control of the nervous system and are thereby able to effect movement of joints.

Bursae—these are small synovial fluid-containing sacs which lie between certain structures and facilitate their movements, e.g. between a tendon and a bone, a bone and overlying skin, or between two muscles. As they are related to the skeletal system, it is convenient to refer later in this section to disease conditions affecting certain of the bursae.

The prefix **osteo-** means pertaining to bone; **chondro-**, pertaining to cartilage; **artho-**, pertaining to joints; and **myo-**, pertaining to muscle.

General Aspects of Diseases of Bones and Joints

Bones may be the subject of congenital disorders, traumatic disorders, infective diseases, neoplasms, and cyst formation. They may also be affected by metabolic diseases, chemical poisons, endocrine and idiopathic diseases.

Many diseases of bone produce secondary effects on neighbouring joints. There are also a number of important primary diseases of joints, among which are certain congenital, traumatic, inflammatory and degenerative conditions.

Bone and joint diseases may give rise to clinical features such as pain, deformity, limitation of movement, bony swelling, soft tissue swelling, secondary wasting of muscles.

X-ray investigation is of great value in the diagnosis and in assessing the response to treatment of many types of bone and joint disease and injury. Bone scanning, using strontium and other radioisotopes is being increasingly employed for the detection of carcinomatous metastases in bone.

Pathological examination (e.g. by bacteriological methods, biopsy, estimation of serum phosphatase levels) is required in several different forms of bone and joint disorder.

Many diseases of the bones and joints, and also of the muscles and tendons, fall within the scope of the orthopaedic surgeon, particularly traumatic diseases (i.e. injuries) and deformities.

The word **orthopaedics** derives from the Greek for straight and child and thus indicates one of the main concerns of this branch of medicine, namely the correction of deformities in children.

The orthopaedic surgeon is concerned both with operative and non-operative treatment. Adams (2) describing non-operative methods of treatment in orthopaedic disorders lists 'rest, support, physiotherapy, local injections, drugs, manipulation and radiotherapy'.

Appliances known as **orthopaedic braces**, or **orthoses**, are widely employed in orthopaedic practice for straightening distorted parts, or as a means of support, and those who are expert in their construction and fitting are termed **orthotists**.

A recently developed technique in orthopaedics is the introduction of a fine telescope into the knee joint and direct inspection of its interior, a procedure called **arthroscopy**.

The work of physiotherapists, occupational therapists and remedial gymnasts frequently plays a very important part in the treatment and rehabilitation of patients suffering from injuries and diseases of the bones, joints and muscles. (*Note:* **rehabilitation** means the process of rendering a disabled person both mentally and physically fit to resume some form of occupation.)

Congenital Abnormalities of Bones and Joints

Congenital abnormalities of the bones and joints are of considerable variety. They range from small isolated developmental errors, affecting a single bone, to gross changes which may be widespread throughout the skeleton. Structural abnormalities are found in some of these disorders unassociated with any upset in the normal processes of ossification, e.g. in polydactyly extra digits are found and these may be normally ossified. In other types, some of which are described as skeletal **dysplasias** and others as skeletal **dystrophies** and as **dysostoses**, there are abnormalities of osteogenesis (bone formation).

Jacobs (3) indicates that some congenital abnormalities are associated with **arthrogryposis multiplex congenita** a lesion characterised by 'congenital failure of muscle development and joint lesions such as club foot, club hand, congenital dislocation of the hip and congenital genu recurvatum.'

Both the nomenclature and the systems of classification used in the description of these disorders are complex and reference here will only be made to some of the commoner, or more interesting, forms of congenital lesions of the skeletal and articulatory systems.

Cervical rib—is an accessory rib and may be formed on one or both sides of the body, articulating with the seventh cervical vertebra. A cervical rib is generally symptomless but, in some instances, may cause pain and disability through pressure on the lowest trunk of the brachial nervous plexus or subclavian artery; thus giving rise to symptoms of **thoracic inlet compression**. Surgical excision of the accessory rib may then be necessary.

Spondylolisis—is an abnormality, thought usually to be congenital but sometimes acquired through injury, in which an affected vertebra has a gap in one or both sides of its posterior arch. The condition is usually confined to a single vertebra—usually the fifth lumbar but sometimes the fourth lumbar vertebra. The importance of this condition is that its presence may result in a forward slipping of the affected vertebra, carrying with it all the spinal vertebrae which lie above. The condition is then referred to as **spondylolisthesis**, i.e. **spondyle**—a vertebra, **listhesis**—slipping.

Spina bifida—is a congenital abnormality in which the two halves of the posterior arch of one or more spinal vertebrae fail to unite. They are thus divided by a cleft, i.e. they are bifid.

If the resultant gap in the posterior arch is large the spinal meninges may protrude through it constituting a **meningocele**, or there may be a protrusion of both meninges and spinal cord, when the condition is called a **meningomyelocele**. Such protrusions are evidenced by a soft-tissue swelling of variable size in the mid-line of the back and over such a swelling the skin may be stretched and thin, and the meninges imperfectly formed.

The underlying spinal cord may also be the subject of developmental abnormality of varying degree. As the cord is developed from the embryonic neural tube, such abnormality may be referred to as **neural tube defect** and may be responsible for various forms of paralysis, and sometimes necessitate operative treatment within the first 24 hours after birth.

Neural tube defect may be predicted by increased amounts of alphafetoprotein in a sample of amniotic fluid obtained by amniocentesis; and it may be possible to demonstrate severe degrees of spina bifida by ultrasound.

The simplest form of spina bifida is often symptomless and not associated with any protrusion of the contents of the spinal cord and is referred to as **spina bifida occulta**; the word **occulta** meaning hidden.

Congenital dislocation of the hip—a **dislocation** is a displacement of bone surfaces which form a joint. In this condition, in addition to dislocation or subluxation (see p 246) of the hip joint on one or both sides, there is usually defective development of the upper part of the acetabulum. Many authorities regard this latter feature as the basis of the disorder and the displacement of the femoral head as secondary to the malformation of the acetabulum, but the cause of the disorder is incompletely understood.

Congenital dislocation of the hip is much commoner in girls than boys.

Early diagnosis is of prime importance in this condition and a simple clinical test can be used to detect the presence of dislocation, or of a predisposition to dislocation, in newborn babies. X-ray examination is used to confirm the diagnosis and in the control of the treatment.

In most cases treatment is by closed reduction and splinting. Some, however, may need an operation.

Achondroplasia—the name of this disease derives from its being due to defective growth (aplasia) of bones that are preformed in cartilage (chondro–meaning pertaining to cartilage). Thus **achondroplasiacs**, i.e. individuals affected with achondroplasia, have abnormally short arms and legs and small skull bases; while the bones of their skull vaults, which are ossified in membrane, grow to a normal size. Their intelligence is normal and their muscular development is usually strong. Many of the dwarfs seen in circuses are achondroplasiacs.

Related to achondroplasia are two other types of congenital bone dysplasia called **Morquio's disease** (chondro–osteodystrophy) and **gargoylism** (Hurler's syndrome). Both these disorders are rare. The latter is associated with disordered metabolism of fat-like substances called lipids.

Osteogenesis imperfecta—this uncommon disease affects the whole skeleton. Owing to defective bone formation, the bones are abnormally fragile and fracture easily when subjected to mild trauma. The liability to fracture may develop in fetal life, or may not occur until early or late childhood. In the course of time the disorder shows a tendency towards spontaneous cure.

Many patients with osteogenesis imperfecta have an intense blue colour of the sclerotic coats of their eyes and may develop deafness in early adult life, due to a condition called otosclerosis.

It is important to distinguish between fractures due to osteogenesis imperfecta and those produced by non-accidental injury (NAI).

Some other congenital abnormalities—these include the following.

- **Arachnodactyly** (spider digits)—in this condition, the fingers, and sometimes the toes, are of abnormal length. In a disorder called **Marfan's syndrome** arachnodactyly occurs in association with congenital heart disease and dislocation of the lenses of the eyes.

● **Cleidocranial dysostosis**—a condition in which defects of ossification occur in the clavicles and skull.

● **Congenital coxa vara**—**coxa** is the Latin term for the hip joint and in this disorder the hip joint is the subject of a **varus deformity**, i.e. a deformity in which the angle between the neck and shaft of the femur is reduced so as to approach a right angle. Varus deformity of the hip joint may be due to causes other than congenital abnormality, e.g. slipping of the femoral head epiphysis (adolescent coxa vara), fracture of the femoral neck in old age.

● **Congenital pes cavus**—congenital claw foot (**pes** means foot).

● **Congenital pes planus**—congenital flat foot. This condition may occur together with **congenital vertical talus**.

● **Congenital talipes equinovarus**—a type of congenital club foot. **Talipes** means club foot and the term **equinovarus** indicates that the foot is both turned inwards (**varus**) and that the anterior part of the foot is dropped with raising of the heel (**equinus**—so called by comparison with a horse's hoof).

● **Congenital torticollis**—congenital wryneck.

● **Hemivertebra**—a condition of failure of development of half of a vertebral body. It is one of the causes of **congenital scoliosis** (lateral curvature of the spine).

● **Craniostenosis**—this is a rare disorder of ossification-in-membrane affecting the bones of the skull vault. It leads to premature fusion of one or more of the sutures which separate these latter bones and consequent deformity of the skull. Such deformity may take various forms according to the suture or sutures involved. The least uncommon variety is known as **oxycephaly** (tower skull). (*Note:* the sutures of the skull vault normally begin to fuse at about 15 years of age.)

● **Hereditary multiple exostoses** (diaphyseal aclasia)—a conditon in which multiple small outgrowths called **exostoses** arise from the growing ends of bones which are preformed in cartilage. The outgrowths are composed of bone with caps of cartilage and are benign tumours of the type called **osteochondromata**.

● **Hypertelorism**—a deformity of the base of the skull resulting in a greatly widened space between the orbits.

● **Osteopetrosis** (Albers–Schönberg disease, marble bones)—an uncommon generalised disease in which affected bones show a greatly increased density on radiographs.

● **Polydactyly**—the presence of extra digits (i.e. fingers or toes).

● **Sacralisation**—a condition of partial or, less commonly, complete fusion between the lowest lumbar vertebra and the first sacral vertebra.

- **Sprengel's shoulder**—congenitally raised scapula.
- **Syndactyly**—web-fingers or web-toes, with which may be associated bony fusion in the affected digits.
- **Amelia** (absent limbs) and **phocomelia** (rudimentary limbs)—two severe forms of developmental error. These two types of malformation were common in offspring of women who had taken the drug thalidomide as a sedative or tranquilliser during pregnancy.
- **Skeletal malformations associated** with **diseases of genetic origin** (see p 319).

Traumatic Disorders of Bones and Joints

These may take the form of fractures of bones, dislocations or sprains of joints, and subperiosteal haematomas.

Fractures—a **fracture** is a break in the continuity of a bone, which usually results from a severe degree of direct or indirect injury, or sometimes from violent muscular contraction (e.g. as in some fractures of the patella and ribs). Rarely, a fracture may occur as a result of repeated minor injuries producing a so-called **stress fracture** (fatigue fracture). The commonest site for a stress fracture is in the shaft of a metatarsal, when it is referred to as a **march fracture**.

A fracture may also occur, with or without violence, through an area of bone weakened by disease, and is then termed a **pathological fracture**. Carcinomatous secondary deposits in bone are a common cause of pathological fracture.

Multiple fractures are a common feature of the so-called **battered baby syndrome** which may be seen in babies and small children as a result of injury inflicted by a parent or guardian. This condition is also termed **non-accidental injury** and denoted by the initials **NAI**.

Fractures are of two main types: (*a*) **simple** (closed)—where no wound connects the fracture site and the surface of the body; and (*b*) **compound** (open)—where there is an external wound which leads down to the fracture site.

Simple or compound fractures may be descibed as **complicated fractures** when associated with injury to nerves, important blood vessels or internal organs, or **comminuted fractures**, when the bone is broken into several fragments.

(*Note:* in all fractures there is injury to small blood vessels with consequent swelling and bruising of adjacent soft tissue.)

Fractures are generally named according to their site, e.g. fracture of neck of the femur. Some, however, are named after surgeons:

Bennett's fracture—a fracture of the base of the first metacarpal, involving its lower articular surface and showing outward displacement of the distal fragment.

Colles' fracture—a fracture of the lower end of the radius about half to one inch above the wrist joint, with outward and backward displacement of the lower fragment. There is often an accompanying fracture of the ulnar styloid process.

Smith's fracture—is often called a reversed Colles. It is a fracture of the lower end of the radius with forward displacement of the lower fragment.

Pott's fracture—this term is nowadays generally used to indicate a variety of fractures, which involve the lower ends of the tibia and fibula in the region of the ankle joint.

Guérin's fracture—a fracture of the maxilla with detachment of the tooth-bearing segment. The injury is usually bilateral.

Clinically, fractures may be evidenced by pain and tenderness over the fracture site, swelling and interference with normal function. If the fracture has caused displacement of the fractured bone ends, there may be visible or palpable deformity. Shock of neurogenic type is also a common associated feature, its degree varying with the severity of the injury.

Radiological examination plays an essential role in the diagnosis of suspected fractures and often in the control of treatment when the diagnosis has been established.

Fracture treatment includes considerations about first aid and the treatment of associated shock, wounds and complications, besides treatment of the injured bone or bones. In most types of fracture the latter consists basically of (i) correcting, as far as possible, any displacement of the fractured bone ends. This is called **reduction** (setting of the fracture). **Closed reduction** consists of manipulative procedures or exerting gradual **traction** to reduce the fracture, i.e. by exerting a pull on the skin (**skin traction**) or on a pin inserted into bone (**skeletal traction**). **Open reduction** involves carrying out a surgical operation to set a fracture; (ii) preventing movement between the fractured bone ends until they are firmly joined together by new bone. This is termed **immobilisation** and may be effected by the use of plaster of Paris splints or casts, metal splints, etc. or after an open reduction by various **internal fixation** methods such as **screwing**, **plateing**, **nailing**, **pinning**, **wiring**, or **bone grafting**; (iii) preserving the function of muscles and joints in the vicinity of the fracture. (*Note:* reduction is not possible in every type of fracture, and it is to be noted that early movements are prescribed for some comminuted fractures. It is also to be noted that in some fractures of the femoral neck in elderly patients reduction is not attempted but the primary treatment is arthroplasty with insertion of a **prosthesis** see p 267).

Fractures heal by production of new bone and, firstly, a rudimentary type of new bone, called **callus** is laid down between the fragments and joins them together. Callus is at first soft but gradually becomes harder. When it is sufficiently hard to prevent any movement between the fragments, union of the fracture is said to have taken place. Callus is gradually converted into mature bone and, when this process is complete, **consolidation** of the fracture is said to have occured.

Fractures, owing to a variety of causes, (e.g. inadequate immobilisation or infection) may be subject to **delayed union**, or to **non-union** with the formation of a **false joint** between fracture bone ends that have not united.

One cause of non-union is known as **avascular necrosis**, a term indicating death of cells in a localised area through loss of their blood supply. This condition is seen when an injury causing a fracture is such as to deprive one of the fragments of the injured bone of an adequate blood supply. This complication occurs most commonly in fractures of the femoral neck and carpal scaphoid. Avascular necrosis also occurs in osteochondritis, after renal transplantation, as a complication of steroid therapy, and in caisson disease. Alternative names for this condition are **avascular osteonecrosis** and **aseptic necrosis**.

Dislocations—a dislocation is a condition of displacement of the ends of bones which form a joint. If the displacement is such that the articular surfaces of these bones retain some degree of contact, the dislocation is described as being **incomplete**, or as a **subluxation**.

Most dislocations result from severe trauma but they can be due to congenital malformation (e.g. congenital dislocation of the hip) or, as in the case of **pathological dislocation**, they may result from disease of a joint or its motor muscles.

Sprains—sprain is a term used to describe a soft tissue injury due to the tearing of the ligaments or articular capsule of a joint.

Traumatic damage to a joint capsule may result in the secretion of excess synovial fluid into a joint, a condition referred to as a synovial effusion or **traumatic synovitis**.

Subperiosteal haematomas—an injury insufficient to cause a fracture may sometimes result in the formation of a haematoma (i.e. a swelling due to a localised collection of blood) beneath the periosteum in the affected part of a bone. Subsequently, calcification or ossification may occur in the swelling.

Minor injury to the skull during labour may result in the formation of a collection of extravasted blood below the *pericranium* (i.e. the periosteum covering the skull) and thus the presence of a palpable swelling beneath the scalp of a newborn infant. Such a swelling is called a **cephalhaematoma** and frequently shows pathological calcification before ultimately resolving.

An **ossifying subperiosteal haematoma** may produce appearances on an X-ray film very similar to those of malignant bone tumour called an osteogenic sarcoma.

Internal derangement of the knee joint (IDK)—is a term used to describe several injuries to the knee joint including sprains due to tearing of the capsule of the knee joint or its collateral ligaments, tearing of the cruciate ligaments within the joint, and tears of the external or internal semilunar cartilages (menisci). Tears of the latter structures are commonly referred to as **torn cartilage** and are especially common in footballers and others who follow athletic pursuits. Arthroscopy and arthrography are both widely used in the diagnosis of IDK.

Infections of Bones and Joints

Infective micro-organisms may invade the soft tissues of the bone marrow causing an inflammatory reaction in these tissues termed **osteomyelitis**. They may also cause inflammation of the periosteum producing **periostitis**. Both these conditions are forms of **osteitis**, a comprehensive term indicating the presence of inflammation in any part of a bone.

In some types of bone infection thrombosis of blood vessels in the affected area may result in fragments of bone undergoing necrosis, through loss of their blood supply. Such dead fragments of bone are called **sequestra** (singular: **sequestrum**). Death of a localised area of bone is called **osteonecrosis**.

When an infective lesion in a bone is situated near a joint, secondary joint infection may result in **infective arthritis** (joint inflammation). Infective arthritis can also start primarily in the synovial membrane of a joint and then develop a secondary spread into adjacent bone.

If a joint infection leads to much destruction of articular cartilage, a common sequel is **ankylosis**, i.e. union of the opposing joint surfaces by fibrous tissue (**fibrous ankylosis**) or by newly formed bone (**bony ankylosis**).

Inflammatory changes in bone may be either acute or chronic. They may result in stimulation of osteoblasts and consequent new bone formation in the cortex of an affected bone and also in its periosteum; or stimulation of osteoclasts with bone destruction in both cortex and medulla. Frequently a combination of both these types of reaction is produced.

New bone formation produces increased bone density on radiographs, and bone destruction results in decreased radiographic density. Such changes are often described as producing, respectively, appearances of **bony sclerosis** and **osteolysis**—although the true meaning of the term sclerosis is hardening.

A combination of new bone formation and bone destruction, together with periosteal bone formation also occurs in conditions other than infections, e.g. malignant neoplasms of bone.

Infection of bones and joints may be (i) haematogenous (i.e. blood-borne), the micro-organisms being carried in the blood from a focus of infection elsewhere in the body; (ii) by direct spread from a focus of infection in nearby tissues; or (iii) via the wound of a compound fracture or a penetrating missile injury.

Some important types of infections of bones and joints are given below.

Acute osteomyelitis (acute suppurative osteomyelitis, acute pyogenic osteomyelitis)—this is an acute suppurative infection of bone usually beginning in the marrow spaces in the medulla but frequently spreading to involve cortical bone and periosteum.

The disease is commoner in children than in adults. It can affect any bone in the body but occurs most frequently in the metaphysis of a long bone, i.e. in the end of the diaphysis just below the epiphyseal plate.

The causal micro-organism is usually a staphylococcus but some cases of osteomyelitis are due to streptococci or other pyogenic (pus-producing) micro-organisms. In most cases infection is haematogenous (bloodborne) from some other infective focus within the body, e.g. a boil in the skin.

The diagnosis is made on clinical grounds in the first instance. Radiographic changes of bone destruction and reactive periostitis do not appear until about seven or more days after the onset of infection and are thus of no value in early diagnosis.

Treatment consists initially of injection of large doses of penicillin or other antibiotics, sometimes followed by surgical measures to release pus from the affected areas of bone.

Sometimes the infection leads to chronic osteomyelitis. Complications include metastatic (secondary) infections in other bones and other tissues, septicaemia, and the formation of infective sinuses which discharge on the skin surface. Sinus formation is associated with the presence of sequestra in the area of bone infection.

Chronic osteomyelitis—chronic infection of bone may occur in the form of a low-grade infection which is of chronic nature from its onset, or as a sequel to an acute osteomyelitis which has failed to resolve. The inflammatory changes in this condition may be diffuse or localised. One form of chronic osteomyelitis occurs in the form of a localised abscess cavity, often containing a small central sequestrum and known as a **Brodie's abscess**.

Acute suppurative arthritis—this is a disease in which pus is formed within a joint either as a result of infection of its synovial membrane by bloodborne pyogenic micro-organisms, spread of infection into a joint from an adjacent area of osteomyelitis, or direct infection of a joint by a penetrating wound.

As with acute osteomyelitis, the commonest causal organism of the condition is the staphylococcus.

Acute suppurative arthritis may lead to bony ankylosis or to **chronic suppurative arthritis**, which may be associated with the formation of infective sinuses, leading from the infected joint to the skin surface.

Tuberculous infections of bones and joints—these are metastatic forms of tuberculosis (see p 55) and produce a chronic inflammatory reaction in affected structures. They are not common nowadays. Tuberculous infection of bone is generally referred to as **tuberculous osteitis**. It occurs more frequently in children and adolescents than in adults. It can, however, affect any bone and develop at any age.

When *tubercle bacilli* infect an area of bone near a joint, spread to this joint with resultant **tuberculous arthritis** is a usual sequel. Conversely, when tuberculous infection occurs in the synovial membrane of a joint, secondary spread to the adjacent bone ends usually follows. Thus tuberculous osteitis in the spine, ends of long bones, and in small bones such as those of the tarsus and carpus, is usually seen with accompanying joint involvement.

The formation of chronic abscesses of a type referred to as **cold abscesses** and sinus formation are common features of skeletal tuberculosis. Pathological calcification is common in old abscess cavities.

Tuberculosis of the spine is an important form of tuberculous osteitis and is frequently referred to as **Pott's disease**. It may cause collapse of vertebral bodies, and changes in adjacent intervertebral discs. It may also lead to formation of abscesses which press on the spinal cord and cause neurological signs and symptoms and also, according to the site of infection, a **retropharyngeal** (cervical spine), **paravertebral** (dorsal spine), **lumbar** or **psoas abscess** (lumbar spine).

Rarely, tuberculous osteitis may occur in the fingers or toes producing **tuberculous dactylitis**; the word **dactyl** meaning a digit.

Tuberculous lesions in bones and joints characteristically produce a persistent aching type of pain. When there is joint infection, limitation of movement of the affected joint and muscle wasting are usually features.

Radiological investigation is an essential procedure in all suspected cases of tuberculous osteitis and arthritis.

Treatment includes giving anti-tuberculosis drugs and immobilisation of the diseased area. Surgical measures are employed to drain abscesses when these have formed.

Syphilitic infection of the bones and joints—syphilitic infection of bone, referred to as **syphilitic osteitis**, occurs in congenital syphilis and in the secondary and tertiary stages of acquired syphilis.

Syphilitic arthritis is very uncommon but may occur in both the congenital and acquired forms of the disease. Syphilitic infection of the nervous system may lead to the development of one or more **Charcot joints** as a result of **neuropathic arthritis**, a condition in which the joint changes are due to involvement of the nerves supplying joints and not to joint infection.

Uncommon infections of bone include: typhoid fever, undulant fever (brucellosis), leprosy, ecchinococcus disease (hydatid disease), actinomycosis and yaws.

Neoplasms of Bone

Bone, as already mentioned, is composed of cells called *osteocytes* and calcified intercellular substances called *bone matrix*. It also contains cells called *osteoblasts* and *osteoclasts*. In addition to bone tissue proper, bones contain in their inner spaces fibrous, vascular, nervous and lymphoreticular tissue. Bones are moreover ensheathed by a fibrous membrane, the *periosteum*, and their articular ends are covered by *articular cartilage*. During early development bones are preformed in either cartilage or membrane.

Bone thus contains a number of different types of tissue from which primary tumours may arise; and is also a common site for metastases from carcinomatous neoplasms arising elsewhere in the body.

Plain X-ray films are extensively employed in the diagnosis of bone tumours and frequently specialised radiological investigations such as tomography, angiography, and bone scanning using radioactive isotopes are also used.

Biopsy is often an essential procedure when a primary malignant neoplasm of bone is suspected.

Neoplasms of bone may be classified as benign or malignant. Malignant neoplasms may be of primary or secondary type. Some of the more important varieties are referred to below.

A classification of tumours and tumour-like lesions of bone, adopted at the Royal National Orthopaedic Hospital, has been given by Murray (4) and can be consulted by those requiring wider information.

Benign Neoplasms

Osteoma—a benign tumour of bone tissue proper. It may consist of cancellous bone (**cancellous osteoma**) or compact bone (**ivory osteoma**). The former type generally arises from a long bone and the latter from a skull or facial bone.

Chondroma—a benign tumour of cartilage. It may be single or multiple. A chondroma which projects from the outer surface of a bone is called an **ecchondroma**, and one growing in the interior of a bone is known as an **enchondroma**.

Osteochondroma—a benign tumour composed of both bone and cartilage. It may sometimes undergo malignant change with the formation of a **chondrosarcoma**.

Osteoclastoma (giant-cell tumour of bone)—a tumour that is composed of cells resembling osteoclasts. This condition holds an intermediate position between the benign and malignant tumours in that, while possessing a number of benign characteristics it may infiltrate widely into surrounding tissues in similar fashion to a malignant tumour. In such cases, it is accordingly described as being **locally malignant**.

Note: An osteoma or osteochondroma may be described as an **exostosis**; a term used to describe any form of localised bony outgrowth and which includes certain conditions which are not of a neoplastic nature (e.g. the condition called **traumatic exostosis** where, as a result of injury, bone is formed in the insertion of a tendon).

Haemangioma (benign angioma)—a benign tumour of blood vessels which may occur in many different tissues, including bone.

Other benign neoplasms—these include **osteoid osteoma**, **benign chondroblastoma**, **chondromyxoid fibroma**, **osteogenic fibroma** (benign osteoblastoma) and **non-osteogenic fibroma**.

Primary Malignant Neoplasms

Osteosarcoma—this is a tumour derived from bone-forming cells. It may also be referred to as an **osteogenic sarcoma** (**osteogenic** means bone forming).

Osteosarcoma is usually highly malignant, local extension being rapid and metastases in the lungs and other organs frequently being early features. Its highest incidence occurs in late childhood and adolescence. A certain number of cases are seen in elderly patients as a result of osteosarcoma developing as a complication of Paget's disease of bone.

The commonest site for the tumour to originate is at the end of a long bone, particularly in the region of the knee joint.

Severe pain in the affected region is usually the first symptom of the disease.

Radiological investigation and biopsy are important complementary diagnostic procedures.

X-ray changes vary considerably with the type of sarcoma present. They are often difficult to differentiate from those caused by certain other conditions, e.g. osteomyelitis, ossifying subperiosteal haematoma. Common radiographic features are the presence of periosteal new bone formation, accompanied by areas of irregular bone destruction and new bone formation in the cortex and medulla.

Treatment is primarily by radiotherapy and chemotherapy, followed subsequently, in some instances, by amputation when the site of tumour renders this operation practicable.

Other bone sarcomas—these include **chondrosarcoma** (formed from cartilage cells), **fibrosarcoma** (formed from fibrous connective tissue cells) and **parosteal sarcoma** (arising from bone forming cells in the periosteum). Also occurring in rare instances are **angiosarcoma** and **liposarcoma**.

Ewing's tumour of bone (Ewing's sarcoma)—a rare malignant neoplasm of bone marrow, named after J. Ewing, an American pathologist. Its exact nature is unknown. Like osteogenic sarcoma it occurs principally in late childhood and adolescence. Unlike this latter condition, however, it usually arises in the middle of a long bone and it may produce metastases in other bones and lymph glands.

Myelomatosis—the word **myeloma** means a tumour of bone marrow. This neoplasm arises from plasma cells (a type of lymphocyte—p 204) in the bone marrow. It is uncommon and whilst it can occur in the form of a single tumour referred to as a **solitary myeloma** or **plasmocytoma**, it usually has a multicentric origin presenting in the form of multiple tumours of the bone marrow when it is referred to as a **multiple myeloma**.

Common sites for the lesions are the bones of the spine, ribs, skull and pelvis (i.e. sites of red marrow in adult life) where they produce areas of bone destruction which may be demonstrated on X-ray films.

The diagnosis may be confirmed by microscopic examination of a fragment of bone marrow tissue obtained by marrow puncture, and by demonstration of immunoglobulins in blood plasma, using an electrical method called **electrophoresis**.

Patients with multiple myeloma often excrete in their urine a type of protein called **Bence-Jones protein**. This protein may be precipitated in the renal tubules causing **myeloma kidney** and lead to chronic renal failure.

Treatment is by radiotherapy and chemotherapy.

Other malignant bone tumours—it is to be noted that some classifications of bone tumours include bone deposits that may occur in the leukaemias, Hodgkin's disease, and non-Hodgkin lymphomas.

Secondary Malignant Neoplasms

Metastases are the commonest neoplasms occurring in bone and develop most frequently from primary carcinomas of the breast, prostate and bronchus. They occur principally in those sites where red bone marrow persists in adult life (see p 237).

Less common primary tumours with a predilection for producing bony metastases are carcinomas of the thyroid, kidney and body of the uterus, and also neuroblastomas of the suprarenal gland.

Metastatic growths in bone may be single, but are more frequently multiple. They may cause bone destruction or may lead to reactive new bone formation, or frequently a combination of both these processes.

Metastases are occasionally painless and evidence of their presence may first be revealed as a result of an X-ray examination or by the patient sustaining a pathological fracture. Usually, however, they cause severe pain and this may be present for a long time before typical X-ray changes can be demonstrated.

Scanning methods after administration of a radioactive isotope are widely used to investigate the presence and distribution of these lesions.

Radiotherapy is extensively used as a form of pallative treatment for bony metastases. Hormone treatment is much employed when such metastases arise from carcinomas of the breast or prostate.

Cysts of Bone

Cysts may occur in bone as a result of various causes, e.g. (i) developmental abnormalities—**simple cysts**, (ii) trauma—**post-traumatic cysts**, (iii) endocrine disease, e.g. **generalised osteitis fibrosa** (due to hyperparathyroidism), (iv) idiopathic disease, e.g. **aneurysmal bone cyst**, **polyostotic fibrous dysplasia**, **osteitis multiplex cystoides** (a manifestation of sarcoidosis).

Metabolic Diseases of Bone

These may be:

(i) due to lack of vitamin C or deficiency of certain types of protein. This form of metabolic bone disease is characterised by generalised **osteoporosis** (see p 238), the bones containing less calcified bone matrix than normal.

(ii) due to vitamin D deficiency, resulting in **osteomalacia**, a metabolic bone disorder in which osteoid tissue is formed in normal amounts but contains less than the normal quantities of calcium salts (see p 238).

(iii) associated with raised amounts of calcium in the blood (i.e. hypercalcaemia). This occurs in a rare but interesting disease of infancy called **infantile hypercalcaemia**. This condition is generally believed to be due to hypersensitivity to vitamin D and, in the more severe cases, areas of increased bone deposition (referred to as areas of **osteosclerosis**) can be demonstrated in radiographs of the bones.

The following are some important clinical types of metabolic bone disease.

Scurvy—a nowadays uncommon disease wherein the formation of osteoid tissue is defective. It is due to deficiency of vitamin C. This vitamin is found chiefly in fresh fruit and vegetables and is essential for the formation of the protein substance collagen, an important constituent of bone matrix and other types of connective tissue. The disease may occur in adults who are deprived of these foodstuffs or in bottle-fed infants who are not given fruit juice to supplement their bottle feeds.

Scurvy is a generalised disease affecting other connective tissues as well as bone. Its principal features are capillary haemorrhages, which are especially common from the gums, in the skin, in joints, and below the periosteum of long bones; anaemia, osteoporosis and delay in the healing of wounds.

Treatment is by giving vitamin C.

Simple rickets—a disease of infancy due basically to deficiency of vitamin D in the diet. Its nature and causation have already been briefly indicated when discussing upsets in the processes of normal ossification (p 238: see under osteomalacia).

It is nowadays rarely seen in the UK other than in children of Asian immigrants.

The condition is a type of osteomalacia and accordingly the bones are softer than normal. As a result, in severe cases marked deformities may develop especially in the lower limbs and pelvis. Deformities of the chest may also occur.

On X-ray, rachitic bones show a diminished density and also widening of epiphyseal lines and splaying of metaphyses, especially at certain sites such as the wrists and ankles.

In some cases of rickets the blood calcium is low and these may show various manifestations of **tetany** (spasmophilia), a condition of hyperexcitability of the nervous system evidenced by various types of intermittent muscular spasms.

Treatment of rickets is by giving vitamin D and a diet with adequate content of calcium and phosphorus.

Dietetic osteomalacia—this disease is the adult form of rickets, the nature and causation of both conditions being similar.

The disease is more frequent in women than in men, and nowadays is rare in its advanced forms, except in some underdeveloped countries.

As in simple rickets the basic pathological feature is defective calcification of bone matrix. This defect in normal maintenance of bony tissue leads to softening of bones and may result in skeletal deformities. These and general rarefaction of bone may be readily demonstrated on radiographs.

In severe cases, localised areas of pronounced rarefaction may simulate fractured bones. Such areas are termed **pseudofractures** or **Looser's zones**. (*Note:* The presence of pseudofractures is the main feature of an unusual type of osteomalacia called **Milkman's syndrome**.)

Other types of rickets and osteomalacia—these are not common but may develop as complications of:

(i) malabsorption syndromes (see p 133) in which there is defective absorption of vitamin D from the bowel: and

(ii) certain renal diseases, when they may be described as forms of **renal osteodystrophy** (renal bone disease), a term indicating bone disorders secondary to renal disease. Such diseases include chronic renal failure (in patients not treated with haemodialysis and also in those receiving long-term haemodialysis); rare tubular disorders such as renal tubular acidosis and Fanconi syndrome; and also another type of tubular disorder which is associated with the passage of large amounts of phosphates in the urine and gives rise to a condition termed **phosphaturic**

rickets which, as it fails to respond to ordinary therapeutic doses of vitamin D, is also referred to as **vitamin D resistant** rickets.

Note: Osteomalacia that is secondary to chronic renal failure may be complicated by bone changes due to secondary hyperparathyroidism, i.e. changes of generalised osteitis fibrosa (p 219).

Idiopathic Diseases

Paget's disease of bone (osteitis deformans)—this disease was so-called after Sir James Paget, a nineteenth century English surgeon. It is a fairly common condition in elderly men and its cause is unknown. It is not an inflammatory condition as might be suggested by its alternative name of **osteitis deformans**.

The pathological changes include a mixture of diffuse absorption of existing bone and the excessive deposition of new bone of spongy type. Affected bones are thickened but are weaker than normal. The changes may be limited to a single bone but usually involve several bones, common sites for the disease being the pelvis, femora, tibiae, lumbar spine and skull.

Pain is often a prominent feature. Deformity of affected bones is common. Pathological fractures are of frequent occurrence and occasionally the development of an osteogenic sarcoma may complicate the disease.

Characteristic changes are seen on radiographs but these are sometimes simulated by carcinomatous metastases especially from carcinoma of the prostate.

Levels of alkaline phosphatase in the blood are often high, reflecting increased activity of osteoblasts.

Treatment with calcitonin, a hormone secreted by the thyroid gland which dimishes the activity of osteoclasts in bone, may be of considerable value in treating Paget's disease as has been described by Doyle (5). Pain may sometimes be considerably relieved by X-ray therapy.

Juvenile osteochondritis (osteochondrosis)—this term describes a condition in which a localised death of bone and cartilage cells (i.e. a necrosis) occurs in the primary or secondary centres of ossification of one or more growing bones.

The necrosis occurring in osteochondritis is thought to result from a defective blood supply to the affected area and hence this condition is described as being a type of **avascular necrosis**. Osteochondritis is not an inflammatory condition as its name suggests and the cause of the deficient blood supply is unknown. It is, however, thought that this latter may, in many cases, be the result of injury, especially of a minor and repeated nature.

Pain and, in some sites, deformity are common clinical features of juvenile osteochondritis.

Radiologically, increased density of the bone in the affected area and later an appearance of fragmentation are usually the principal signs. Juvenile osteochondritis is found in a variety of ossific centres. The different types are named either by the name of the person who first described them, or better, according to their site of occurrence. Examples are given below.

Site of osteochondritis	*Alternative name*
Vertebral epiphyseal plates	Scheuermann's disease (anterior marginal epiphysitis)
Semilunar bone of carpus	Kienböck's disease
Epiphysis of femoral head	Perthes' disease (pseudocoxalgia)
Epiphysis of the tibial tubercle	Osgood–Schlatter's disease
Navicular bone of tarsus	Kohler's disease
Apophysis of os calcis	Sever's disease
Second and third metatarsal head epiphysis	Freiberg's disease

Juvenile osteochondritis bears a resemblance to other conditions seen in adults and known collectively as **adult osteochondritis**. It is thought probable, however, that many of these latter are the results of minor undiagnosed, and consequently untreated, fractures.

Note: The majority of secondary centres of ossification are at the growing ends of bones where they take part in the formation of joints and are known as **epiphyses**. Secondary centres of ossification which take no part in the formation of joints are called **apophyses** (singular: apophysis.)

Osteochondritis dissecans—this is a disorder in which a small localised area of necrosis of articular cartilage, and bone lying immediately beneath it, develops at a joint surface. Like juvenile osteochondritis (see above) the condition is thought to be a type of avascular necrosis, probably resulting from injury.

The dead area of bone and cartilage gradually separates from the surrounding live tissue and may ultimately become completely detached to form a **loose body** within the joint.

On radiographs both the loose body and the defect in the bone in the area from which it has separated are usually demonstrable, but special positioning may be required.

Osteochondritis dissecans is seen most frequently in adolescents and young adults and usually occurs in the larger joints, especially the knee joint. It gives rise to pain, effusion of synovial fluid and when a loose body has formed it may produce a condition of sudden fixation of an affected joint called **locking**.

Slipped upper femoral epiphysis (adolescent coxa vara)—in this conditon, which may affect one or both hips, the *capital epiphysis* (epiphysis of the head of the femur) slips downwards and backwards on the neck of the femur. The disorder develops in adolescence and causes pain and a limp. It occurs more frequently in males than in females. Its cause is unknown. Some authorities consider that it is of traumatic origin and others that endocrine factors play a part in its causation.

Irritable hip—a condition in which there is pain in the hip and a limp, raising a suspicion of early tuberculous infection or of osteochondritis. With rest, the signs and symptons usually resolve in a few days or weeks. The cause of the disorder is unknown although it has been suggested it is due to a synovitis caused by either slight injury or mild infection. X-ray findings are negative.

Idiopathic scoliosis—the term **scoliosis** denotes a lateral curvature of the spine. (*Note:* an abnormal backward spinal curvature is called a **kyphosis** and a forward curvature, a **lordosis**.) Scoliosis may be due to many causes (e.g. congenital abnormality, disease of the vertebral bodies, muscular paralysis following anterior poliomyelitis) but the majority of cases develop in childhood or adolescence and form a group of unknown origin, called **idiopathic scoliosis**.

Hypertrophic pulmonary osteopathy—an uncommon condition in which periosteal new bone formation occurs around short and long bones in the upper and lower limbs. Its cause is unknown but it develops in association with certain lung diseases and bronchial carcinoma, usually accompanied by finger clubbing (see p 92).

Chronic Arthritis

It is to be noted that while the term **arthritis** strictly speaking means joint inflammation, it is also employed to indicate certain joint conditions of a degenerative nature. The latter are better described as **arthroses** (singular: arthrosis). Both types of disorders may be referred to as **arthropathies**, **arthropathy** being a term used to describe any type of joint disease.

Chronic suppurative arthritis may develop as a sequel to acute suppurative arthritis (see p 248) and **tuberculous arthritis** is another important type of chronic arthritic disorder (see p 249). Other important types of chronic arthritis include **osteoarthrosis (osteoarthritis)** which is a degenerative disorder, **rheumatoid arthritis** and **ankylosing spondylitis**, which are inflammatory diseases, and the **gouty arthritis** due to a metabolic disease called gout. These latter four types of chronic joint inflammation are often referred to as **chronic rheumatic diseases**.

As was stated by Duthie (6) 'the term 'rheumatism' has been loosely applied to all conditions causing pain and stiffness of the muscles and joints'.

Osteoarthritis (osteoarthrosis, hypertrophic arthritis, degenerative arthritis) is a common type of chronic arthritis, occurring predominantly in middle and old age and commoner in men than in women.

It may develop in a single joint but often affects a number of joints. Malalignment of joint surfaces, as a result of injury or disease, and the pursuit of occupations causing strain on joints appear to be important contributory factors in the causation of many cases. Obesity appears to predispose to osteoarthritis in weight-bearing joints.

The chief pathological features of the condition are degenerative changes and destruction of articular cartilage of affected joint surfaces; reactive new bone formation in areas of bone underlying destroyed articular cartilage; and the formation around joint margins of projecting spurs of new bone referred to as **osteophytes**.

Osteophytes are readily demonstrable on radiographs. Radiographs may also show loss of joint space (due to the destruction of articular cartilage) and increased density of bone ends (due to the reactive new bone formation).

The chief clinical features are pain, stiffness, deformity and decreased movement in affected joints.

There is no curative treatment as the joint changes are permanent. Pain relieving drugs, physiotherapy, and manipulation together with the injection of hydrocortisone are employed to produce some relief of symptoms. Surgical measures (e.g. arthrodesis or arthroplasty) may be necessary in cases with severe pain and disability.

Rheumatoid arthritis—this term describes a common inflammatory disorder of connective tissue, the principal clinical manifestations of which result from an arthritis which affects multiple joints and is referred to as a **polyarthritis**. Anaemia is also a common feature in the established disease and other features which may develop include subcutaneous nodules called **rheumatoid nodules**, **pleurisy** or **pleural effusion** and lung changes, the different varieties of which are sometimes referred to as **rheumatoid lung**.

The chronic inflammatory changes start in the synovial membranes of affected joints and are reversible in their early stages, but later often lead to much destruction of articular cartilage and underlying bone. Muscle wasting is frequently severe around affected joints and pathological dislocations are not uncommon.

When damage to articular cartilage is severe, opposing joint surfaces may become united by fibrous tissue, formed as a result of the inflammation. This is termed **fibrous ankylosis**. Subsequently, osteoblasts may deposit bone in the fibrous tissue converting the condition into one of **bony ankylosis**.

The cause of rheumatoid arthritis is unknown. It shows certain features resembling those of an infection but no infective microorganism has ever been established as its cause. As indicated by Harrison (7), it may be an autoimmune disease due to the presence of an abnormal globulin (**rheumatoid factor**) in the blood. This acts as an antigen and causes connective tissue damage as a result of its provoking antigen-antibody reactions with immunoglobulins in the patient's blood plasma.

The disease usually starts in early adult life and shows a much higher incidence in female subjects than in males. Common sites for its onset are the small joints of the hands and feet which become painful, stiff and swollen. Later it may spread to include the larger joints of the limbs and the trunk.

Periodic attacks of active inflammation and remissions are common in the course of the disease. During the former, some degree of fever and increase in pulse rate may occur. Psychological stress possibly plays some ill-understood role in many patients.

X-ray investigation is of value in the demonstration of joint changes, the earliest sign of which is osteoporosis around affected joints. Later loss of joint space, joint deformity, bone erosions and evidence of bony ankylosis may be demonstrated.

Examination of the blood will show the anaemia resulting from the disease and tests such as the **Rose–Waaler agglutination test** and the **latex fixation test** may show the rheumatoid factor to be present in the blood serum during the active stages of rheumatoid arthritis.

As in many other inflammatory disorders, a test called the **erythrocyte sedimentation rate** (**ESR**) shows increased values in phases of activity of the disease.

Treatment includes (i) measures to improve general health, (ii) physiotherapy with measures designed to try to prevent deformities from developing, (iii) giving drugs such as asprin, phenylbutazone, gold salts, or corticosteroids, (iv) occupational therapy.

An operation called **synovectomy** (excision of the synovial membrane of a joint) is sometimes employed in the treatment of acutely inflamed joints in the early stages of rheumatoid arthritis.

When the active phase of the disease has subsided surgical treatment may correct or improve residual deformities. This may sometimes include arthroplasty.

A type of rheumatoid arthritis which occurs in children is called **Still's disease**, after Sir George Frederick Still, an English paediatrician, and is associated in many cases with enlargement of lymph glands and the spleen.

Ankylosing spondylitis—ankylosis is a term indicating fusion of joints and **spondylitis** means inflammation of a vertebra or vertebrae.

Ankylosing spondylitis is an inflammatory disorder which begins in the sacroiliac joints, where it produces destruction of articular cartilage and subsequent bony ankylosis. As the disease progresses, arthritic changes develop in other joints of the spine and the costovertebral joints between the spine and ribs. These changes are also of inflammatory nature and involve the ligaments of affected joints leading to varying degrees of **ligamentous ossification** (i.e. the formation of bone within ligaments). In advanced cases resultant immobility and rigidity of the spine produces a condition known as poker-back. The lesions in the sacroiliac joints and spine may sometimes be accompanied by arthritic changes in limb joints. In some cases, spontaneous arrest of the disease may occur in its earlier stages.

The cause of ankylosing spondylitis is unknown. Its onset is usually in early adult life and its incidence is much higher in men than in women.

Radiology is of great value in the early diagnosis of the condition and in assessing its progress. In the advanced stages, ossification of ligaments may give rise to an X-ray appearance referred to as bamboo-spine.

Treatment is mainly by non-steroid anti-inflammatory drugs (NSAIDs).

An arthritis resembling ankylosing spondylitis may occur in Reiter's syndrome (see p 59), and also in so-called **colic arthritis**, which develops as an infrequent complication of ulcerative colitis.

Gouty arthritis—the development of inflammatory changes in joints, first of acute type but later becoming chronic, is one of the outstanding features of a disorder of purine metabolism called **gout**.

Note: purines are derivatives of a class of proteins which are constituents of cell nuclei and are called *nucleoproteins*. One of the end products of purine metabolism is an acid called *uric acid*.

Gout is an uncommon condition which rarely develops before middle age, although hereditary factors are important in its causation. It occurs much more frequently in men than in women. It is characterised during its active phases by **hyperuricaemia** (i.e. increased amounts of uric acid in the blood), as can be shown by **estimation of the serum uric acid** salts, and by the deposition of crystals of uric acid salts, called **urates** in soft tissues around joints, in cartilage and bone in the vicinity of joints, in the cartilage of the external ear, and in bursae, especially the olecranon bursa.

Deposits of urate crystals produce nodules called **tophi**. These produce palpable swellings in the subcutaneous tissues and may lead to ulceration of overlying skin. In the bones they produce localised areas of bone absorption demonstrable on radiographs.

Hypertension and renal disease are frequent accompaniments of gout.

Gout has to be distinguished from another disease, called **pseudo-gout (chondrocalcinosis, pyrophosphate arthropathy)** in which pyrophosphate crystals are deposited in joints.

Neuropathic arthritis—this term describes the occurrence in joints of chronic arthritic changes which are secondary to some form of **neuropathy**, i.e. disease of the nervous system. Joints affected by neuropathic arthritis are frequently referred to as **Charcot joints** after Jean Martin Charcot, a nineteenth century French physician. They develop most frequently as a complication of tabes dorsalis or syringomyelia, but are sometimes due to diabetic neuropathy.

Owing to pathological changes in the nerves supplying it, a neuropathic joint is characteristically painless although severe joint disorganisation frequently develops. Either single or multiple joints may be the subject of this condition in the same individual. Large joints are more often affected than small joints.

Disorders of the Intervertebral Discs and Spondylosis

The intervertebral discs act as shock absorbers in the spinal column. They may be the subject of congenital abnormality or involvement by infective lesions in adjacent vertebral bodies (e.g. as in spinal tuberculosis), or they may undergo degenerative changes or be damaged by trauma. Disc disorder is of greatly varying severity but in the more serious cases it may result in a portion of a disc slipping out of the space between the vertebral bodies. A condition of **prolapsed disc**, or **slipped disc**, is then said to be present.

Prolapsed disc is commonest in the lower lumbar and lower cervical regions of the spine, but may occur elsewhere in these regions and also in the dorsal region.

Lumbar disc prolapse—in this condition the protruding portion of the disc may press on nerves or nerve roots causing a type of pain in the lumbar region of the back called **lumbago** and pain in the distribution of the sciatic nerve referred to as **sciatica**.

The commonest site for lumbar disc prolapse is the lumbosacral disc space.

The diagnosis is made principally on the clinical features.

Plain radiography is limited in value to excluding some other cause of the symptoms, such as spinal tuberculosis, metastases in the spine, ankylosing spondylitis, etc. Evidence that a disc is damaged may be revealed in plain films by narrowing of the disc space. It cannot, however, be said from such examination whether or not the damage has resulted in actual prolapse of the damaged disc. It is also well recognised that demonstration of a normal disc space on conventional film does not exclude there being prolapse of the disc which lies within it. Prolapsed discs can, however, be demonstrated by myelography and this examination may be employed when the clinical features are equivocal.

The lumbar discs may also be examined by discography.

There are various forms of treatment for this condition, e.g. manipulation, traction, immobilisation by a spinal corset. Operative treatment to remove the protruding portion of the affected disc is occasionally necessary. Access to the affected disc is obtained by removing one or both of the laminae of the overlying vertebral arch. This operation is called **laminectomy**.

Cervical disc prolapse—this condition occurs most frequently in the lower cervical region and may affect either a single disc or several discs. The disc protrusion may press on cervical nerves, causing among other features pain in the arm or shoulder. Less commonly, pressure may be exerted on the spinal cord itself, causing nervous signs and symptoms in the lower limbs.

As in the lumbar region, plain radiography may be of value in indicating disc damage and excluding other vertebral conditions. Among these latter is the presence of a cervical rib. Cervical disc protrusions may be shown by myelography.

Initial treatment may be by manipulation, traction or immobilisation by some form of support. Laminectomy is occasionally necessary in cases which fail to respond to non-operative measures.

Spondylosis

This term is used to describe degenerative changes of osteoarthritic type occurring in the spinal column. It is characterised by the presence of bony spurs (osteophytes) which develop as outgrowths from the margins of the vertebral bodies. Spondylosis is thought to develop as a secondary result of degenerative changes in the intervertebral discs. It is extremely common in older people of both sexes. It is often symptomless unless, as may happen particularly in the cervical region, the bony outgrowths develop so as to press on nerve roots or, as described by Lodge (8), on the spinal cord itself.

Pressure by osteophytes on the roots of the brachial plexus may cause a condition known as **brachial radiculitis**, in which there is pain and other evidence of nerve root irritation.

As stated by Brain (9), **cervical spondylosis** is an important cause of headache and can intensify the symptoms of **vertebrobasilar ischaemia**. In this last condition atheroma of the vertebral and basilar arteries causes interference with the blood supply to the brain stem, with resultant symptoms such as dizziness, disturbances of vision and gait, etc.

In one type of spondylosis, termed **senile ankylosing hyperostosis** or **Forestier's disease**, large osteophytes develop and form bridges of bone between the anterior aspects of adjacent vertebral bodies.

Some Other Bone and Joint Diseases and Deformities

Loose bodies in joints—loose bodies, composed of bone and cartilage, may be found in joints as a result of injury; in osteochondritis dissecans (see p 256); in association with osteoarthritis: or in a condition of unknown origin called **synovial osteochondromatosis**. Locking of an affected joint (see p 256) is a common indication of the presence of a loose body.

Chondromalacia patellae—an uncommon disorder in which degenerative changes occur in the articular cartilage covering the posterior surface of the patella. It is sometimes secondary to recurrent dislocation of the patella.

Metatarsalgia—a term used to describe pain in the forefoot arising from a variety of causes including pes planus and march fracture.

Hallux valgus—a common deformity, especially in females, in which the great toe deviates outwards. It is often associated with varus deformity (inward deviations) of the first metatarsal. This latter condition is known as **metatarsus primus varus**.

Hallux rigidus—a condition due in its chronic form to osteoarthritis of the first metatarsophalangeal joint and causing pain and stiffness of this joint.

Subungual exostosis—an **exostosis** is an outgrowth of bone and **subungual** means beneath the nail. This condition principally occurs in the great toe.

Genu valgum (knock-knee) and **genu varum** (bowlegs)—in both these disorders the great majority of cases in the UK are due to unknown causes which operate during childhood and usually the deformity rights itself during growth. A small proportion of cases, however, result from disease (e.g. rickets) or bony injury in the region of the knee joint.

Hammer toe—a name used to describe a toe with flexion deformity at either its proximal or distal interphalangeal joint. This condition occurs most commonly in the second toe. Its cause is unknown.

Mallet finger—a condition of flexion deformity of the distal interphalangeal joint of a finger due to an injury causing detachment of the extensor tendon from its insertion into the base of the terminal phalanx.

Coccydynia—a condition of chronic pain in the region of the coccyx which usually develops as a sequel to an injury in this region.

Baker's cyst—a cystic swelling, containing synovial fluid and due to herniation of a section of the capsule of the knee joint through the posterior ligament of this joint. It usually occurs in connection with either osteoarthritis or rheumatoid arthritis.

Skeletal Muscles

Pathological conditions of the skeletal muscles may be due to primary diseases of muscle, or occur secondary to (i) diseases and injuries to bones and joints, (ii) diseases and injuries primarily affecting the nervous system, or (iii) disease of other structures.

Atrophy (wasting) and weakness or paralysis (loss of function) of muscles are common features of many muscle disorders. In some types of disorder, an investigation called **electromyography** (EMG) may be employed to differentiate between primary muscle disease and disease of muscle occurring secondary to lesions in the nervous system.

Muscle biopsy is another type of investigation sometimes used to investigate lesions in skeletal muscles.

Diseases of the skeletal muscle include the following.

Traumatic conditions—injuries of a certain type may produce marked tearing of fibres resulting in a condition of partial or complete loss of continuity of tissue in a tendon, or less commonly in muscle fibres. This is referred to as a partial or complete **rupture** of tendon or muscle, e.g. rupture of the Achilles tendon.

After injury to a muscle or tendon bone may occasionally be laid down in the area of tissue damage producing a condition known as **traumatic myositis ossificans**. This occurs most frequently in the brachialis muscle, following a fracture in the region of the elbow joint or dislocation of this joint.

Inflammations—these may result from infection of muscular tissue with pathogenic micro-organisms, parasitic infestations such as **cysticercosis** (see p 313) and **trichiniasis**, a disease due to a worm called the muscle worm, or as a manifestation of certain **connective tissue diseases** (see p 307).

Inflammation of muscular tissue is called **myositis**. Pain of muscular origin is called **myalgia**. The disease called variously **epidemic myalgia**, **epidemic pleurodynia**, or **Bornholm disease** is characterised by severe pain in the chest as a result of inflammatory changes in intercostal muscles. It is believed to be due to a Coxsackie virus infection.

Inflammation of a tendon is termed **tendinitis**. Tendon sheaths possess an inner synovial lining and outer fibrous sheath. As indicated by Adams (10) inflammatory changes in the former are referred to as **tenosynovitis**, and in the latter as **tenovaginitis**. Tenosynovitis may be of traumatic causation or due to infection. Tenovaginitis is a condition of unknown origin.

Inflammation of fascia is known as **fasciitis**. Inflammatory changes occurring in the plantar fascia, in the sole of the foot, in the region of its attachment to the os calcis produce a painful disorder called **plantar fasciitis**.

Note: the use of the term **rheumatism** to describe conditions causing pain and stiffness in muscles and joints has already been referred to (see p 257).

It was formerly widely held that besides being due to various forms of acute and chronic arthritis, symptoms of rheumatism also frequently resulted from non-specific inflammatory changes in muscles and surrounding soft tissues. Hence rheumatic symptoms were often ascribed as being due to **muscular rheumatism**, **non-articular rheumatism** or **fibrositis** (inflammation of fibrous connective tissue). Such diagnoses are made infrequently nowadays; modern opinion in general ascribing such clinical features as due to muscular spasms, strains or tearing of ligaments or tendons, and minor injuries to intervertebral discs and the interfacetal joints of the spine.

Neoplasms—of rare occurrence is a malignant tumour of striated muscle tissue called a **rhabdomyosarcoma**. Also of infrequent incidence are benign and malignant **synoviomas** which may arise from the synovial sheaths of tendons and also from the synovial lining of joint capsules.

Myopathies—as defined by Simpson (11), **myopathy** is a generic term that includes all primary diseases of muscle.

According to Govan *et al* (12) the muscle abnormalities of the myopathies 'are essentially disturbances of metabolism'. Such disturbances result in atrophy of affected muscles (usually those of proximal groups), and this may progress to destruction of muscle fibres and their replacement by fat. Clinically, muscle wasting and weakness are the chief features.

Myopathies may be inherited or acquired. **Inherited myopathies** are also termed **muscular dystrophies** and include the conditions called **pseudohypertrophic muscular dystrophy** (Duchenne-type dystrophy); **facioscapulohumeral dystrophy**; and **myotonic dystrophy**, one form of which is called **myotonia congenita** (Thomsen's disease). **Myotonia** is a condition in which sustained muscular contraction is followed by slow relaxation.

Acquired myopathies develop in association with various other diseases e.g. endocrine disorders, connective tissue diseases, or may be induced by steroids or certain other drugs. Included in this group is an inflammatory form of myopathy called **polymyositis**, in which inflammatory lesions develop in affected muscles, and sometimes in the skin and subcutaneous tissues as well, when the condition is referred to as **dermatomyositis**. Polymyositis and dermatomyositis are believed to be autoimmune diseases and may in some cases be associated with an occult (hidden) carcinoma.

Electromyography, muscle biopsy and biochemical tests may be used to diagnose myopathies. A valuable biochemical test includes measurement of the concentration of *creatine kinase* in the blood serum, increased levels of this enzyme indicating destruction of muscle fibres.

Myasthenia gravis—the name of this disease means severe muscular weakness and it is characterised by a rapid onset of fatigue in voluntary muscles. The muscles involved vary, but those responsible for movements of the eyes and limbs and those concerned with speech are often affected.

The cause of myasthenia has not been established but in many cases there is some associated disorder of the thymus gland. In some, this latter takes the form of a tumour called a **thymoma** and in others there is hypertrophy of the gland.

The drugs called neostigmine and pyridostigmine are extensively used in treatment. Selected patients may derive considerable benefit from thymectomy or irradiation of thymus, or from a combination of both these procedures.

Volkmann's ischaemic contracture—this is an uncommon disorder in which as a result of ischaemia (localised deficiency in blood supply) there occurs a replacement of muscular tissue by fibrous tissue, in the flexor muscles of the forearm. Contraction of the fibrous tissue leads to deformity of the wrist and fingers.

The condition usually occurs as a complication of injuries around the elbow joint which interfere with the blood supply to the flexor muscles of the forearm.

Tennis elbow (lateral epicondylitis)—a condition of incompletely understood nature characterised by pain in the region of the common tendon of origin of the extensor muscles of the forearm.

Ganglion—this term is used to describe a cystic swelling developing in connection with a tendon sheath or joint capsule. Ganglia occur most commonly on the dorsum of the wrist and may require surgical excision. They are unrelated to nervous ganglia (see p 269).

Supraspinatus calcification—a condition in which pain on movement of the shoulder joint is associated with the deposition of calcium in the tendon of the supraspinatus muscle, close to its insertion into the greater tuberosity of the humerus. The pain may sometimes occur only during partial abduction of the shoulder joint and this type of pain is described as being due to **painful arc syndrome**, an abnormality of which there are a number of other causes.

Frozen shoulder—a condition in which there is a general limitation of shoulder joint movements and pain on movement. It is attributed to changes of unknown causation in the capsule of the joint and is also referred to by Adams (13) as **adhesive capsulitis**.

Bursitis

Bursitis, i.e. inflammation of a bursa (see p 239) may be acute or chronic and may occur as a result of mechanical irritation, e.g. as in **prepatellar bursitis** (housemaid's knee), or as a result of infection, e.g. pyogenic infection or tuberculous infection.

Olecranon bursitis is sometimes seen as a complication of gout.

Some Orpthopaedic Operations

Arthrodesis—operative fusion of a joint.

Arthroplasty—operative reconstruction of a joint, designed to provide a movable joint. It may take the form of an **excision arthroplasty** or a **replacement arthroplasty**. The latter involves replacement of one of the joint surfaces (e.g. Austin–Moore hip arthroplasty) or both joint surfaces (e.g. **total hip replacement**) by a **prosthesis**, i.e. an artificial component inserted into or attached to the body as a replacement for some absent or defective structure.

Arthrotomy—making an opening into a joint.

Bone grafting—a procedure in which a portion of bone (i.e. a graft) is transferred from another bone in the patient's body (or sometimes from a bone of another person) and inserted into, or fixed, to a bone which is the site of some defect, e.g. a fracture that has not united, or a cavity produced by removal of a tumour or cyst.

Internal fixation operations employed in fracture treatment—e.g. fixation of a fracture of the femoral neck by a metallic pin and plate (see also p 245).

Laminectomy—removal of the lamina from one or both sides of the posterior arch of a spinal vertebra to gain access to the spinal canal.

Osteotomy—cutting through a bone.

Reimplantation operations—involving replacement of a structure detached from the body (e.g. a digit or limb) in its former site.

Synovectomy—excision of the synovial membrane of a joint.

Tenotomy—cutting through a tendon.

Tendon transplant (tendon transfer)—the operative detachment of a tendon from its normal site of insertion and its transfer to another site of insertion.

REFERENCES

(1) and (12) Govan, A. D. T., Macfarlane, P. S., Callander, R. (1981). *Pathology Illustrated*. Edinburgh: Churchill Livingstone.

(2), (10) and (13) Adams, J. C. (1981). *Outline of Orthopaedics*, 9th Edn. Edinburgh: Churchill Livingstone.

(3) Jacobs, P. (1980). *A Textbook of Radiology and Imaging*, 3rd Edn. (Sutton, D., ed.) Edinburgh: Churchill Livingstone.

(4) Murray, R. O. (1980). *A Textbook of Radiology and Imaging,* 3rd Edn. (Sutton, D., ed.) Edinburgh: Churchill Livingstone.

(5) Doyle, F. H. (1975). *Recent Advances of Radiology*, 6th Edn. (Lodge, T., Steiner, R. E., eds.) Edinburgh; Churchill Livingstone.

(6) Duthie, J. J. R. (1966). *The Principles and Practice of Medicine*, 8th Edn. (Davidson, S., ed.) Edinburgh: Livingstone.

(7) Harrison, R. J. (1980). *Textbook of Medicine*. London: Hodder and Stoughton.

(8) Lodge, T. (1955). *Recent Advances in Radiology*, 3rd Edn. (Lodge, T., ed.) London: Churchill.

(9) Brain, W. R. (1963). *British Medical Journal*; **1**: 771.

(11) Simpson, J. A. (1984). *Davidson's Principles and Practice of Medicine*, 14th Edn. (Macleod, J., ed.) Edinburgh: Churchill Livingstone.

THE TEETH

The diagnosis and treatment of diseases of the teeth is principally the concern of those engaged in the dental profession, but understanding some of the terms referring to such diseases is of importance to members of other professions allied to medicine. Some important dental disorders are as follows.

Developmental abnormalities of the teeth—these include the presence of (i) extra teeth called **supernumerary teeth**, (ii) a deficiency in the number of teeth, (iii) delay or failure in the eruption of teeth, (iv) misplaced teeth, (v) abnormally formed teeth.

Misplaced teeth frequently develop so as to become wedged against adjacent teeth in such a manner that they are unable to erupt normally through the gums. This condition is termed **impaction** and occurs most commonly in the lower third molar teeth (wisdom teeth).

The treatment of many forms of developmental abnormality is the concern of a branch of dentistry called **orthodontics**, the name of which derives from the Greek words meaning straight and tooth.

Fractures of the teeth—these may occur in either the crown, neck or roots of an affected tooth.

Inflammatory disorders.

(i) **Dental caries**—an infective disorder, also referred to as dental decay.

(ii) **Periapical infection**—a condition resulting in spread of infection from a tooth whose pulp has been killed by caries, into the bony tissues of the tooth socket. It results in the formation of either an **acute** or **chronic apical abscess** (dental abscess) in the part of the socket around the apex of the root or roots of the dead tooth or, less commonly, in certain other types of infective process (e.g. root absorption).

> A dental abscess presents radiographically as a translucent area around the apex of an affected tooth, resulting in bone destruction. There is also characteristically a loss of continuity in the white line which represents the *lamina dura*, the cortical bone lining the tooth socket. When the abscess is of acute type the radiographic changes do not usually appear for about 7–10 days after the onset of the infection.

(iii) **Pyorrhoea** (paradontal disease, periodontal disease)—a disease of unknown origin in which inflammatory changes first appear in the gums (**gingivitis**) and later spread to the underlying bony margins of the mandible and maxilla.

Odontomes—these are certain neoplasms and malformations which arise in connection with dental tissues. There are various types, e.g. **adamantinoma** (ameloblastoma), and **dentigerous cyst** (associated with an unerupted tooth).

Dental cyst—a cyst which usually arises in connection with an infected tooth root and develops in the mandible or maxilla.

Buried tooth roots (retained roots)—these may result from breaking a tooth during extraction or destruction of the distal part of a tooth by severe caries.

NERVOUS SYSTEM

Some Anatomical and Physiological Considerations

The nervous system consists of (i) the *central nervous system* (the *brain* and *spinal cord*), often referred to as the CNS, (ii) the *peripheral nervous system* (the *cranial* and *spinal nerves*), (iii) the *autonomic nervous system* (the *sympathetic* and *parasympathetic nervous systems*).

Nervous tissue is composed of units called *neurons* which consist of *nerve cells* together with processes called *dendrites* and other elongated processes which are called *nerve fibres (axons)*.

In the brain and spinal cord, nervous tissue is arranged in the form of *grey matter* which mainly comprises collections of nerve cells, and *white matter* which consists of nerve fibres. Also found within the nervous system is a specialised type of supporting tissue called *neuroglia* containing cells of three types: *astrocytes*, *oligodendrocytes*, and phagocytic cells called *microglial cells*.

Outside the central nervous system are found collections of nerve fibres arranged in cord-like structures referred to as *nerve trunks*, or *nerves*. In certain sites, composite arrangements of nerve-trunks, resembling a network, constitute what are termed *nervous plexuses* (e.g. the brachial plexus).

All nerve fibres are surrounded by *nerve sheaths* and according to whether or not this sheath contains a fatty substance called *myelin*, they are referred to as *medullated* or *non-medullated nerve fibres*.

In addition to the nerve cells in the grey matter, small collections of nerve cells are found in certain sites outside the central nervous system in structures called *ganglia* (singular: *ganglion*). These latter occur in association with certain cranial nerves and the dorsal roots of spinal nerves, and also in the sympathetic and parasympathetic nervous systems.

The brain and spinal cord are completely surrounded by membranous structures called *meninges*. These consist of three membranes known as the *dura mater*, *arachnoid mater* and *pia mater*, the dura mater providing the outer covering and the pia mater the inner covering of the central nervous system. The *cerebrospinal fluid (CSF)*, which is formed in the *ventricles of the brain*, circulates in the *subarachnoid space* (i.e. between the arachnoid and pia mater). The portion of the meninges covering the spinal cord is referred to as the *spinal theca*, the word theca meaning a sheath.

Functionally, the nervous system consists of:

(i) *sensory (afferent) neurones*—concerned with the reception and appreciation of sensory impulses from both the external environment and the interior of the body;

(ii) *motor (efferent) neurons*—which control the movements of both voluntary and involuntary muscle tissue; and

(iii) *connector neurones*—linking the sensory and motor components of the system.

By this arrangement of neurones, the nervous system can regulate and co-ordinate the activities of all the other systems of the body and control the processes by which the individual adapts to his external environment.

The prefix **neuro-** means pertaining to the nervous system and the branch of medicine which is concerned with diseases of the nervous system is termed **neurology**.

The adjective **cerebral** means pertaining to the brain and the prefix **encephalo-** has the same meaning. **Myelo-** means pertaining to the spinal cord but it is to be noted that this prefix is also used in other contexts with reference to the bone marrow (e.g. a myeloma is a tumour of the bone marrow).

Some General Aspects of Diseases of the Nervous System

Diseases of the nervous system may be congenital, traumatic, infective, neoplastic, or degenerative. They may also occur as a result of vascular disorders or be due to other causes.

They are evidenced by a wide variety of signs and symptoms arising from disturbances in the functions of the sensory and motor neurones of the system, and the resultant effects of these disturbances in other tissues.

Among the many clinical features of nervous diseases, therefore, are found disorders of smell, vision, hearing, balance and speech; abnormalities of sensibility to touch, temperature and pain; defects of positional sense; pain in the course of nerve trunks; weakness or paralysis and subsequent wasting of muscle groups, supplied by nerves which are the subject of injury or disease; abnormal muscular contraction and incoordination of muscular actions; disorders of bladder and

bowel control; abnormalities of reflexes; associated mental changes.
Note: **reflexes** are involuntary reactions produced automatically by certain stimuli, e.g. the tendon reflex called the **knee jerk**, which is an involuntary contraction of the quadriceps muscle in response to a sharp tap over the lower part of its tendon just below the patella.

The following are some of the terms used to indicate clinical signs and symptoms which may arise from different types of diseases of the nervous system:

amnesia—loss of memory;

anaesthesia—loss of sensation, particularly loss of sensibility to pain, but the term can be used to indicate loss of sensibility to temperature (**thermal anaesthesia**) and touch (**tactile anaesthesia**) (see also p 26);

aphasia—this term is used to refer to disorders in which the power of speech is partially or completely lost. Such loss may be due to inability to understand spoken and/or written words (**sensory aphasia**), or from inability to express thought in the form of articulated speech and/or in writing (**motor aphasia**);

ataxia—an absence of proper co-ordination of muscular action;

Babinski sign—also referred to as an **extensor plantar response**—consists of an upward movement of the great toe (the normal movement is downwards) when the outer side of the sole of the foot is stroked with a blunt object. It is a sign of great value in indicating disease affecting certain motor neurones in the central nervous system;

coma—a state of unconsciousness from which the sufferer cannot be aroused;

convulsions—attacks of involuntary contractions of muscles which may be of localised or widespread distribution;

dementia—impairment of mental faculties due to organic disease of the brain;

diplegia—motor paralysis of the same members on both sides of the body (e.g. both legs);

dysarthria—a defect of articulated speech resulting from lack of co-ordination or paralysis of the muscles which produce the spoken voice. It thus differs from the disorders of speech described above as being due to aphasia;

dyslexia—difficulty in understanding written words;

fit—a term used widely to indicate various types of organic and functional disorders of sudden onset and often of periodic occurrence. In neurology this term is commonly used as a synonym for convulsion (see above);

hemianaesthesia—loss of sensation in one side of the body;

hemiplegia—motor paralysis of one side of the body;

neuralgia—pain of severe type in the distribution of a sensory nerve;

nystagmus—a variety of abnormal involuntary movements of the eyes;

palsy—a synonym of paralysis (see below);

photophobia—dislike of light;

papilloedema—swelling of the optic disc as a result of oedema of this structure, a condition observed on examination of the interior of the eye by an ophthalmoscope. It is also referred to as **choked disc**;

paraesthesiae—abnormal sensations such as feeling of numbness and tingling and the sensations described as pins and needles;

paralysis—loss of function. Used without qualification this term indicates **motor paralysis**, i.e. a loss of the power of movement. Loss of sensation is sometimes, however, described as **sensory paralysis**. Loss of function in motor nerves results in paralysis and wasting of the muscles which they supply. According to the site of the nerve lesions the muscular paralysis may occur in the form of **spastic muscular paralysis** or **flaccid muscular paralysis**;

paraplegia—a term used commonly to indicate paralysis of both lower limbs, often together with paralysis of the lower part of the trunk;

paresis—a condition of partial paralysis;

quadriplegia—motor paralysis of all four limbs;

spasm—a sudden involuntary contraction of a muscle or group of muscles;

stupor—a condition of partial unconsciousness;

syncope—fainting;

tinnitus—a sensation of ringing or noises in the ears;

tremor—abnormal coarse or fine movements of a vibratory nature in voluntary muscles;

vertigo—a sensation of giddiness.

Special Examinations

These include the following.

Examinations of cerebrospinal fluid, e.g. by taking pressure readings; by examining specimens of this fluid by microscopy and taking differential cell counts; and by various other pathological procedures; chemical (e.g. measurement of protein and glucose concentrations, Lange's colloidal gold test), and bacteriological. Such specimens are most commonly obtained by **lumbar puncture**; a procedure which involves insertion of the tip of a needle into the subarachnoid space within the spinal theca. The puncture is made in the lower lumbar region, well below the termination of the spinal cord, the lower limit of which lies at the lower border of the first lumbar or upper border of the second lumbar vertebra.

In certain conditions **cisternal puncture** is used as an alternative to lumbar puncture, the needle being inserted between the occipital bone and first cervical vertebra into the *cisterna magna*, a part of the subarachnoid space lying just below the brain and just above the posterior part of the foramen magnum.

Radiological Procedures

(i) *Plain radiography*—to show changes in the skull, spine and other structures secondary to or associated with diseases of the nervous system. In suspected space-occupying lesions within the cranium, one important procedure is taking film to demonstrate any displacement of the *pineal gland* (pineal body) which lies in the midline behind the upper part of the third ventricle of the brain. This gland, particularly in older individuals, often shows calcium deposits in its substance thus rendering it visible on skull radiographs.

(ii) *Specialised radiological investigations*—such as investigation of the brain by **computed tomography (CT)**, also termed **computerised axial tomography (CAT)**; demonstration of the ventricles of the brain by **ventriculography** or **encephalography**; demonstration of the cerebral blood vessels by **carotid** or **vertebral angiography** or **arch aortography**; investigation of the spinal cord and theca by **myelography**, and the lumbosacral nerve roots by **radiculography**.

The indications for cerebral angiography and air studies of the ventricular system have greatly diminished since the introduction of CT into clinical practice in 1972.

Nuclear magnetic resonance (NMR) is likely in future to play an increasing role in the investigation of some disorders of the central nervous system.

(iii) *Investigations employing radioactive isotopes*.

Electroencephalography (EEG)—a procedure whereby tracings of electrical discharges from the brain are recorded in wave–form.

Echoencophalography—a method employing ultrasound to investigate displacement of midline structures of the brain by intracranial space-occupying lesions (see p 283).

Electromyography—investigation of the electrical responses in muscle groups supplied by damaged motor nerves (see p 264).

Congenital Abnormalities

These include the following.

Spastic diplegia (Little's disease)—this is one type of a group of disorders known collectively as **cerebral palsy**. Thomson and Cotton (1) state 'it may possibly be due to birth trauma but more probably is a developmental abnormality of the brain tissue'. Its principal clinical feature is spasticity of muscle groups in the legs (spastic paraplegia), or in both legs and both arms (spastic quadriplegia), resulting in various degrees of paralysis of the affected limbs.

Sufferers from this condition and other forms of cerebral palsy are commonly known as **spastics**.

Anencephaly (see p 189).

Microcephaly—a condition in which there is defective development of the brain and the cranium is abnormally small.

Abnormalities associated with spina bifida—meningocele, meningomyelocele and neural tube defect (see p 241).

Downs syndrome—a congenital disorder associated with an abnormality of chromosomes and resulting in a severe degree of defective development of mental processes.

Sufferers possess flat faces and obliquely-set eyes, resulting in this condition being called mongolism, a designation now largely discarded. A proportion of those affected suffer from congenital heart disease.

Congenital hydrocephalus—hydrocephalus is a condition of excessive accumulation of cerebrospinal fluid in the cranium, resulting in varying degrees of cranial enlargement. The congenital variety is due to factors present during intrauterine existence and may develop in fetal life (**fetal hydrocephalus**—see p 189) or shortly after birth. It results from some form of obstruction to the normal circulation of cerebrospinal fluid and may be produced by developmental defects or certain infective conditions which affect the fetus. Hydrocephalus can also occur as an acquired condition in postnatal life, e.g. secondary to meningitis or an intracranial neoplasm.

Treatment of hydrocephalus may sometimes be by a shunt operation, inserting a tube with a Spitz-Holter valve to drain cerebrospinal fluid from a lateral ventricle into the internal jugular vein, or other shunt or bypass operation.

Arnold-Chiari malformation—a developmental abnormality in which there is protrusion of parts of the cerebellum and medulla oblongata, through the foramen magnum into the upper part of the spinal canal. This condition is one of the causes of congenital hydrocephalus.

Traumatic Disorders

Injuries to the brain—traumatic injury to the brain may occur with or without associated **fracture of the cranium** (i.e. the part of the skull which contains the brain). Compound fractures with brain damage may lead to infection in the meninges and underlying brain tissue.

In all cases of suspected brain injury it is important to determine, if possible, whether or not a fracture is demonstrable by radiography, particularly with reference to demonstrating or excluding a depressed fracture of the skull. A comprehensive account of the indications for radiological examination of head injuries and the principles concerned is given by Du Boulay (2).

In its simplest form, brain injury may be evidenced by an instantaneous but temporary loss of consciousness termed **simple concussion**. This condition is frequently accompanied by a loss of memory (**amnesia**) for incidents immediately before the causal trauma and for subsequent happenings over a variable period of time.

A more serious injury may lead to haemorrhage from blood vessels supplying the meninges or brain tissue (**intracranial haemorrhage**) and the formation of an **intracranial haematoma** (i.e. a swelling composed of blood) which constitutes what is termed an **intracranial space-occupying lesion**. Such a lesion causes a rise in intracranial pressure and thus causes compression of brain tissue, evidenced by a clinical condition known as **cerebral compression**.

Severe injuries may also lead to **contusion** (bruising) or **laceration** (tearing) **of the brain** and these conditions may occur together with or in the absence of haematoma formation within the cranium.

Simple concussion usually recovers without causing any long-lasting after–effects. In cases in which there is contusion or laceration of the brain, concussion may be followed by signs and symptoms of brain damage termed **cerebral irritation**, which may last several weeks before recovery ensues. This latter condition is evidenced by features such as stupor, restlessness, mental irritability.

More serious degrees of contusion or laceration may be evidenced immediately after the causal trauma by signs and symptoms of more severe neurological disorders and may produce after–effects such as permanent paralyses and **traumatic epilepsy** (Jacksonian epilepsy).

In cases with intracranial haemorrhage, concussion may be followed directly by evidence of compression but commonly these two states are separated by an interval during which consciousness is regained. This interval is called the **lucid interval** and while it lasts, a time of varying length, there is frequently little or no clinical evidence of brain injury.

With the development of compression, however, there appear signs such as abnormalities of pulse rate, respiration and body temperature; abnormalities of the pupils of the eyes, drowsiness, mental confusion and unconsciousness; disordered reflexes; muscular paralyses. (*Note:* cerebral compression may also be caused by conditions other than trauma, see 'space-occupying lesions in the cranium'.)

As noted above, one result of traumatic intracranial haemorrhage is the formation of a localised collection of blood referred to as a **haematoma**. According to the site of the haemorrhage, intracranial haematomas are described as **extradural haematomas** (between the dura and overlying skull); **subdural haematomas** (between the dura and arachnoid mater) and **intracerebral haematomas** (within the brain).

Extradural haematomas are frequently the result of injury to the middle meningeal artery and associated with a fracture of the temporoparietal region of the skull. Subdural haematomas occur in both acute and chronic form, the latter sometimes being the result of a relatively minor injury which results in a slow leakage of blood into the subdural space.

Radiological investigations, especially CT and ultrasonic methods, frequently play an important role in the diagnosis of these disorders.

Intracranial haematomas are treated surgically, the skull being opened and the haematoma evacuated.

Injuries to the spinal cord—these usually, but not invariably, occur in association with fracture dislocations or dislocations of the vertebrae. They may take the form of **contusions** or **lacerations of the spinal cord substance**, or of **compression of the spinal cord** as a result of haemorrhage (cf cerebral compression) or pressure of displaced bony parts on the cord (see p 284).

According to its extent and severity, injury to the cord may cause varying degrees of temporary, or permanent, motor paralysis; sensory loss below the level of the damage to the cord tissue; and accompanying disorders of bowel and bladder function. Injuries which tear through the substance of cord or cause irreversible damage involving part or the whole thickness of the cord at the site of injury are referred to as causing **partial** or **complete transection of the spinal cord**.

Peripheral nerve injuries—these consist of **contusion** (bruising), **compression**, **partial division** and **complete division of nerves** and result in a loss of nervous function in affected nerves. This loss may affect motor or sensory functions, or both, according to whether an injured nerve is of motor, sensory or mixed type. The resultant effects may be temporary or permanent according to the nature of the injury. Damage to motor nerve fibres results in paralysis of muscles supplied by such fibres and subsequent muscle wasting.

Damaged nerve fibres possess certain powers of regeneration and eventual complete recovery is common in injuries in which there is no actual division of nerve fibres (i.e. in contusion and compression nerve injuries). In these, treatment is directed to the care of paralysed muscles with various forms of physiotherapy, while recovery of nervous function is proceeding.

In order to obtain restoration of function in cases of partial or complete division, when practicable the cut nerve ends must be stitched together; the operation being called **nerve suture**. In some instances it is necessary to fill in a gap between the nerve ends by a short segment obtained from another nerve in the patient's body. This procedure is called **nerve-grafting**.

Various investigations are made in cases of nerve injury to estimate the degree of nerve damage and also the progress of regeneration when this occurs. Included among these are the testing of the responses to galvanic and faradic currents of muscles supplied by the affected nerve and an investigation called electromyography.

Infective Diseases

Inflammatory changes in the various structures of the nervous system are denoted by the following terms: brain tissue—**encephalitis**; meninges—**meningitis**; brain and meninges—**meningo-**

encephalitis; spinal cord tissue—**myelitis**; brain and spinal cord—**encephalomyelitis**; grey matter of spinal cord—**poliomyelitis**; nerves—**neuritis**.

Meningitis—inflammation of the meninges may be due to various causes including bacterial infections and infections with viruses (viral meningitis).

Infective bacteria may reach the meninges (i) by the bloodstream as in meningococcal meningitis (see p 53), tuberculous meningitis, and meningitis occurring as a complication of streptococcal infections elsewhere in the body, (ii) by direct spread from infective processes in sites such as the frontal sinuses and mastoid air cells, and (iii) as a result of pentrating wounds of the skull.

Viral meningitis may occur rarely as a complication of virus infections such as mumps and measles, or sometimes as a primary infective condition of the meninges.

In addition to general signs and symptoms of infection, e.g. headache, pyrexia, increase of pulse rate, patients with meningitis show signs due to **meningeal irritation** such as limitation of the movements of the neck due to muscle spasm (neck rigidity), and a sign called **Kernig's sign** which consists of inability to extend the knee when the thigh is flexed to a right angle on the trunk. In severe cases there may also be a condition of marked extension of the neck called **head retraction**. **Photophobia** (dislike of light) is also common in meningitis.

Signs of meningeal irritation due to meningitis have to be differentiated from similar signs occurring in a condition called **meningism**, which may occur during the course of pneumonia and other acute febrile infections, especially in childhood.

Examination of the cerebrospinal fluid is an important diagnostic procedure in meningitis. Antibiotics are widely used in the treatment of meningeal infections.

Encephalitis—inflammation of brain tissue may result from infection with pyogenic (pus-producing) bacteria (see brain abscess), spirochaetes (see neurosyphilis), and viruses. Encephalitis also occurs in the form of malaria called **cerebral malaria** and in another infection called **toxoplasmosis**, which is also due to a protozoan parasite.

In rare cases bloodborne infection of brain tissue with tubercle bacilli may occur and lead to the formation of a solitary lesion called a **cerebral tuberculoma**.

Among the types of encephalitis due to viruses are diseases called **encephalitis lethargica** which may cause a condition called **Parkinsonism** (see p 285); **rabies** (hydrophobia) a virus infection transmitted to humans by dogs or, less commonly, other animals; and encephalitis occurring as an unusual complication of acute infectious fevers such as chickenpox and smallpox, or very rarely consequent on vaccination against smallpox or whooping cough.

Brain abscess—infection of brain tissue with pyogenic

microorganisms may result in the formation of a brain abscess (i.e. a cavity containing pus), which constitutes a space-occupying lesion within the cranium and results in raised intracranial pressure. The infection may be bloodborne or derived from a neighbouring focus such as an infected frontal sinus or infected mastoid air cells, or due to a penetrating wound of the skull.

A brain abscess occurs most commonly in one of the cerebral hemispheres or in the cerebellum and may be demonstrated by CT. Treatment is by aspiration or surgery.

Infective sinus thrombosis (infective cerebral venous thrombosis)— this condition is a serious complication which occurs when a nearby infective process spreads to involve venous sinuses lying in the dura mater. With the increased use of antibiotics in the treatment of infections it is nowadays uncommon. The principal types of sinus thrombosis are **cavernous sinus thrombosis**, which may occur secondary to a carbuncle of the face, and **lateral sinus thrombosis** which may complicate mastoid infection.

Neurosyphilis, i.e. syphilis of the nervous system is not nowadays common but can develop in the tertiary and quaternary stages of acquired syphilitic infection.

In the tertiary stage it presents in the form of **meningovascular syphilis**, so called because in this disorder the infective lesions chiefly affect the meninges and blood vessels of the brain and spinal cord. A variety of clinical pictures may result from this condition and these may not infrequently mimic those of other diseases of the central nervous system.

The manifestations of quaternary syphilis may take the form of a condition called **general paralysis of the insane**, when the lesions affect the brain, or **tabes dorsalis** when they chiefly involve the spinal cord and the posterior roots of the spinal nerves.

General paralysis of the insane (dementia paralytica), as indicated by its name, is associated with severe mental changes and the development of weakness and paralysis in various groups of muscles.

Tabes dorsalis is also called **locomotor ataxia** and one of its features is a staggering gait as a result of a lack of coordination of muscular action (ataxia) in the muscles of the legs. Other features include pains around the chest referred to as girdle pains; bladder and bowel disturbances; areas of sensory loss which may lead to painless ulcers developing in the feet and legs; and Charcot joints.

The term tabes means wasting and the name tabes dorsalis refers to degenerative changes which occur in structures composed of white matter called the *posterior (dorsal) columns* of the spinal cord.

In tabes and other forms of neurosyphilis the lesions may also affect the nerve supply of the pupils of the eyes producing a condition referred to as **Argyll Robertson pupils**, i.e. pupils which possess normal powers of accommodation but show a loss of normal reflex reaction to light (**accommodation** is the mechanism by which adjustments are effected in the lens of the eye to permit clear visualisation of objects at different distances).

Acute anterior poliomyelitis—this is an infection due to a virus called the *poliovirus*. It is thought to be carried by droplet infection and also in contaminated food and water, and thus to gain access to the bloodstream, and thence to the central nervous system via the nasopharynx and alimentary tract.

The disease starts with a febrile illness known as the **preparalytic stage** of the disease. In so-called **non-paralytic cases**, the infection does not progress beyond this stage. In others, however, it proceeds to a **paralytic stage** as a result of involvement and resultant inflammatory changes in structures within the grey matter (polio) of the spinal cord called the *antorior horns*. These changes give the disease the name of **anterior poliomyelitis**.

Poliomyelitis not infrequently occurs in adults below middle age, but its chief incidence is in childhood and it is therefore sometimes referred to as **infantile paralysis**.

The inflammatory changes affect not only motor nerve cells in the spinal cord but sometimes motor nerve cells in the brain as well (**polioencephalitis**), causing muscular paralysis of variable distribution.

Poliomyelitis occurs both in the form of isolated cases and epidemics. The extent of the muscular paralysis varies greatly from patient to patient as does the degree of permanent damage caused, so during the **convalescent stage** of the disorder, which can last about two years, the paralysis may recover completely, improve to a varying extent, or alternatively show no evidence of recovery at all.

There is no specific treatment for poliomyelitis but the patient should rest and measures should be taken to prevent deformity in the acute phase of the disease, and intensive physiotherapy given to help recovery of muscle function during convalescence. Special methods of feeding are required in patients with paralysis of the muscles used in swallowing, and those with paralysis of the respiratory muscles need tracheostomy and some form of artificial ventilation of the lungs.

Protection against poliomyelitis may be given by oral administration of poliovaccine.

Herpes zoster (shingles)—is an infection of the nervous system in which inflammatory lesions develop in sensory ganglia of cranial nerves, or the posterior root ganglia of spinal nerves. It is caused by the chickenpox virus. The lesions occur on only one side of the body.

Severe pain may be experienced in sensory nerve fibres connected with affected ganglia and a vesicular rash (i.e. a rash consisting of small blisters) appears in areas of skin supplied by such fibres. The pain may persist long after the rash has disappeared, the condition then being referred to as **postherpetic neuralgia**.

Neoplasms

Intracranial Neoplasms

These commonly produce the signs and symptoms of a space-occupying lesion within the cranium (see p 283). They are of the following main types.

Gliomas—these tumours arise from the neuroglia (i.e. the specialised supporting connective tissue of the central nervous system). They tend to be locally malignant but never produce metastases outside the central nervous system. There are various types of glioma distinguished by names such as **astrocytoma**, **glioblastoma multiforme**, **oligodendroglioma** and **ependymoma**. The tumours called **medulloblastomas** and **spongioblastomas** are also often classified as gliomas, but more strictly are regarded as originating from the precursors of the nerve cells rather than being of glial origin.

Medulloblastomas are common in childhood. They may spread via the subarachnoid space producing secondary deposits which involve the spinal cord.

Few gliomas are amenable to surgical removal and radiotherapy is extensively used in their treatment.

Meningioma—a benign tumour arising from the meninges. Surgical removal of this tumour is frequently possible. Inoperable cases are treated by radiotherapy.

Pituitary tumours—these have already been referred to in connection with diseases of the endocrine system (see p 215).

Acoustic neurofibroma (auditory nerve tumour, acoustic neuroma)—a benign tumour arising from the fibrous sheath of the eighth cranial nerve (acoustic or auditory nerve). It causes deafness on the affected side and vertigo (giddiness). This neoplasm sometimes occurs in association with generalised neurofibromatosis (see p 281).

Angioma—the term angioma means a tumour of blood vessels but many authorities regard angiomas of the brain as congenital malformations rather than true neoplasms. Rupture of abnormal blood vessels within an angioma may cause intracranial haemorrhage.

Cerebral metastases—carcinomatous metastases in the brain develop most frequently from primary carcinomas of the breast and bronchus, but may be secondary to carcinomas in other sites and rarely to sarcomas.

Tumours in the Spinal Canal

These are tumours of the spinal cord, the spinal meninges, the spinal nerve roots and their sheaths, and blood vessels and soft tissues within the spinal canal.

The spinal cord is sometimes referred to as the **spinal medulla** and tumours arising within the cord are known as **intramedullary tumours**, while the other tumours arising within the spinal canal are termed **extramedullary tumours** (**intradural** and **extradural** tumours).

These tumours are not common but the most frequently seen of the intramedullary variety are gliomas, arising from the neuroglia and of the same nature as those which occur in the brain. Among the different types of extramedullary tumours encountered are meningiomas, neurofibromas, cauda equina tumours, and neoplasms arising in the spinal vertebrae (e.g. metastases, chordoma).

A **meningioma** arises from the meninges and a **neurofibroma** from a nerve sheath. A **cauda equina tumour** arises in the collection of nerve roots which lie in the lower part of the spinal canal below the termination of the spinal cord.

A **chordoma** is a rare tumour caused by remnants of an embryonic structure called the notochord. It arises most frequently from the base of the skull or the sacrococcygeal region, but can develop anywhere in the spinal column.

Generalised Neurofibromatosis

A **neurofibroma** is a benign tumour which arises in a nerve sheath from cells, called Schwann cells, and hence is sometimes referred to as a **Schwannoma**. This type of neoplasm, as has already been noted, may develop from the sheath of the acoustic nerve (acoustic neurofibroma), or arise from a nerve sheath within the spinal canal. In either of these sites it may be solitary or occur as part of a disorder wherein multiple neurofibromata arise in the same patient. In this latter instance the disorder is known as **generalised neurofibromatosis** or **von Recklinghausen's disease**.

The tumours produce rounded nodules in the course of both superficial nerves and deep nerves and are associated with areas of brown pigmentation in the skin, referred to as *café au lait* patches. In some sites they may also cause a mixture of bone destruction and reactive new bone formation as a result of pressure on neighbouring bony structures.

Other Tumours of Nervous Tissue

These include **ganglioneuromas** and **neuroblastomas** which arise from the tissues of the autonomic nervous system or from the suprarenal medulla which is derived from nervous tissue of similar origin to that of the sympathetic nervous system.

Cerebral Vascular Disease

The term cerebral vascular disease is generally taken to refer to disorders of the blood vessels of the brain and its covering meninges other than those occasioned by traumatic injury (e.g. extradural and acute and chronic subdural haematomas—see p 275).

Arterial disorders have a much greater incidence than disorders of veins and their commonest cause is cerebral atheroma (see p 81). Their causes include congenital and acquired aneurysms in the cerebral circulation (see p 82), malformations of the type known as angiomas (see p 280) and syphilitic infection of the cerebral and meningeal arteries (see p 276).

The clinical effects of cerebral vascular disease are in the main due to either rupture of diseased blood vessels resulting in **cerebral haemorrhage** or **subarachnoid haemorrhage**; or to inadequacy of arterial blood supply to an area or areas of brain tissue. This latter condition is referred to as **cerebral ischaemia** or **cerebral vascular insufficiency**.

CT is extensively used to investigate cerebral vascular disease, supplemented by appropriate forms of cerebral angiography when indicated.

Intracerebral haematomas, infarcts of brain tissue, and cerebral atrophy with resultant ventricular enlargement due to cerebral vascular disease can be demonstrated by CT, but angiography is commonly required for the demonstration of cerebral aneurysms and angiomas.

Cerebral haemorrhage (intracerebral haemorrhage)—this is a condition of spontaneous bleeding into the brain substance which is usually due to rupture of an arterial vessel; atheroma of the cerebral arteries and hypertension (high blood pressure) being important predisposing factors in such rupture.

In its more severe forms the onset of cerebral haemorrhage, and also subarachnoid haemorrhage and cerebral thrombosis, is frequently marked by what is termed a **cerebral vascular accident** (CVA) causing **apoplexy** (**stroke**). Mann (3) states 'by apoplexy is meant the abrupt cessation of the function of the brain as a consequence of interference with blood supply, an event commonly known as a stroke'.

Various different forms of motor paralysis and sensory loss may follow the occurrence of a non-fatal stroke. Disturbances of speech and hemiplegia (paralysis of one half of the body), of either a transient or permanent nature, are not uncommon sequels.

It has already been noted that occasionally a large haemorrhage into the brain tissue may cause an intracerebral haematoma, and this latter condition gives rise to the signs and symptoms of an intracranial space-occupying lesion.

Subarachnoid haemorrhage—is a condition in which bleeding occurs into the subarachnoid space between the arachnoid mater and pia mater. It is most commonly due to rupture of a congenital aneurysm of one of the arteries forming the circle of Willis, which lies in the sub-arachnoid space at the base of the brain. It may, however, develop as a complication of cerebral atheroma or other vascular disease.

As with intracerebral haemorrhage, subarachnoid haemorrhage is often first evidenced as a cerebral vascular accident (see above) but when the bleeding is subarachnoid the diagnosis may be confirmed by performing a lumbar puncture to disclose the presence of blood in the cerebro-spinal fluid.

CT is used in investigation, but cerebral angiography is an important procedure to determine whether an aneurysm of a cerebral artery can be demonstrated.

Cerebral ischaemia (cerebral vascular insufficiency)—this is a con-dition in which, as a result of narrowing or blockage of the cerebral carotid, basilar or vertebral arteries, there is a localised deficiency of blood supply to a part or parts of the brain. It develops most frequently as a result of atheroma.

Blockage of a cerebral artery may lead to death of an area of brain tissue, such an area then being referred to as a **cerebral infarct**. This may occur as a result of **cerebral arterial thrombosis**, i.e. thrombus (clot) formation in cerebral arteries (developing most frequently secon-dary to atheroma), and **cerebral embolism**—resulting in occlusion of cerebral vessels by emboli derived from the heart, aorta, carotid arteries or cerebral arteries.

Clinically, cerebral ischaemia may present either in the form of: (i) **transient ischaemic attacks** which are of short duration and from which recovery is complete, leaving no residual signs of neurological disorder; (ii) a slow development of various forms of motor paralysis and sensory disturbance; or (iii) the sudden occurrence of a cerebrovas-cular accident (see p 382).

Cerebral infarcts are demonstrable by CT.

Intracranial Space-Occupying Lesions

In the foregoing account of diseases of the nervous system, certain pathological conditions were mentioned as constituting what are ter-med **space-occupying lesions** within the cranium. Such lesions, by causing an increase in the amounts of fluid or tissue, or both, within the restricted space contained by the walls of the cranium cause a rise in intracranial pressure. They thus commonly produce general signs and symptoms, due to this increase of pressure, such as headache; vomiting; **papilloedema** (i.e. swelling of the optic discs which may be detected with an instrument called an ophthalmoscope) and convulsions. In addition, they frequently also produce localising signs and symptoms resulting from pressure on or involvement of structures in the vicinity of the lesion, e.g. paralysis of muscles supplied by cranial nerves, paralysis of limbs, loss of sensation in various parts of the body, mental changes, disturbances of speech, vision and hearing, vertigo, and abnormalities of posture and gait.

The following are some of the principal types of intracranial space-occupying lesions: intracranial tumours and cysts; brain abscesses; intracranial haematomas (e.g. chronic subdural haematomas); large blood clots within the brain due to haemorrhage from a cerebral artery; large intracranial aneurysms; cerebral tuberculomas.

Special investigations employed in the diagnosis of space-occupying lesions include plain radiography, CT, electroencephalography, echoencephalography and scanning with radioactive isotopes. Rarely, cerebral angiography and air studies of the ventricles may be indicated.

Plain radiographs are normal in a high proportion of space-occupying intracranial lesions. When, however, radiographic abnormalities are present they may include features such as calcification in neoplasms and aneurysms, enlargement of the pituitary fossa and/or destruction of its walls, displacement of the shadow of the calcified pineal gland, and separation of the cranial sutures in infants and children.

Note: lumbar puncture is seldom carried out in these disorders because it may be dangerous when there is raised intracranial pressure.

Spinal Cord Compression

It was noted when discussing traumatic injuries that these could cause compression of the spinal cord as a result of haemorrhage within the spinal canal, or pressure from displaced bony parts of the spinal column due to dislocations or fracture-dislocations.

More commonly, however, the clinical signs and symptoms of compression are of gradual development and non-traumatic origin. Among the conditions responsible for this condition may be mentioned: central protrusion of an invertebral disc; pressure from a bony outgrowth in cervical spondylosis; metastases in the spine, primary neoplasms arising within the spinal canal, and tuberculosis of the spine.

The radiological investigation of these disorders consists of plain films in the first instance, frequently supplemented by tomography. These often need to be followed by myelography to demonstrate the exact site and extent of the lesion.

The effect of spinal compression is to cause muscular weakness or paralysis, and sensory disorders below the level of the lesion, the extent of these varying considerably according to the site and severity of the lesion responsible for the cord compression. There is often pain at the level of the lesion. Disorders of bowel and bladder function are common with compression at certain sites.

Some Other Disorders of the Central Nervous System

Idiopathic epilepsy—the name epilepsy is derived from a Greek verb meaning to seize hold of and derives from the fact that, in ancient times, the disease was attributed to possession of the sufferer's body by evil spirits.

Epilepsy is a functional disorder of the brain which may be of unknown causation (**idiopathic epilepsy**) or develop secondary to some other disease which affects the brain (**symptomatic epilepsy**), e.g. due to brain injury or cerebral tumour. It may present as a generalised disturbance of cerebral function (**general epilepsy**) or as a localised disturbance of such function (**focal epilepsy**).

Hereditary factors play a part in some but not all cases of idiopathic epilepsy.

In general epilepsy, and some forms of local epilepsy, patients are subject to attacks in which consciousness is partially or completely lost.

The severe forms of general epilepsy are known as **major epilepsy** (grand mal) and in them loss of consciousness is accompanied by muscular convulsions producing what are termed **epiletic fits** or **epileptic seizures**. Such fits do not occur in the milder forms of the disease which are termed **minor epilepsy** (petit mal).

Radiological investigations and electroencephalography are valuable aids in differentiating between idiopathic and symptomatic epilepsy.

Idiopathic epilepsy is treated by the daily administration of anticonvulsant drugs (e.g. phenobarbitone, phenytoin) with the object of preventing the attacks or diminishing their severity and frequency.

Migraine—this is a condition characterised by the occurrence of severe periodic headaches which are preceded by some form of temporary disturbance of vision or other sensation known as an **aura**, and are frequently accompanied by nausea and vomiting. The headache is frequently experienced in only one side of the head.

Sufferers from migraine are often highly conscientious individuals and given to worrying excessively about their affairs. They themselves may describe their symptoms as being due to **bilious attacks**.

Parkinsonism—a condition in which tremors and rigidity develop in the muscles of face, trunk and limbs as a result of degenerative or inflammatory lesions in structures called the *basal ganglia* (basal nuclei) which lie in the lower parts of the cerebral hemispheres.

It may occur as a primary disease of degenerative type when it is known as **paralysis agitans**, or as a secondary manifestation of various other diseases which affect the central nervous system. Among these latter is the virus infection called **encephalitis lethargica** and a rare hereditary disorder of copper metabolism called **Wilson's disease**, or **hepatolenticular degeneration**. In this latter disorder accumulation of copper occurs in the basal ganglia of the brain, the renal tubules, the eye and the liver where the resultant cellular damage leads to the development of cirrhosis.

Treatment is principally by drugs (e.g. levadopa, benzhexol) but stereotactic surgical procedures may be employed in selected cases to destroy certain parts of the basal ganglia.

Chorea—this condition may occur in a form known as **Sydenham's chorea**, when it is a manifestation of acute rheumatism (see p 70) due to inflammatory changes in the central nervous system. Chorea of this type was formerly called **St Vitus dance** after the patron saint of dancers.

The chief feature of chorea is the occurrence of abnormal jerky involuntary movements, described as **choreiform** movements.

Huntington's chorea, the other main type of chorea is an inherited disease in which choreiform movements occur in association with dementia.

Multiple sclerosis (disseminated sclerosis)—this is a common disease in which widespread lesions develop in the brain and spinal cord causing patchy destruction of myelin in nerve sheaths (a process termed **demyelinisation**), reactive proliferation of surrounding neuroglia, and later some destruction of nerve fibres.

The names of the disease derive from the multiple and disseminate (widespread) nature of the lesions and the areas of sclerosis (i.e. hardening) which develop in the central nervous system as a result of the overgrowth of neuroglia.

The cause of multiple sclerosis is unknown. Its maximum incidence is in early adult life. It pursues an intermittent course in its early stages, the first symptoms often disappearing completely and then reappearing, sometimes after the lapse of years. In accordance with the disseminate nature of the lesions, the clinical features are variable and may mimic those of many other disorders of the nervous system.

The diagnosis of multiple sclerosis may, however, be made by demonstrating unusual protein patterns in the cerebrospinal fluid, using sophisticated techniques of high resolution electrophoresis.

> Although the disease produces no radiological signs, patients with multiple sclerosis are frequently referred for X-ray examination, to exclude some other lesions (e.g. spinal tumour, cervical disc lesion) as being the cause of the signs and symptoms.

Among the many clinical features which may result from multiple sclerosis are disturbances of vision, speech and hearing; disturbances of gait; disturbances of bladder function; various forms of muscular paralysis and sensory disturbance; and mental changes. Mental changes often lead to an unwarranted feeling of well-being termed **euphoria**.

There is no specific treatment.

Syringomyelia—an uncommon disease of unknown origin which develops in adult life. Its basic feature is overgrowth of neuroglia in certain regions of the spinal cord and sometimes in the medulla oblongata; the latter changes being referred to as being due to **syringobulbia**. Proliferation of neurological tissue results in degeneration and destruction of nerve cells in affected areas resulting in clinical features such as wasting and weakness in the muscles of the hands and arms, spastic weakness of the lower limbs and characteristic sensory disturbances in the upper limbs (i.e. loss of sensibility to heat, cold and pain without loss of sensibility to touch, so-called **dissociated anaesthesia**).

The name of the disease derives from the occurrence of cavitation in areas of proliferation of the neuroglia, because in such areas the spinal cord bears some resemblance to a hollow tube (cf syringe, a type of hollow tube).

Complications of syringomyelia include the development of Charcot joints in the upper limbs, pes cavus (claw foot) and painless ulceration of the soles of the feet.

Subacute combined degeneration of the cord (vitamin B12 neuropathy)—this disorder develops as a complication in about 10% of patients with pernicious anaemia and is due to deficiency of vitamin B12. Sensory and motor changes develop in this condition as a result of degenerative changes in structures called *dorsal (posterior)* and *lateral columns* of the spinal cord (hence the name of combined degeneration), and also in peripheral nerves.

Treatment is by the administration of vitamin B12.

Hereditary ataxias—these are a group of uncommon hereditary disorders, degenerative in nature, in which **ataxia** (uncoordinated muscular movements) is the most prominent feature. In the type called **Friedreich'a ataxia** there is usually associated bilateral pes cavus (claw foot) and a scoliosis. The ataxia results in an unsteady gait, uncoordinated movements of the upper limbs and disordered speech.

Motor neurone disease—this term describes a rare group of diseases of unknown causation in which muscle wasting develops as a result of degenerative changes in motor neurones in the spinal cord and brain. The individual diseases of the group are named **progressive muscular atrophy**, **amyotrophic lateral sclerosis** and **progressive bulbar palsy**.

Alzheimer's disease—a disorder of unknown causation in which **dementia** (impairment of mental faculties due to organic brain disease) occurs as a result of diffuse cerebral atrophy. It is most common in the elderly and middle aged, but can occur in younger people.

According to Houston *et al* (4) about 50% of elderly patients with dementia have Alzheimer's disease, about 15% have cerebrovascular disease alone and about 20% have a combination of these two degenerative diseases.

Other Disorders of the Peripheral Nervous System

The peripheral nervous system consists of the cranial and spinal nerves. Some reference has already been made to certain **traumatic peripheral nerve injuries** and to the benign tumours called **neurofibromas** which arise from the sheaths of cranial and spinal nerves. Some of the other disorders which may affect such nerves include the following.

Optic neuritis—a disorder due to inflammatory or degenerative changes in the second cranial (optic) nerve. It may lead to atrophy of this nerve, a condition referred to as **optic atrophy**.

Trigeminal neuralgia (tic douloureux)—a disorder of unknown origin in which periodic attacks of severe pain occur within the distribution of the fifth cranial (trigeminal) nerve, i.e. in the face, forehead, teeth, jaws, and anterior part of the tongue.

Facial palsy (Bell's palsy)—a condition of unknown origin and sudden onset which affects the seventh cranial (facial nerve) causing a unilateral paralysis of the facial muscles.

Radiculitis—a term used to indicate inflammatory conditions and other disorders of the roots of the spinal nerves. Pressure on nerve roots from prolapsed intervertebral discs, bony spurs occurring in spondylosis, and carcinomatous metastases in the spine are common causes of radiculitis.

Pressure on certain roots of the brachial plexus by a cervical rib or other abnormalities in the region of the thoracic inlet (e.g. prolapsed intervertebral disc) may cause disturbances of motor and sensory function in the neck and forearm. These, sometimes together with associated disturbances of the blood supply resulting from pressure on the subclavian artery, produce clinical signs and symptoms described as being due to **thoracic inlet syndrome**. (*Note:* some authorities refer to this condition as **thoracic outlet syndrome**.)

Mononeuritis—a term used to indicate inflammatory conditions or other disorders affecting a single spinal or cranial nerve. Examples of these conditions are **optic neuritis**; **neuritis of the median nerve** due to compression of this nerve at the wrist in the disorder called **carpal tunnel syndrome**; and **ulnar neuritis**, due to compression of the ulnar nerve in the region of the medical epicondyle of the humerus (e.g. as a result of a fracture in this region).

Note: where a condition similar to mononeuritis affects several nerves it may be referred to as **multiple neuritis**. The term **neuritis** is also applied to certain disorders of nerve plexuses, e.g. **brachial neuritis**—a condition of acute onset causing pain in distribution of nerves arising from the brachial plexus and paralysis of muscles around the shoulder girdle. The term **polyneuritis** (see below) is applied to another type of disorder which affects many of the peripheral nerves and which usually produces lesions with a symmetrical distribution.

Peripheral neuropathy—a great many diseases may be complicated by degenerative changes (in most instances of non-inflammatory nature) in peripheral nerves producing a disorder described as peripheral neuropathy, or alternatively as **polyneuropathy, peripheral neuritis**, or **polyneuritis**.

The term **neuropathy** means a disease of nervous tissue. The prefix **poly-** indicates that a number of nerves are affected simultaneously.

The degenerative changes occur most commonly in the nerves of the limbs, especially the lower limbs, and tend to have a symmetrical distribution. Common features resulting from the disorder are muscular weakness, various forms of sensory disturbance and loss of normal reflexes in the areas supplied by the affected nerves.

Among the many causes of peripheral neuropathy may be mentioned: diabetes, diphtheria, various forms of chemical poisoning (e.g. lead poisoning, arsenical poisoning); nutritional deficiency diseases (e.g. **beriberi** due to lack of vitamin B1, chronic alcoholism, malabsorption syndromes); **malignant neuropathy** (due most commonly to bronchial carcinoma); and the uncommon disorder called **acute infective polyneuritis** (Guillain-Barré syndrome).

Peripheral neuropathy may also occur as a manifestation of **hereditary porphyria**, a rare disorder the other features of which include mental disturbances, the development of skin lesions as a result of exposure to sunlight, and the passage of urine which is dark red owing to the presence of pigments called porphyrins.

Menière's disease—see p 302.

Some Neurosurgical Operations

Surgical methods of opening the cranium.
These include the following.
  (i) Drilling one or more **burr holes**, e.g. for ventricular puncture to decompress the brain or introduce radiological contrast medium, or for aspiration of a cerebral abscess.
 (ii) **Trephining**—cutting out one or more circular discs of bone, which can subsequently be replaced, by means of an instrument called a **trephine**, e.g. for biopsy of a tumour or raising a depressed fracture.
(iii) **Craniotomy**—an operation which is performed when it is thought that an intracranial lesion (e.g. an operable type of neoplasm) can be dealt with by surgery. A large flap of scalp, bone and dura mater is cut and turned back in such a manner that it can be replaced at the end of the operation. This flap is known as an **osteoplastic flap**.

Laminectomy—removal of one or more vertebral laminae in order to gain access to the interior of the vertebral canal, e.g. to remove a spinal tumour or protrusion of an intervertebral disc.

Nerve suture and nerve grafting—see p 276.

Rhizotomy—cutting through the root of a spinal nerve in the spinal canal.

Sympathectomy—division or resection of a part of a sympathetic trunk or other part of the sympathetic nervous system, e.g. for chronic pain or peripheral arterial disease.

REFERENCES

(1) Thomson, A. D., Cotton, R. E. (1983). *Lecture Notes on Pathology*, 3rd Edn. Oxford: Blackwell.
(2) Du Boulay, G. H. (1980). *Principles of X-ray Diagnosis of the Skull*, 2nd Edn. London: Butterworths.
(3) Mann, W. N. (1975). *Conybeare's Textbook of Medicine* (Mann, W. N., Lessof, M. H., eds.). Edinburgh: Churchill Livingstone.
(4) Houston, J. C., Joiner, C. L., Trounce, J. R. (1982). *A Short Textbook of Medicine*. London: Hodder and Stoughton.

THE EYE

Some General Considerations

The *eye* is the organ of vision. Each *eyeball* is contained within a bony cavity called the *orbit*, which also contains the *orbital muscles* and *orbital fat*. Three coats of tissue surround the eyeball: (i) an outer fibrous coat consisting in its posterior two-thirds of the *sclera*, and anteriorly of a transparent layer called the *cornea*, (ii) a middle pigmented vascular coat called the *uveal tract*, consisting of the *choroid*, *ciliary body* and *iris*, (iii) an inner coat of nervous tissue called the *retina*.

The *optic nerve*, which is the nerve of vision, transmits visual stimuli from the retina to the brain. Its fibres leave the retina at the *optic disc*.

In the interior of the eye are the *anterior* and *posterior chambers*, partially separated by the iris and containing a liquid substance called *aqueous humour*, the *crystalline lens* and its *suspensory ligament* and, posteriorly, a jelly-like substance called the *vitreous humour*.

The amount of light entering the eyeball is controlled by the action of muscle fibres in the iris which can contract or dilate the *pupil*, i.e. the central aperture in the iris.

Within the eyeball light rays are bent to focus on the retina and form clear images of objects from which they are reflected. This process of bending light rays is called **refraction**. In order that the focus of the eye may be adjusted to view objects at different distances the eye possesses a property called **accommodation**, whereby alterations in focusing are made by altering the convexity of the anterior surface of the lens. Such alterations are effected by the action of muscle fibres in the ciliary body which can tighten or relax the suspensory ligament of the lens.

Under normal conditions, impulses are received by both eyes and slightly differing images are formed on each retina and then made into a single image by the brain. This is termed **binocular single vision**. (*Note:* vision with one eye is called **monocular vision**.)

Associated with the eyeball are several accessory structures such as the *orbital muscles* and *fascia*, *orbital fat*, *eyebrows*, *eyelids* and *eyelashes*, *conjunctiva* and *lacrimal apparatus*.

The *conjunctiva* is a mucous membrane which covers the exposed anterior portion of the white of the eye and the cornea and lines the inner surfaces of the eyelids.

The *lacrimal apparatus* of each eye consists of the *lacrimal gland* and its *ducts*, which secrete and carry tears into the conjunctival sac; and the *lacrimal passages*, i.e. the *lacrimal canaliculi*, *lacrimal sac* and *nasolacrimal duct*, through which the tears are conveyed from the conjunctival sac into the nasal cavity.

The prefixes **ophthalmo-** and **oculo-** both refer to the eye while **opto-** may refer to the eye or to vision. **Optics** is a branch of science relating to light and to vision. **Ophthalmology** is the branch of medicine concerned with disorers of the eye and its accessory structures.

Methods of investigation in ophthalmology include ordinary visual inspection; inspection of the interior of the eye with an **ophthalmo-scope**; visual inspection with magnifying devices and special illuminat-ion, e.g. **slit lamp microscopy**; investigation of visual acuity by **Snellen's test types**; **perimetry**, i.e. measurement of the extent of the field of vision; **refraction** (see p 294); **radiological investigations** such as plain radiography, orbital angiography, orbital venography, orbital pneumography, dacryocystography; CT; and **ultrasono-graphy**.

In the succeeding account it will be possible to indicate only a limited number of the many medical terms that refer to various disorders encountered in ophthalmic practice.

The treatment of ophthalmic conditions may involve local applications in the form of eye drops (guttae), eye lotions and eye ointments (oculenta); the internal administration of various drugs; surgical measures, and photocoagulation by laser beams.

The name **laser** stands for light amplification by stimulated emission of radiation. Conditions in which laser treatment may be used include retinal detachment, diabetic retinopathy, and melanoma of the eyeball.

Diseases of the Eyeball

These may be congenital, traumatic, infective, neoplastic, or of other types. The most important are given below.

Intraocular foreign body—this may be metallic or less commonly non-metallic. It is a serious condition as it may result in permanent visual damage, particularly if the lens is injured, and in other serious complications. Among these latter is the development of chronic **iridocyclitis** (inflammation of the iris and ciliary body) in the injured eye which may later be followed by a condition called **sympathetic ophthalmia** (sympathetic iridocyclitis) in which iridocyclitis also develops in the uninjured eye.

Ophthalmia is a term used to indicate certain forms of inflammation affecting the eyeball or conjunctiva.

X-rays are of great value in demonstrating and locating metallic foreign bodies in the eyeball and those that are magnetic may be removed with the aid of a hand magnet or giant magnet, according to their position. Ultrasound may be used to locate and help in the removal of non-metallic foreign bodies.

Inflammatory disorders—terms used to indicate inflammatory disorders occurring in various parts of the eyeball include the following: **keratitis** (cornea), **scleritis** (sclera), **iritis** (iris), **iridocyclitis** (iris and ciliary body), **uveitis** (uveal tract, i.e. iris, ciliary body and choroid), **choroiditis** (choroid), **retinitis** (retina), **papillitis** (optic disc), **panophthalmitis** (inflammation affecting all the tissues of the eyeball).

Corneal ulceration is a common result of inflammatory processes, due to trauma or other causes which affect the cornea. **Hypopyon** is a condition in which an inflammatory exudate is found in the anterior chamber of the eye and may develop as a complication of corneal ulceration.

Chronic inflammation of the cornea occurs in the condition called **interstitial keratitis**, usually a manifestation of congenital syphilis.

Iritis, usually accompanied by inflammatory changes in the ciliary body and thus generally more correctly referred to as **iridocyclitis**, is a not uncommon condition. It may occur in association with dental abscesses, infected paranasal sinuses or infective lesions elsewhere in the body, as a manifestation of sarcoidosis, tuberculosis, gonorrhoea or syphilis, or it may be due to other causes. In patients with sarcoidosis, lesions in iris and ciliary body are frequently associated with lesions in the parotid gland (**uveoparotid sarcoidosis**).

> Patients with iritis are frequently referred for chest X-rays to exclude tuberculosis and pulmonary sarcoidosis, dental and sinus X-rays to exclude infection around the roots of the teeth and in the paranasal sinuses; and also radiographs of the sacroiliac joints to exclude ankylosing spondylitis or other forms of sacroiliitis.

The term **retinitis** is used to include not only true inflammatory disorders of the retina, but also a number of degenerative and other disorders.

As stressed by Martin-Doyle and Kemp (1) it is less misleading to use the term **retinopathy** to describe various retinal manifestations of general disease in which the retinal changes are essentially of a degenerative nature. As described by the same authors, retinopathy may occur as a complication of arteriosclerosis (**arteriosclerotic retinopathy**), certain forms of renal disease (**renal retinopathy**), diabetes (**diabetic retinopathy**), leukaemia (**leukaemic retinopathy**), and as **toxaemic retinopathy** in pregnancy.

Neoplasms—these are all rare. They include **melanomas** (see p 131) which arise most frequently from the choroid; **retinoblastomas** malignant tumours of retinal cells which usually develop in childhood and are often bilateral; **gliomas of the optic nerve**; and **carcinomatous metastases** from primary tumours elsewhere in the body, e.g. the breast.

Vascular disorders of the retina—these include:
  (i) **retinal haemorrhages**—these may be due to a variety of causes including trauma and retinopathies (see above);
 (ii) **occlusion of the central artery of the retina**—due to thrombosis or embolism;
(iii) **thrombosis of the central vein of the retina**.

Glaucoma—a condition in which accumulation of fluid and a consequent rise in pressure occurs in the fluid in the anterior chamber of the eyeball. Causation of glaucoma is a complex subject for an understanding of which reference should be made to a textbook of ophthalmology. Primary and secondary varieties of the disorder are described. The latter may develop as a result of iridocyclitis, haemorrhage into the eyeball, etc.

A history of glaucoma is an important contraindication to the use of anticholinergic drugs such as hyoscine–N–butylbromide (Buscopan) in radiological procedures (e.g. to prevent muscle spasm during barium enemas).

The treatment of glaucoma may be medical or surgical.

Papilloedema—see p 283.

Detached retina—a disorder in which, due to different causes, an area of dissolution is formed within the retina and leads to detachment of a part of the retina, of varying extent, from the underlying choroid. Retinal detachment may occur as a result of trauma or complicate certain diseases of the retina, choroid, or iris and ciliary body. The condition is diagnosed by examination with the ophthalmoscope and treatment is surgical or by laser beam photocoagulation.

Toxic amblyopias—these are conditions in which a type of defective vision called **amblyopia** develops as a result of the action of certain toxic substances on the optic nerve or retina. Drinking methylated spirits or other drinks containing methyl alcohol is a well known cause of toxic amblyopia. Other forms of this disorder may occur as a result of excessive consumption of ordinary alcoholic drinks (ethyl alcohol) and excessive smoking of pipe tobacco.

Cataract—a fairly common disorder in which the crystalline lens of the eye, or its capsule, becomes partially or completely opaque. It may be of congenital or acquired type. Maternal rubella (German measles) developing in early pregnancy is one cause of the congenital variety. The variety of the acquired disorder, called **senile cataract**, is a common disorder of old age. Among the other types of acquired cataract may be mentioned cataract occurring as a complication of diabetes (**diabetic cataract**) and cataract due to excessive exposure to ionising radiation.

Operative removal of a cataract is called **cataract extraction**.

Optic atrophy—this is a degenerative disorder of the optic nerve leading to impairment of vision and sometimes to complete blindness. It may be due to certain diseases which affect the retina or optic disc (e.g. toxic amblyopias, papilloedema), neuritis of the optic nerve, see p 288), or to involvement of the optic nerve in certain diseases of the central nervous system (e.g. tabes dorsalis, or pressure from an intracranial neoplasm).

Senile macular degeneration—a common cause of defective vision in elderly people. It is due to a localised vascular lesion of the choroid beneath the macula.

Retrolental fibrodysplasia—a retinal disorder in which there occurs an overgrowth of retinal blood vessels leading to haemorrhages and formative of fibrous bands behind the lens of the eye. It is caused by administering excessive amounts of oxygen to premature infants.

Errors of Refraction

The process of refraction of light rays within the eye has been referred to on p 290. The term **ametropia** indicates a condition in which the refractive power of the eyeball is defective. The most commonly encountered types of ametropia are given below.

Hypermetropia (long sight)—a condition in which the eyeball is short and entering light rays are brought to a focus behind the retina. It is correctable by spectacles with convex lenses.

Myopia (short sight)—a condition in which the eyeball is long and entering light rays are brought to a focus in front of the retina. It may be corrected by spectacles with concave lenses.

Presbyopia (old sight)—a defect affecting near vision which develops with increasing years. It is due to defective accommodation (see p 290) resulting from loss of the normal elasticity of the crystalline lens of the eye.

Astigmatism—a condition in which rays of light coming from a point are imperfectly refracted and do not form a point image on the retina. It is most commonly due to an abnormality of the curvature of the cornea.

Strabismus (Squint)

An abnormality resulting from a lack of coordination of the orbital muscles which are responsible for the movements of the eyeballs. In this condition the visual axes of the two eyeballs, which are normally parallel, either converge or diverge. In some types of strabismus, there is **diplopia**, i.e. double vision, a condition in which single objects form two visual images. This, however, does not obtain in all types of strabismus because the brain may be able to suppress one of the two images.

Martin-Doyle and Kemp (2) describe two main forms of strabismus: **paralytic strabismus**, due to paralysis or weakness of one or more of the muscles which move the eyeballs, and **concomitant strabismus** which is due to a functional disorder affecting one or both of the eye balls.

Strabismus may occur in association with refractive error.

The main types of treatment employed singly or in combination in cases of squint are the correction of refractive errors, orthoptic treatment (see p 24) and operative treatment.

Conjunctivitis

Inflammation of the conjunctiva may present in acute or chronic form and may result from a variety of causes, among which are bacterial and viral infection, exposure to irritant gases and dusts, eyestrain, foreign body in the eye, allergy (e.g. hay fever).

Clinical features include **lacrimation** (excessive secretion of tears), discomfort in the eye, a mucopurulent or purulent discharge from the eye, and redness of the conjunctiva due to vascular congestion.

A special form of conjunctivitis which affects the newborn is called **ophthalmia neonatorum** and is due to infection of the eyes derived from the tissues of the maternal birth canal. Some cases are due to gonococcal infection. The disease may be prevented by instillation of antibiotic eye drops into the eyes of a newborn infant shortly after delivery.

Trachoma is a specific type of conjunctivitis which is very common in the tropics and subtropics and is due to infection with *Chlamydia trachomatis*.

An uncommon type of conjunctivitis occurs in association with urethritis and arthritis in **Reiter's syndrome** (see p 59).

The Orbit

Diseases of the orbit include:
 (i) **fractures of the bony walls of the orbit**;
 (ii) **orbital cellulitis**—an inflammation of the soft tissues of the

orbital cavity, due to infection with pyogenic bacteria and most commonly secondary to infection in the paranasal sinuses;

(iii) **benign** and **malignant neoplasms growing within the orbit**.

The eyeball may be pushed forward as a result of inflammatory or neoplastic processes within the orbit, a displacement referred to as **exophthalmos** or **proptosis**. Bilateral exophthalmos occurs as a feature of the disorder of the thyroid gland called exophthalmic goitre (see p 218).

Fractures of the orbit may occasionally result in displacement of the eyeball backwards into the cavity of the orbit. This condition is known as **enophthalmos**.

Diseases of the Eyelids

Traumatic conditions—these may take the form of bruising and haematoma formation (black eye), wounds or burns. Wounds and burns may result in the formation of scar tissue within the eyelids and various resultant deformities of these structures (see later).

Blepharitis—inflammation of the eyelids. This condition is usually of infective origin and may occur as an acute or chronic disorder.

Stye (hordeolum)—a condition due to pyogenic infection of sebaceous glands associated with the roots of the eyelashes.

Meibomian cyst (tarsal cyst)—a swelling in the eyelid arising from one of the *tarsal glands*. These latter are sebaceous glands lying between the conjunctival lining of the eyelids and the *tarsal plates*, which are plates of dense connective tissue within the eyelids.

Neoplasms—both benign and malignant neoplasms occur in the eyelids, the most common of the former being **papillomas**, and of the latter type, **rodent ulcers**.

Deformities of the eyelids—these may be congenital or due to traumatic, inflammatory or neoplastic disease, or spasm or paralysis of the muscles which move the eyelids. Some terms used in the description of these deformities are: (i) **coloboma**—a congenital defect in the margin of an eyelid; (ii) **entropion**—a turning inwards of an eyelid; (iii) **ectropion**—a turning out of an eyelid; (iv) **ptosis**—drooping of the upper eyelid; (v)v **symblepharon**—adhesion of an eyelid to the eyeball.

Diseases of the Lacrimal Apparatus

These diseases may affect the lacrimal glands or the lacrimal passages. The former group are rare. Inflammation of the lacrimal glands is termed **dacryoadenitis** and acute dacryoadenitis may occasionally occur as a complication of mumps.

Diminished secretion of the lacrimal glands, together with diminished secretion of the salivary glands is found in a disorder called **Sjogren's syndrome**, which occurs predominantly in middle-aged women and is frequently accompanied by chronic arthritis.

Rarely, the lacrimal glands may be enlarged as a result of tumour formation, and enlargement of the lacrimal and parotid glands occurs in **Mikulicz's syndrome**, a rare condition which may develop as a result of sarcoidosis and certain other generalised diseases.

The lacrimal passages may be obstructed as a result of congenital malformations; or traumatic inflammatory disorders resulting in **epiphora**, a condition in which the tears are unable to drain away normally and thus flow out of the conjunctival sac and down the cheek. One cause of this condition is **dacryocystitis**, i.e. inflammation of the lacrimal sac. Acute inflammatory changes in this latter structure may progress to the formation of an abscess in the sac termed a **lacrimal abscess**.

Obstruction of the lacrimal passages which is not relieved by simpler measures may necessitate **dacryorhinostomy**, an operation in which a permanent communicaton is made between the lacrimal sac and the nasal cavity.

The site of a chronic obstructive lesion in the lacrimal passages may be demonstrated by a form of contrast radiography called **dacryocystography**.

Some Ophthalmic Operations

Brief reference has already been made to the operations of **cataract extraction** and **dacryorhinostomy** and the use of lasers, and it has been indicated that operative measures may be employed in the treatment of glaucoma and strabismus.

Three terms referring to surgical procedures not included in the foregoing account are: (i) **iridectomy**—removal of a portion of the iris; (ii) **corneal grafting** (corneal transplantation—keratoplasty), an operation in which a portion of the cornea is excised from a patient's eye and replaced by a portion of cornea of similar size taken from a donor eye; (iii) **enucleation of the eyeball**—removal of the eyeball from its socket.

REFERENCES

(1) and (2) Martin-Doyle, J. L. C., Kemp, M. H. (1976). *A Synopsis of Ophthalmology*, 5th Edn. Bristol: Wright.

THE EAR

Some General Considerations

The ear is the organ of hearing and of balance. Each ear consists of three parts:

(i) **the external ear**, consisting of the *pinna (auricle)* and *external auditory meatus*;

(ii) **the middle ear** (tympanic cavity, tympanum), which is separated from the external ear by the *tympanic membrane (eardrum)* and contains the three *auditory ossicles*, the *malleus*, *incus* and *stapes*. The middle ear contains air at atmospheric pressure as its cavity communicates with the nasopharynx via the *Eustachian tube*. This cavity also communicates with the *mastoid air cells*.

During part of its course the *seventh cranial nerve (facial nerve)* lies in bony canal called the *facial canal*, which runs through the medial and posterior walls of the middle ear. The *chorda tympani* (nerve of taste) joins the motor portion of the facial nerve in the facial canal;

(iii) **the inner ear** (labyrinth) consists of several cavities in the petrous portion of the temporal bone, i.e. the *cochlea*, *vestibule* and *semicircular canals*, which constitute the *bony labyrinth*, and a number of membranous structures contained in these cavities, i.e. the *duct of the cochlea* (containing the *organ of Corti*), the *utricle* and *saccule*, and the *membranous ducts* of the *semicircular canals*, these latter structures forming the *membranous labyrinth*.

A fluid called *endolymph* circulates within the membranous labyrinth and another fluid called *perilymph* circulates in the space between this structure and the surrounding walls of the bony labyrinth.

The inner ear is separated from the middle ear by a bony partition in which lie two openings, the *oval window (fenestra vestibuli)* into which fits the footplate of the stapes, and the *round window (fenestra cochleae)* which is closed by a fibrous membrane.

The *cochlear division* of the *eighth cranial nerve (acoustic nerve, auditory nerve)* transmits impulses concerned with hearing to the brain from the hair cells in the organ of Corti. Impulses concerned with balance also pass to the brain, from end-organs in the membranous ducts of the semicircular canals and in the utricle and saccule, being transmitted by the *vestibular division* of this nerve.

The inner part of the external auditory canal. the middle ear, the inner ear, and the mastoid air cells are all contained within the temporal bone.

In its course from the inner ear to the brain the eighth cranial nerve traverses the petrous portion of the temporal bone through a bony canal called the *internal auditory meatus*. Before entering the facial canal, the seventh cranial (facial nerve) also lies in the internal auditory meatus. (*Note:* the word **meatus** may indicate either a canal or an opening.)

The branch of medicine concerned with diseases of the ear is called **otology**, a name of Greek derivation. The adjectives **otic** and **aural** are both used with reference to the ear, the latter word being of Latin derivation. The surgery of the ear is sometimes called **aural surgery**. The adjective **auditory** may be used to refer to the ear or to the sense of hearing, and the adjective **acoustic** to indicate the sense of hearing.

Pathological conditions that affect the organs of hearing may be congenital, traumatic, infective, neoplastic or due to high intensity noises. Among their clinical features may be mentioned the following: **deafness** (impairment or loss of the sense of hearing), **otorrhoea** (discharge from the ear), **otalgia** (pain in the ear), **tinnitus** (ringing in the ears), **vertigo** (giddiness).

Methods of investigation used in the investigation of disorders encountered in otology include: (i) visual examination of the external ear and tympanic membrane with an instrument equipped with a magnifying lens and an illuminating device, called an **auriscope** or **otoscope**; (ii) examination by means of an **operating microscope**; (iii) bacteriological examination of discharges from the ear; (iv) radiological investigation of the ear and temporal bone by plain films and tomography, conventional and computed; (v) **hearing tests**. These test the patient's ability to hear whispered and normal speech at different distances, ability to hear the sound produced by a tuning fork, and investigate hearing by a method termed **audiometry**. This is carried out with an electronic instrument called an **audiometer** which enables a record, called an **audiogram**, to be made.

Some of the disorders of the organs of hearing will now be discussed.

Diseases of the External Ear

Congenital disorders—these include various malformations of the pinna and complete or partial failure of development of the external auditory meatus.

Cauliflower ear—a condition of enlargement and deformity of the pinna due to trauma which causes the formation of a haematoma within this structure.

Otitis externa—a term used to indicate inflammatory changes in the external auditory meatus, arising usually as a result of infection of the skin lining this structure. The infection may be primary or occur secondary to otitis media complicated by perforation of the eardrum. One form of external otitis is the so-called **meatal furuncle** (boil) which is due to staphylococcal infection of a hair follicle in the meatus.

Otitis externa is often a painful disorder and causes a discharge from the ear.

Neoplasms—these include **osteoma** arising from the bony wall of the external auditory meatus; **epithelioma** (squamous cell carcinoma) arising from the skin of the pinna or external meatus; and **rodent ulcer** (basal cell carcinoma) of the skin of the pinna.

Impacted wax in the meatus—this condition results from excessive accumulation of wax (cerumen) produced by the *ceruminous glands* in the outer cartilaginous part of the meatus. It may cause conductive deafness (see later) which can be relieved by softening the wax by eardrops and subsequent syringing.

Diseases of the Tympanic Membrane

Myringitis—i.e. inflammation of the tympanic membrane (eardrum), occurs most commonly in association with otitis media (inflammation of the middle ear) and may result in spontaneous perforation of the membrane. Spontaneous perforation may be avoided by **myringotomy**, an operation in which a small incision is made through the tympanic membrane to permit infective discharges to escape from the middle ear.

Myringitis may also develop as a complication of otitis externa.

Traumatic rupture of the tympanic membrane—McNab Jones (1) gives the following examples of the causes of this condition: direct trauma, blast and fractured skull.

Diseases of the Middle Ear

Otitis media—this term means inflammation of the middle ear. Such inflammation is usually due to pathogens (e.g. streptococci, staphylococci) which reach the middle ear via the Eustachian tube and derive from some infective process in the upper respiratory tract. Otitis media may thus develop as a complication of conditions such as coryza, tonsillitis, sinusitis, enlarged adenoids; and from secondary bacterial infections of the upper respiratory tract complicated by virus diseases such as measles and influenza. A much less common route of infection is from the external auditory meatus via a traumatic perforation in the tympanic membrane.

Otitis media may be of acute, subacute or chronic type. It is a common disease, especially in children, and is often bilateral.

Acute suppurative otitis media is a serious condition in which pus forms in the middle ear and, if not controlled by treatment, or if untreated, may result in complications such as the following:

- **perforation of the tympanic membrane** and resultant otorrhoea;
- spread of infection to the mastoid antrum and mastoid air cells causing **mastoiditis**;
- rarely, spread of infection to the inner ear causing **labyrinthitis**;
- spread of infection to air cells which are sometimes present in the petrous bone, causing **petrositis**;

- thrombosis in neighbouring veins which may spread to reach the lateral (sigmoid) venous sinus of the dura mater causing **lateral sinus thrombosis**;
- spread of infection through the temporal bone causing **extradural abscess**, **meningitis**, or **cerebral abscess**;
- formation of adhesions between the auditory ossicles and resultant permanent **defect of hearing**;
- **chronic otitis media** (see below).

Severe pain in the ear together with general signs of infection and deafness are common features of acute otitis media. If the tympanic membrane ruptures or myringotomy is performed, there is also a purulent discharge from the external meatus. When mastoiditis complicates the disease there is then pain in the mastoid process and tenderness of this structure. Swelling of soft tissues over the mastoid process, or in front of the pinna, may also develop.

Treatment is by administration of systemic penicillin or other antibiotic and analgesic drugs. Myringotomy may also be indicated. When acute mastoiditis complicates the disease it may be necessary to drain the pus from the mastoid process by an operation termed **cortical mastoidectomy** (conservative mastoidectomy).

Chronic suppurative otitis media may develop as a sequel to acute suppurative otitis media, or may be the result of an infective process which is chronic from the outset. It is frequently associated with chronic mastoid infection and also with chronic sinusitis and enlarged adenoids. In this type of infection there is a permanent perforation of the eardrum and destructive changes may occur which affect the bony walls of the middle ear, and often involve the mastoid process as well. In addition there may be considerable destruction of the auditory ossicles resulting in permanent impairment of hearing.

The chief clinical features are otorrhea and deafness.

The complications of chronic otitis media include (i) overgrowth of granulation tissue (see p 38) within the middle ear leading to the formation of a polypoid swelling called an **aural polyp** which may protrude through a perforation of the eardrum; (ii) formation of a **cholesteatoma**, a tumour-like mass of dead epithelial cells, bacteria and cholesterol crystals which develops in the middle ear as a result of inflammation, and may extend into the mastoid process; (iii) involvement of the facial nerve and resultant **facial paralysis** as a result of involvement of the walls of the facial canal (see p 298) in the infective process; (iv) **labyrinthitis**; (v) **intracranial spread**.

Surgical treatment, designed to eradicate the infection in the middle ear and mastoid, by the operations of **modified radical mastoidectomy** or **radical mastoidectomy** may be necessary in chronic otitis media. In suitable cases, the perforation in the tympanic membrane associated with the disease may subsequently be repaired by a plastic operation called **tympanoplasty** (myringoplasty).

Secretory otitis media—is another form of otitis media and is associated with Eustachian tube obstruction and the formation of a thick exudate in the middle ear. This latter has led to the disorder being termed **glue ear**. It is common in childhood.

Myringotomy, suction, and drainage with a grommet-type or other type of ventilation tube are measures employed in treatment.

Neoplasms—these are rare. They include **carcinoma of the middle ear** (which often spreads into the external ear) and a very rare neoplasm called a **glomus tumour**. This is a benign neoplasm but may grow so as to invade and destroy the middle ear and the inner ear. It belongs to a class of tumours called **chemodectomas**. These may arise at several sites in the body in minute structures which are called *chemoreceptors* and are sensitive to certain types of chemical change in the circulating blood. (*Note:* another example of a chemodectoma is the **carotid body tumour**, a rare neoplasm arising from the carotid body at the bifurcation of the common carotid artery.)

Otosclerosis—a disease of unknown cause in which the formation of new bone occurs within the bony labyrinth and involves the oval window, first limiting and then preventing movement of the stapes (the innermost of the auditory ossicles). Loss of mobility of the stapes interferes with the normal conduction of sound waves through the middle ear and thus causes progressive deafness of a type called conductive deafness (see later).

Otosclerosis tends to run in families. It affects both ears, is commoner in females than in males, and its onset is usually in adolescence or early adult life.

Surgery, in the form of an operation called **stapedectomy**, may relieve the deafness. This operation involves removal of the stapes bone and implantation of a Teflon piston or other form of prosthesis in its place.

Diseases of the Inner Ear

Labyrinthitis—as has been noted the inner ear is also known as the labyrinth and the term labyrinthitis hence indicates inflammation of the inner ear. This condition occurs most commonly as a result of spread of an acute or chronic infection from the middle ear but may be due to other causes (e.g. sensitivity to the drug streptomycin; virus infection limited to the labyrinth alone). Labyrinthitis causes impairment of hearing, vertigo and other disorders of balance. Another feature of this condition may be the presence of abnormal eye movement termed **nystagmus**.

Menière's disease—a disease of unknown cause affecting the labyrinth of one or sometimes both sides and characterised by violent attacks of sudden vertigo (giddiness), tinnitus (ringing in the ears) and progressive loss of hearing. It is associated with an increase in tension of the fluid circulating in the semicircular canals. In the first instance treatment is medical, but if this fails surgical measures of various types may be advocated or ultrasound may be used to destroy the labyrinth.

Diseases of the Auditory Nerve

Traumatic—the eighth cranial (auditory, acoustic) nerve may be damaged by fractures of the skull involving the petrous portion of the temporal bone. There may be concomitant injury to the facial nerve.

Infective—various forms of meningeal infection and certain virus infections may affect the auditory nerve.

Neoplastic—acoustic neurofibroma—see p 280.

Types of Deafness

Foxen (2) describes conductive; sensorineural and mixed deafness.

Deafness is a condition of impairment or loss of the sense of hearing.

The normal mechanism of hearing is the passage of atmospheric vibrations, called sound waves, along the external auditory meatus and their transmission through the tympanic membrane and the auditory ossicles of the middle ear to the oval window. Here they set up pressure waves in the perilymph (see p 298). These latter are transmitted to the endolymph through the membranous walls of the duct of the cochlea, where they produce stimuli which are received by the nervous end-organs in the organ of Corti. These stimuli are then transmitted to the brain by nerve fibres in the cochlear division of the acoustic (auditory) nerve, where they produce sensations of hearing.

Interference with the transmission of sound waves by the tympanic membrane or the ossicles causes **conductive deafness**. Interference with reception of stimuli by the organ of Corti, as a result of diseases of the labyrinth which affect the cochlea or, alternatively as a result of lesions of nerve fibres which transmit hearing impulses along the acoustic nerve, cause **sensorineural deafness**. **Mixed deafness** is due to a combination of factors responsible for conductive and sensorineural deafness.

Examples of conditions which cause conductive deafness are impacted wax in the ear, otitis media of both suppurative and secretory type, traumatic rupture of the ear drum, and otosclerosis. Among the diseases causing sensorineural deafness are various forms of labyrinthitis; fractures of the petrous portion of the temporal bone causing damage to the labyrinth or acoustic nerve; acoustic neurofibroma; Meniére's disease; and certain disorders of the central nervous system.

The treatment of deafness is directed, where possible, to the treatment of its cause by conservative or surgical measures. The disability resulting from deafness that cannot be adequately relieved by such measures may be alleviated by learning **lip reading** or using **hearing aids.**

REFERENCES

(1) McNab Jones, R. (1980). *Surgery*. (Robinson, J. O., Brown, A., eds.). London: Heinemann.
(2) Foxen, E. H. M. (1980). *Lecture Notes on Diseases of the Ear, Nose and Throat*. Oxford: Blackwell.

THE MIND

The Greek word psyche means the soul or mind and the science concerned with the study of the mind and mental processes is called **psychology**.

The branch of medicine concerned with disorders and disabilities of mental processes is termed **psychiatry** or **psychological medicine**.

A detailed description of terms used in psychiatry is beyond the scope of this book but it may be noted that among the important type of conditions encountered in psychiatric practice are the following.

Mental handicap (formerly termed subnormality)—a condition in which development of the mind is arrested or incomplete and intelligence is below normal.

Mental handicap may result from hereditary factors, or disease or injury affecting the developing brain during fetal life or childhood.

Psychoneuroses (neuroses)—these are disorders of mental function which affect large numbers of the population. While they do not produce any complete breakdown of mental processes and affected patients often possess considerable insight into their own psychological problems, they may produce serious effects, both mental and physical, and impairment of work efficiency.

Some examples of disorders classified as psychoneuroses are: **anxiety states**, **obsessive-compulsive neuroses**, **post-traumatic neuroses**, **hysteria**, **anorexia nervosa** (a condition, seen predominantly in young single women, of immature personality, who refuse to take food of all types and consequently develop severe wasting. There is often also amenorrhoea and other endocrine changes), **phobic neuroses** (persistent unjustified or irrational fears), and **behaviour disorders of childhood**.

Psychoses—severe disorders of mental function in which the patient's insight into his own psychological problems may be impaired or lost. They produce a marked breakdown in mental processes, which in some of these conditions is temporary but in others is permanent.

Psychoses are often accompanied by hallucinations, delusion and impulsive behaviour.

Important types of psychoses are:

• **schizophrenia**—a disease whose name means 'split mind' and in which disintegration of personality occurs. A major problem in psychiatric practice;

- **affective disorders** (disorders of mood)—**mania** and **depression**;
- **melancholia of involutional type**;
- **organic psychoses**—i.e. in which the mental disorder develops secondarily to some organic disorder of the brain (e.g. traumatic, infective, neoplastic, toxic effects arising from chronic alcoholism; or idiopathic, as in Alzheimer's disease—see p 287);
- **psychoses of the elderly**, e.g. **senile dementia, senile confusional states, senile mania, senile melancholia**.

Aberrations of sexual behaviour, e.g. **homosexuality** and **sexual perversion**.

Disorders resulting from defective development of personality, e.g. **psychopathic personality**, a disorder in which immaturity of personality prevents the patient from adapting himself to normal social relationships. Common features of this condition include irresponsible and often aggressive behaviour, a lack of moral principles and an inability to form lasting friendships.

Addiction to alcohol or drugs, e.g. morphine, cocaine, heroin, amphetamines, barbiturates, cannabis (marihuana), lysergic acid diethylamide (LSD25).

Psychosomatic disorders, i.e. disorders in which there is thought to be a significant association between mental factors and structural changes in organs and tissues other than those of the nervous system. Authorities who accept the concept of psychosomatic disorders differ as to the diseases which should be so regarded. Among the conditions described by some writers as being of this nature are eczema, neurodermatitis, bronchial asthma, primary thyrotoxicosis, peptic ulceration and ulcerative colitis.

A brief reference to some forms of treatment for psychiatric illness was made on p 23.

The legal provisions regarding the care and treatment of patients with mental illness have been the subject of change as a result of the coming into force in September 1983 of the Mental Health Act 1983 which repeals many, but not all, the provisions of the Mental Health Act 1959. The new Act gives legal definitions of mental disorder, mental and severe mental impairment, and psychopathic disorder.

PART V

Certain Other Types of Diseases

CONNECTIVE TISSUE DISEASES

Connective tissue is composed of cells and of ground substance called *matrix*. Bone, *cartilage* and *white fibrous tissue* are all types of connective tissue.

Most types of this tissue contain *fibres* within their matrix of types known as *white, elastic,* or *reticular fibres*.

White fibres are composed of *collagen*, a protein substance which is an important constituent of white fibrous tissue, areolar tissue, cartilage and bone.

The term **connective tissue diseases** describes a diverse group of conditions which show widespread lesions in the connective tissues of various structures and organs, often associated with changes in the collagen content of these tissues. Many of these diseases are thought to be due to autoimmune factors.

Thomson and Cotton (1) include in their description of these disorders: **rheumatoid arthritis**, **rheumatic fever**, and several other conditions among which are the following.

Systemic lupus erythematosus (SLE)—also known as disseminated lupus erythematosus. Its features include fever, inflammatory lesions in bones and joints, arteritis, skin rashes, pleural and pericardial effusions and disorders of the central nervous system. Characteristic LE cells may be shown in the blood.

Scleroderma—also called **progressive systemic sclerosis**—characterised by (as indicated by its name which means hard skin) areas of skin thickening. Lesions may also occur in the joints, tendons, lungs, gastrointestinal tract and kidneys.

Dermatomyositis—see p 265.

Polymyalgia rheumatica—a condition of unknown origin in which persistent pain and stiffness develop in muscle groups, usually those of the shoulder and pelvic girdles and upper part of the limbs. There is often associated fever, and temporal arteritis (giant-cell arteritis) sometimes develops as a complication (see p 84).

Polyarteritis nodosa—in which widespread inflammatory changes develop in the walls of small and medium arteries. These may include arteries supplying the joints, retina, gastrointestinal tract, and nervous system. Haemorrhages and aneurysm formation may occur.

Wegener's granulomatosis—characterised by ulcerative lesions in the nasal passages, chronic inflammatory changes in the lungs and glomerulonephritis.

REFERENCES

(1) Thomson, A. D., Cotton, R. E. (1983). *Lecture Notes on Pathology*, 3rd Edn. Oxford: Blackwell.

TROPICAL DISEASES

Certain diseases which show their greatest incidence in warm climates (but sometimes also occur in temperate and cold climates) are classified as **tropical diseases**.

Many tropical diseases are in the nature of infections or infestations. Nutritional disorders, although frequently showing a high incidence among the inhabitants of many of the developing countries in the tropics and subtropics, are not generally classified under the heading of tropical diseases.

The condition of **tropical sprue** has already been referred to when discussing terms describing various forms of malabsorption syndromes.

Some reference has been made when describing various diseases of the blood, to **sickle-cell anaemia** and **thalassaemia** (Cooley's anaemia or Mediterranean anaemia), two forms of haemolytic anaemia whose maximum incidence occurs among the natives of certain countries with warm climates.

Discussion in this section will be limited to terms indicating certain important infections and infestations that occur predominantly in the tropics and subtropics.

Infections

These may be due to bacteria, viruses, fungi, or protozoa.

Dysentery—this term indicates a condition of disordered bowel action. The predominant feature of conditions described as dysentery is an infective colitis (inflammation of the large bowel) resulting in diarrhoea, often accompanied by the passage of blood and mucus in the stools. The causal organisms of dysentery are excreted in the faeces of infected individuals and transmitted to other individuals by contaminated food and water.

Bacillary dysentery, as indicated by its name, is a bacterial infection with bacilli called *Shigellae*. According to the nature of the causal bacilli it may take the form of **Shiga, Flexner** or **Sonne dysentery**. The disease begins as acute colitis and may occasionally result in chronic infection of the colon. Complications are rare but include a form of arthritis termed **colitic arthritis**. Bacillary dysentery is of worldwide distribution but has a considerably higher incidence in warm climates than in temperate climates.

Chronic bacillary dysentery may cause ulceration of the colonic mucosa and fibrosis of the colonic walls. It may thus produce appearances at barium enema similar to those seen in chronic ulcerative colitis (see p 127).

Amoebic dysentery (intestinal amoebiasis)—may be contracted outside the tropics but is predominantly a tropical disease. It is due to infection with a protozoon called *Entamoeba histolytica*. It can cause acute colitis which subsequently becomes chronic in nature but, more commonly, causes colonic inflammation which is chronic from its onset. Chronic amoebic colitis may be complicated by spread of infection to the liver, causing **amoebic hepatitis** (hepatic amoebiasis) or **amoebic liver abscess** and, less commonly, to the lungs resulting in **pulmonary amoebiasis**.

Like chronic bacillary dysentery (see above) chronic amoebic colitis may produce appearances at barium enema similar to those seen in chronic ulcerative colitis.

Giardiasis, also known as **lambliasis**, is a type of dysentery due to infection with a protozoan *Giardia lamblia*. As well as occurring in the tropics it is found in temperate climates. It is much less common than either bacillary or amoebic dysentery.

Malaria—this is the commonest of all tropical infections. It is caused by a protozoon called the *malaria parasite*, which undergoes part of its life cycle in a species of mosquito called *anopheles*. A human becomes infected with malaria as a result of malaria parasites gaining access to his bloodstream through the bite of an infected female anopheline mosquito. Within the human body the life cycle of the parasites is continued, firstly in the liver and then in red blood cells in the circulating blood. The red blood cells which contain the parasites rupture at a certain stage of development of the parasites and these latter are then set free within the bloodstream. The characteristic attacks of malarial fever develop at the times of such release of malaria parasites into the bloodstream. The coincident destruction of red cells may result in the development of anaemia of the haemolytic type.

There are four different types of malaria parasite, the two most commonly encountered being *Plasmodium vivax* and *Plasmodium falciparum*. The former causes a clinical form of disease called **benign tertian malaria**, in which bouts of fever occur every third day.

Plasmodium falciparum also tends to produce attacks of fever with a three-day periodicity but the infection is more severe and is known as **malignant tertian malaria**. This latter condition may be complicated by brain involvement causing **cerebral malaria**, or by extensive destruction of red cells within the circulation causing a disorder termed **blackwater fever**, in which haemoglobin is set free in the blood plasma (haemoglobinaemia) and is consequently passed in the urine (haemoglobinuria).

Splenomegaly (enlargement of the spleen) is a frequent development in patients with chronic or recurrent malarial infections.

Benign tertian malaria is subject to recurrences of infection which may persist for up to about two years after the infected individual has left a malarious area.

The clinical diagnosis of malaria is confirmed by demonstration of the causal parasites in a blood smear.

Quinine has been used for many centuries in the treatment of malaria but, in recent times, modern synthetic drugs such as chloroquine and primaquine have been extensively used in its therapy. Chloroquine, and other drugs such as proguanil, may also be used by those living in malarious areas in order to suppress the clinical features of malarial infection in the so-called **suppressant therapy of malaria**.

The incidence of infection in malarious areas may be largely controlled by precautions taken by individuals to avoid mosquito bites and measures designed to destroy anopheline mosquitoes and prevent their breeding.

Cholera—is a bacterial infection of the small intestine, due to a pathogen called the *Vibrio cholerae* or *comma bacillus*, which causes inflammatory changes in the large bowel. These result in severe diarrhoea with typical rice-water stools, vomiting and dehydration. This disease occurs most commonly in the Far East, where it appears from time to time in epidemic form, sometimes with high mortality. It is spread by food and water contaminated by the excreta of sufferers from the disease. There is no specific treatment but protection against the disease may be given by prophylactic vaccination.

Plague—is a bacterial infection which is endemic in some tropical and subtropical countries and sometimes appears in epidemic form. The causal pathogen is called *Pasteurella pestis*; the name *Pasteurella* deriving from that of the nineteenth century French bacteriologist Louis Pasteur.

There are three clinical types of plague called **bubonic**, **pneumonic** and **septicaemic plague**, the first-named being the most common. Infection is derived from infected rats and other rodents and transmitted to man by the bite of rat fleas.

Bubonic plague is so-called from the fact that the regional lymph glands draining the area of the flea bite form enlarged tender swellings called **buboes**.

Plague in former times was not confined in its occurrence to countries with warm climates, and in mediaeval times was referred to as the **Black Death**.

The incidence of plague may be diminished by measures to destroy rats and fleas and by protective vaccination of subjects living in infected localities.

Brucellosis—the type of this infection called **Malta fever** is classified as a tropical disease (see p 62).

Leprosy—this chronic bacterial infection only develops as a result of prolonged contact with other individuals who are suffering from the disease. The lesions of leprosy develop in the nerves, skin, subcutaneous tissues and mucous membranes and sometimes also affect the skeleton.

There are two principal clinical types of the disorder known as **nodular (lepromatous) leprosy** and **maculo–anaesthetic leprosy**.

Yaws—this is a granulomatous condition which develops in stages and shows certain clinical similarities to syphilis. It also gives rise to a positive Wasserman reaction in the blood but is not of venereal origin. The causal organism is a spirochaete called *Treponema pertenue*.

Bone and joint lesions occur in yaws and appearances on radiographs, due to periostitis and osteomyelitis, strongly resemble those of syphilic infection.

Tropical ulcer—a type of sloughing ulceration of the skin, which occurs in hot countries and appears to be associated with malnutrition and general ill health. Ulceration of this type is most commonly seen in the lower limb, below the knee.

Other tropical infections—some of these and their mode of transmission are given below.

    Bacterial—**typhoid fever** (see p 52), **relapsing fever** man to man by ticks or lice). **rat–bite fever** (usually rat direct to man).

- **Rickettsiae**—**typhus fever**, **Q fever**, **Rocky Mountain spotted fever** and **trench fever** (see p 60).
- **Viral**—**dengue** (man to man by *aedes* mosquitoes), **sandfly fever** (man to man by sandflies), **yellow fever** (man to man by *aedes* mosquitoes), **Lassa fever** (mode of transmission uncertain, infection also occurs in rats); **Marburg disease** (mode of transmission unknown; infection known also to occur in green monkeys); **Japanese B encephalitis** (animals and birds to man by culicine mosquitoes).
- **Protozoal**—**cutaneous leishmaniasis** or **oriental sore** (man to man by sandflies); **visceral leishmaniasis** or **kala-azar** (man to

man by sandflies); **African trypanosomiasis** or **sleeping sickness** (from man to man, or from cattle or antelopes to man, by *tsetse* flies); **South American trypanosomiasis** or **Chagas' disease** (from man to man, or certain animals to man, by winged bugs).

• **Fungal**—these include the infections named **blastomycoses**, **coccidioidomycosis**, **histoplasmosis**, **mycetoma** (Madura foot), and **sporotrichosis**. (*Note:* fungal infections may be referred to as **mycotic infections** or **mycoses**.)

Infestations

These disorders are due to the presence in the body of organisms called *helminths* or *worms* which are **parasitic** in nature, i.e. they live in or on the tissues of another organism, referred to as a **host**, from which they draw their nutriment. Some worms require only one host for the completion of their life cycle; others undergo the earlier stages of their development in a so-called **intermediate host**, and the adult stages in a second host known as a **definitive host**.

There are three main types of helminths: *nematodes* (e.g. *roundworms*), *cestodes* or *tapeworms*, and *trematodes* or *flukes*. Some nematodes have only a single host but tapeworms and flukes require both an intermediate and a definitive host.

Infestations with parasitic helminths occur with much greater frequency in the tropics and subtropics than in temperate regions.

Some important disorders due to such infestations are as follows:

Ascariasis—a common infestation, of wide distribution and due to a round worm called *Ascaris lumbricoides*. This worm, which may be as much as ten inches long, goes through its life cycle within a human host and its ova are excreted in the faeces. The infestation is spread to other humans by food or water contaminated with ascaris ova.

During their development within the body, the parasites pass through the lungs where they may cause inflammatory changes. The adult worms live in the small bowel of the host where they may be demonstrated by a barium meal follow-through examination.

Oxyuriasis—(threadworm infestation)—a condition due to nematodes called *threadworms* which live in the intestine of the human host. Threadworm infestation is of worldwide distribution and particularly common in children. It frequently leads to pruritus (itching) and inflammatory changes in the region of the anus and vulva. The ova are excreted in the faeces.

Ankylostomiasis (hookworm infestation)—an infestation due to a nematode called the *hookworm* or *Ankylostoma duodenale*, which has a very high incidence in many tropical countries. The adult worms live in the intestine causing inflammatory changes and bleeding from the intestinal wall. This bleeding frequently results in severe anaemia. The ova of the parasites are excreted in the faeces and, when they are deposited in warm soil, develop into embryos which can invade the body of another human host by penetrating his skin. They then reach his intestine via the venous circulation, lungs, oesophagus and stomach.

Other nematode infestations—these include **trichiniasis** (muscle worm infestation) in which the pig is the intermediate host and man, the definitive host; **dracontiasis** (Guinea-worm infestation) in which a small fresh water organism of the crustacean variety is the intermediate host and man the definite host; and **filariasis** in which the parasites are transmitted from man to man by mosquito bites. The commonest form of filariasis is due to a parasitic worm called *Wuchereria bancrofti* and is associated with blockage of lymphatic channels in affected tissues, leading to **elephantiasis**, a condition of marked thickening of the skin and subcutaneous tissues.

The diseases called **loa-loa** and **onchocerciasis** (river blindness) are other varieties of filariasis, and the disorder called **tropical pulmonary eosinophilia** is thought to be an allergic reaction to the presence of certain types of filariae within the lungs.

Tapeworm infestations—the principal of these in man are infestations with the pork tapeworm, *Taenia solium*, and the beef tapeworm, *Taenia saginata*, and the disorder called hydatid disease.

Cattle are the intermediate hosts in beef tapeworm infestation.

In human infestation with the pork tapeworm the pig is usually the intermediate host and man the definitive host. Occasionally, however, a human subject may become the intermediate host of this parasite by ingesting its ova and develop a disorder called **cysticercosis**; characterised by the development of epilepsy and the presence of pathological calcification within the bodies of parasitic embryos which, have settled and subsequently died in the tissues of the skeletal muscles. Such calcification may readily be demonstrated on radiographs.

Hydatid disease (Echinococcus disease) is due to the *Taenia echinococcus*. This tapeworm is a parasite of dogs. If its ova are ingested by a human being, embryos which develop from them may enter the circulation, and reaching sites such as the liver, lungs, kidneys and bones may then produce **hydatid cysts**. Sufferers from hydatid disease usually give positive reactions to a blood test called a **complement fixation test** and a skin test called the **Casoni test**.

Schistosomiasis (bilharziasis)—this is the name given to a group of diseases caused by members of a species of fluke called *Schistosoma*. The intermediate host is a fresh-water snail. Man, the definitive host, contracts the disorder from contact with water contaminated with immature forms of the parasite called **cercariae**. These enter the human body by penetrating the skin or the mucous membrane of the mouth. The adult worms live in the portal venous system but, according to the type of infestation, the females deposit their eggs in the walls of the host's urinary bladder—causing inflammation and haematuria—or in the wall of the bowel, causing inflammation and bleeding from the rectum. Chronic infestation may lead eventually to the development of carcinoma of the bladder or rectum.

In some cases of schistosomiasis, calcification in the bladder wall is demonstrable on plain radiographs. Other bladder changes and evidence of complicating carcinoma may be demonstrable by contrast urography.

Other infestations with flukes—these include infestations with *liver flukes* (*Fasciola hepatica* and *Clonorchis sinensis*, the Chinese liver fluke), and **paragonimiasis** due to *lung flukes*.

NUTRITIONAL DISORDERS

Nutritional disorders may be due to (i) inadequate food consumption resulting in various degrees of **starvation**, (ii) excessive food consumption resulting in pathological degrees of **obesity**, a condition in which there is excessive deposition of fat within the body, (iii) deficiency of essential food constituents; or defective absorption (e.g. as in malabsorption syndromes) or utilisation of these essential food constituents by the body. This latter disorders are often referred to as **deficiency diseases** and include conditions resulting from deficiencies of protein, minerals, and vitamins.

As discussed by Truswell (1) the most important dietary deficiency disease in the world is **protein-energy (calorie) malnutrition (PEM)**, a condition of high incidence among children in developing countries. This author describes the clinical disorders of **nutritional marasmus**, **kwashiorkor**, **marasmic kwashiorkor** as manifestations of PEM and also the adaptation of some children to PEM by **nutritional dwarfism**.

The term marasmus means wasting.

A common example of a nutritional disease due to mineral deficiency is **iron deficiency anaemia**.

Some examples of clinical disorders due to deficiency of the essential accessory food factors called vitamins are as follows:

Type of Vitamin Deficiency	*Principal Clinical Disorders*
Vitamin A (retinol–fat soluble)	Night blindness
Vitamin B complex (water soluble)	Xerophthalmia (an eye disease)
(i) Vitamin B1 (thiamin, aneurin)	Wet beri-beri (chief feature—heart disease with oedema)

Type of Vitamin Deficiency	*Principal Clinical Disorders*
	Dry beri-beri (chief feature —polyneuritis)
(ii) Vitamin B2 (riboflavine)	Vascularisation of the cornea Angular stomatitis
(iii) Nicotinic Acid	Pellagra
(iv) Vitamin B12 (cyanaco-balamin)	Pernicious anaemia (see p 208) Subacute combined degeneration of the cord (see p 287)
(v) Folic Acid	Megaloblastic anaemia (see p 209)
Vitamin C (ascorbic acid–water soluble)	Scurvy (see p 253)
Vitamin D (fat soluble)	Rickets (see p 254) Dietetic osteomalacia (see p 254)
Vitamin K (fat soluble)	Dietetic osteomalacia (see p 000) Hypoprothrombinaemia (resulting in diminished coagulability of the blood)

Note: It is important to note that several types of vitamin deficiency may occur together in the same patient.

REFERENCE

(1) Truswell, A. S. (1984). *Davidson's Principles and Practice of Medicine* (Macleod, J., ed.) 14th Edn. Edinburgh: Churchill Livingstone.

POISONING

The term **poisoning** describes a condition in which tissue damage, sometimes resulting in a fatal outcome, is caused by the entry into the body of a variety of harmful solid, liquid or gaseous substances termed **poisons**. Poisoning may be accidental or the result of attempted suicide or homicide.

The commonest type of poisoning is **food poisoning** which is due to eating food contaminated by certain types of infective bacteria and is evidenced by symptoms of gastritis or gastroenteritis.

Self-poisoning with drugs is nowadays unfortunately very common, Aspirin, paracetamol, hypnotic and antidepressant preparations, and barbiturates are frequently used in attempted self-poisoning.

In the two former instances levels of salicylates or of paracetamol in the blood may be measured, thus affording a valuable guide to treatment and prognosis.

Some other well-known forms of poisoning include those due to

carbon monoxide (coal gas); drugs such as **opium; arsenical** and **lead poisoning; corrosive poisoning** (e.g. due to lysol and phenol); **snakebite poisoning; alcoholic poisoning; strychnine poisoning; hydrocyanic acid (prussic acid) poisoning**; poisoning from **paraquat** (used as a weedkiller) and **parathion** (used as a pesticide).

The branch of science concerned with the study of poisons is called **toxicology**.

DISORDERS DUE TO PHYSICAL AGENTS

These disorders include the following.

Disorders due to heat, e.g. **heatstroke**—a condition in which hyperpyrexia develops as a result of failure of the normal mechanisms of body temperature control; and **heat exhaustion**—a condition of severe weakness, leading sometimes to circulatory collapse, and often associated with salt (sodium chloride) deficiency in the blood plasma.

Disorders due to cold, e.g. **frostbite**—a condition due to exposure of the extremities to severe cold with resultant diminution of blood supply and development of gangrene in severe cases; and **hypothermia** a condition of general lowering of body temperature which may occur when heat loss by the body exceeds heat production. (*Note:* the use of artificial hypothermia with general anaesthesia was noted when discussing surgical operations on the heart in Part IV.)

Disorders due to abnormal atmospheric pressures, e.g. **altitude sickness** experienced at high altitudes as a result of oxygen deficiency; and **caisson disease**, a disorder which occurs in those who work under high atmospheric pressure (e.g. divers) when subjected to too rapid decompression, during the return to normal atmospheric conditions.

RADIATION HAZARDS AND RADIATION INJURY

As is widely known, radiation of the type known as ionising radiation (see p 318) can, in high doses, cause damage to the tissues of the body. Such radiation in lower doses can cause changes in transmissible hereditary material contained in **genes** (units of hereditary material).

Two different types of hazard are thus associated with the use of man made ionising radiation in medicine, industry or warfare: the risk of causing **somatic damage**, i.e. damage to the tissues of an irradiated individual; and the risk of causing **genetic damage**, i.e. damage to hereditary material contained within the genes of an irradiated individual.

Somatic damage—*serious somatic damage is produced only by high amounts of radiation* but may develop as a result of the tissues receiving such amounts in a short period of time, or the cumulative effect of numerous small doses of radiation, producing a high total dosage over a lengthy period (e.g. after many years).

When tissue damage occurs it varies greatly in severity according to the amount and penetrating power of the causal radiation, and the extent and site of the irradiated area. Thus radiation injuries vary from slight reactions, which affect only a localised area of skin, to the extensive tissue damage that results from high doses of whole-body radiation.

While any tissue in the body may be injured by excessive exposure, ionising radiation tends to produce its effects mainly in certain radiosensitive tissues where cell multiplication is most active, i.e. in the lymphatic system and bone marrow, gastrointestinal tract, skin, gonads (testes and ovaries); and, in early fetal life, the central nervous system. Thus, radiation injury may be evidenced by effects such as: lowered white and red blood cell and platelet counts and resultant clinical features of agranulocytosis and anaemia; inflammatory changes in the skin referred to as **radiation dermatitis**; severe skin damage, manifested by **radiation burns**; inflammatory changes in the gastrointestinal tract, producing nausea, vomiting and diarrhoea; and impaired fertility.

Illnesses due to the more immediate effects of somatic damage may be referred to as **acute radiation syndrome** or, in general, as **radiation sickness**, particularly when manifested by signs and symptoms of gastrointestinal disorder.

Late effects of radiation injury include the development of leukaemia and also sometimes the growth of malignant tumours (e.g. skin carcinomas) in areas of tissue damage.

In view of the high doses of radiation which must often be employed in the radiotherapy of malignant neoplasms, and the small differences that may exist between an adequate treatment dose and the amount of radiation that will damage normal tissue cells in the vicinity of the treatment area, some minor damage to normal tissues may be inevitable in patients undergoing radiotherapy. A correct application of modern methods of protection against ionising radiations will, however, obviate somatic hazards to patients undergoing diagnostic radiological investigations and to staff working in diagnostic X-ray and radiotherapy departments.

Genetic damage—as noted above, this type of radiation injury may be produced by doses of radiation lower than those required to produce somatic damage.

Genetic damage results in alterations in genes known as **mutations**. Mutations occurring in genes in reproductive cells of an individual will be transmitted to his or her offspring. The production of mutations within the reproductive cells of large numbers of individuals carries the risk of causing the appearance of undesirable inherited defects after several generations. This potential hazard makes it important that when any person of, or below, childbearing age is exposed to ionising radiation, in the course of medical investigation or treatment or as a result of his or her occupation, irradiation of the gonads should be avoided or limited to such an extent as is practicable.

Measures for protection of patients and staff against hazards arising from the use of ionising radiation in medical and dental practice are set out in the 'Code of Practice fo the Protection against Ionising Radiations arising from Medical and Dental Use' (HM Stationery Office, 1972). It is to be noted, however, that this code of practice is soon to be replaced by the Ionising Regulations which, unlike the 1972 code will carry the force of law. The new regulations will be supported by Approved Codes of Practice and Guidance Notes.

(Note: Ionising radiations are so-called because, when they pass through matter, they cause a process called **ionisation** whereby neutral atoms acquire a temporary electric charge.

These forms of radiation consist of *electromagnetic radiation*—X-rays and gamma rays (γ-rays) and *corpuscular radiation*—alpha particles (α-particles), beta particles (β-particles), neutrons and protons.

X-rays are electromagnetic waves of short-wave length produced in X-ray tubes, by bombarding a heavy metal target with fast-moving electrons.

Atoms are composed of a central nucleus, around which revolve negatively-charged particles called *electrons*. The central nucleus contains particles called *protons*, which are positively charged, and *neutrons* which have no charge. Atomic nuclei which contain high numbers of neutrons relative to protons are unstable and disintegrate forming stable nuclei of simpler elements.

Beta-particles (β-particles) which are fast-moving electrons; *alpha-particles* (α-particles) which are the nuclei of helium atoms; and *gamma-rays* (γ-rays) which are electromagnetic waves of very short wave-length, are all forms of radiation which may be emitted when the nuclei of atoms undergo disintegration.

The spontaneous emission of ionising radiation which accompanies nuclear disintegration is termed *radioactivity*. This property is possessed by a few naturally occurring elements which have unstable nuclei (e.g. radium) and by some man–made isotopes. *Isotopes* are differing forms of the same element, all of which have identical chemical properties and the same atomic number, but possess different atomic weights. Some isotopes have unstable nuclei which disintegrate with the emission of ionising radiation, and these are thus known as *radionuclides* or *radioactive isotopes*; or more simply as *radioisotopes*.)

DISEASES OF GENETIC ORIGIN

Genes are units of hereditary material. They are of particulate nature and are composed of the chemical compound called deoxyribonucleic acid (DNA).

Genes are carried on chromosomes in precisely determined positions, and are normally transmitted from one generation to another without undergoing any substantial change. As a result of circumstances, for the most part unknown, a gene may undergo a transmissible change. Such a gene may then be termed a **mutant gene**; the change being referred to in genetic science as a **mutation**.

All cell nuclei possess *chromosomes* (a name meaning coloured bodies and referring to their staining reactions with certain dyes used in cytology). They are arranged in pairs, numbered downwards in accordance with their size, the number varying in different species.

In the human body all the cells, other than germ cells (sperms and ova), possess 46 chromosomes; 44 of these are of identical type and are called *autosomes*; the other two are *sex chromosomes*. In females there are two identical *X-chromosomes*, while males possess one *X-chromosome* and one *Y-chromosome*.

The process whereby the normal number of chromosomes is halved during the development of male and female germ cells is called **meiosis**. Each germ cell possesses 22 *autosomes* and one *sex chromosome*.

Changes in genetic material may occur as a result of mutations or of numerical or structural abnormalities of the chromosomes, in which such material is carried, and give rise to clinical disorders which are of wholly genetic origin. Clinical disorders may also be of partially genetic origin when both genetic and environmental factors both appear to operate in their causation.

Emery (1), who gives a detailed and interesting account of genetic factors in disease, refers to these disorders as **unifactorial**—due to single gene defects, **chromosomal disorders**, and **multifactorial disorders** —due partially to genetic factors and partially to environmental factors.

A few examples of these three types of genetic disease are as follows.

Unifactorial disorders—(i) **haemophilia**, which is described as an X-linked recessive inherited disease because the responsible gene is carried on the X-sex chromosome; (ii) **achondroplasia**—an autosomal dominant inherited disease; (iii) **Duchenne muscular dystrophy**, an X-linked recessive disorder.

Chromosomal disorders—(i) **Down's syndrome** (formerly also called mongolism) in which chromosome 21, instead of being paired, is triplicated and an affected individual therefore has an extra chromosome. Such an abnormality is termed **trisomy**; (ii) **Turner's syndrome** (ovarian dysgenesis) in which only one X-chromosome is present and the chromosomes total 45, a condition known as **monosomy**; (iii) **Klinefelter's syndrome**, a disorder of males in which there are one or more extra X-chromosomes, or sometimes also an extra Y-chromosome.

Multifactorial disorders—congenital heart disease and various other congenital diseases and malformations, schizophrenia, essential hypertension, some types of diabetes and epilepsy, some types of cancer.

Antenatal diagnosis by chromosome analysis of fetal cells present in amniotic fluid and by biochemical tests on such fluids (e.g. measurement of alphafetoprotein in amniotic fluid and also in maternal serum) is possible in some types of disorder.

In genetic medicine an important preventive measure is **genetic counselling** for those considered to be at risk in producing children affected by genetic disease.

REFERENCE

(1) Emery, A. E. H. (1984). *Davidson's Principles and Practice of Medicine* (Macleod, J., ed.) 14th Edn. Edinburgh: Churchill Livingstone.

Appendix

Standard works and journals consulted by the author

Anatomy and Physiology

McNaught, A. B. (1983). *Companion to 'Illustrated Physiology'*. Edinburgh: Churchill Livingstone.

Pearce, E. (1980). *Anatomy and Physiology for Nurses*. London: Faber and Faber.

Warwick, R. (1961). *Whillis's Elementary Anatomy and Physiology*. London: Churchill.

Warwick, R., Williams, P. L. (eds.). (1973). *Gray's Anatomy*, 36th Edn. Edinburgh: Churchill Livingstone.

Medicine (including Dermatology, Gastroenterology, Genetics, Neurology, Paediatrics and Psychological Medicine)

Altschul, A. (1977). *Aids to Psychiatric Nursing*. London: Baillière Tindall.

Brimblecombe, F., Barltrop, D. (1978). *Children in Health and Disease*. London: Baillière Tindall.

Carter, C. O. (1977). *Human Heredity*. Harmondsworth, Mdx: Penguin Books.

Forster, F. M. (1966). *Synopsis of Neurology*. St. Louis, Missouri: Mosby.

Harrison, R. J. (1980). *Textbook of Medicine*. London: Hodder and Stoughton.

Houston, J. C., Joiner, C. L., Trounce, J. A. (1982). *A Short Textbook of Medicine*. London: Hodder and Stoughton.

Hutton, J. H. (1966). *Practical Endocrinology*. Springfield, Illinois: Thomas.

Macleod, J., (ed.). (1984). *Davidson's Principles and Practice of Medicine* Edinburgh: Churchill Livingstone.

Mann, W. N., Lessof, M. H., (eds). (1975). *Conybeare's Textbook of Medicine*. Edinburgh: Churchill Livingstone.

Meadow, S. R., Smithells, R. W. (1981). *Lecture Notes on Paediatrics*. Oxford: Blackwell.

Oswald, N. C., Fry, J. (1962). *Diseases of the Respiratory System*. Oxford: Blackwell.

Percival, G. H. (1967). *An Introduction to Dermatology*. Edinburgh: Livingstone.

Read, A. E. A. (1981). *Basic Gastroenterology*. Bristol: Wright.

Richardson, J. (ed.). (1960). *The Practice of Medicine*. London: Churchill.

Rodger, T. F., Ingram, I. M., Timbury, G. C., Mowbray, R. M. (1967). *Lecture Notes on Psychological Medicine*. Edinburgh: Churchill Livingstone.

Sneddon, I. B., Church, R. E. (1976). *Practical Dermatology*. London: Arnold.

Obstetrics and Gynaecology

Barnes, J. (1983). *Lecture Notes on Gynaecology*. Oxford: Blackwell.

Clayton, S. G., Lewis, T. L. T., Pinker, G. (eds). (1980). *Gynaecology by Ten Teachers*. London: Arnold.

Clayton, S. G., Lewis, T. L. T., Pinker, G. (eds). (1980). *Obstetrics by Ten Teachers*. London: Arnold.

Clayton, S. G., Newton, J. R. (1983). *A Pocket Gynaecology*. Edinburgh: Churchill Livingstone.

Clayton, S. G., Newton, J. R. (1983). *A Pocket Obstetrics*. Edinburgh: Churchill Livingstone.

Phillip, E. E. (1970). *Obstetrics and Gynaecology*. London: Lewis.

Pathology (including General Pathology, Biochemistry, Haematology and Microbiology)

Boyd, W. A., Sheldon, H. (1980). *An Introduction to the Study of Disease*. Philadelphia: Lea and Febiger.

Boyd, W. A. (1970). *A Textbook of Pathology*. Philadelphia: Lea and Febiger.

Dible, J. H. (1950). *Dible and Davie's Pathology*. London: Churchill.

Gibson, J. M. (1979). *Modern Microbiology and Pathology for Nurses*. Oxford: Blackwell.

Gillies, R. R. (1978). *Lecture Notes on Medical Microbiology*. Oxford: Blackwell.

Govan, A. D. T., Macfarlane, P. S., Callander, R. (1981). *Pathology Illustrated*. Edinburgh: Churchill Livingstone.

Montgomery, R., Dryer, R. L., Conway, R. W., Spector, A. A. (1980). *Biochemistry*. Saint Louis, Missouri: Mosby.

Thompson, R. B. (1979). *A Short Textbook of Haematology*. London: Pitman.

Thomson, A. D., Cotton, R. E. (1983). *Lecture Notes on Pathology*. Oxford: Blackwell.

Turk, D. C., Porter, I. A., Duerdon, B., Reid, T. M. S. (1983). *A Short Textbook of Medical Microbiology*. London: Hodder and Stoughton.

Pharmacology

Dale, J. R., Appelbe, G. E. (1979). *Pharmacy Law and Ethics*. London: Pharmaceutical Press.

Sears, W. G., Winwood, R. S. (1980). *Materia Medica for Nurses*. London: Arnold.

Radiology and Medical Imaging (including Diagnostic Radiology, Radiotherapy and Oncology, Nuclear Medicine and Ultrasound)

Barnes, P. A., Rees, D. J. (1972). *A Concise Textbook of Radiotherapy*. London: Faber and Faber.

Caffey, J. (1978). *Paediatric X-Ray Diagnosis*. Chicago: The Year Book Medical Publishers.

Capra, L. G. (1972). *The Care of the Cancer Patient*. London: Heinemann.

Chesney, D. N., Chesney, M. O. (1978). *Care of the Patient in Diagnostic Radiography*. Oxford: Blackwell.

Du Boulay, G. H. (1980). *Principles of X-Ray Diagnosis of the Skull*. London: Butterworths.

Emmett, J. L. (1971). *Clinical Urography*. Philadelphia: Saunders.

Gershon-Cohen, J. (1970). *Atlas of Mammography*. Berlin: Springer-Verlag.

Goldberg, B. B., Wells, P. N. T. (1983). *Ultrasonics in Clinical Diagnosis*. Edinburgh: Churchill Livingstone.

Hancock, B. W., Bradshaw, J. D. (1981). *Lecture Notes on Clinical Oncology*. Oxford: Blackwell.

Jefferson, K., Rees, S. (1980). *Clinical Cardiac Radiology*. London: Butterworths.

Kreel, L. (ed.). (1979). *Medical Imaging*. Aylesbury, Bucks: H. M. & M. Publishers.

Lodge, T. (1955). *Recent Advances in Radiology*. 3rd edn. London: Churchill.

Lodge, T. (1964). *Recent Advances in Radiology*. 4th edn. London: Churchill.

Lodge, T., Steiner, R. E. (eds). (1964). *Recent Advances in Radiology*. 5th edn. Edinburgh: Churchill Livingstone.

Meire, H. B., Farrant, B. (1982). *Basic Clinical Ultrasound*. London: British Institute of Radiology Teaching, Series 4.

McLaren, J. W. (ed.). (1960 & 1970). *Modern Trends in Radiology*. London: Butterworths.

Middlemiss, H. (1961). *Tropical Radiology*. London: Heinemann.

Pugh, D. G. (1951). *Roentgenologic Diagnosis of Diseases of Bone*. Baltimore: Wilkins and Wilkins.

Saxton, H. M., Strickland, B. (1972). *Practical Procedures in Diagnostic Radiology*. London: Lewis.

Shanks, S. C., Kerley, P. (eds). *A Textbook of X-Ray Diagnosis*, 4th edn. (Vol. I, 1969; Vol. II, 1972; Vol. III, 1973; Vol. IV, 1969; Vol. V, 1970; Vol. VI, 1971). London: Lewis.

Steiner, R. E. (ed.). (1983). *Recent Advances in Radiology and Medical Imaging* – 7. Edinburgh: Churchill Livingstone.

Sutton, D. (ed.). (1980). *Textbook of Radiology and Imaging*. Edinburgh: Churchill Davidson.

Wagner, H. N. (ed.). (1975). *Principles of Nuclear Medicine*. Philadelphia: Saunders.

Surgery (including Ophthalmology, Orthopaedics, Otorhinolaryngology andUrology)

Adams, J. C. (1981). *Outline of Orthopaedics*. Edinburgh: Churchill Livingstone.

Blandy, J. (ed.). (1976). *Urology*. Oxford: Blackwell.

Foxen, E. H. M. (1980). *Lecture Notes on Diseases of the Ear, Nose and Throat*. Oxford: Blackwell.

Illingworth, C. (1972). *A Short Textbook of Surgery*. Edinburgh: Churchill Livingstone.

Martin-Doyle, J. L. C., Kemp, M. H. (1975). *A Synopsis of Ophthalmology*. Bristol: Wright.

Miller, A., Slade, N., Leather, H. M. (1966). *A Synopsis of Renal Diseases and Urology*. Bristol: Wright.

Newsam, J. E., Petrie, J. J. B. (1981). *Urology and Renal Medicine*. Edinburgh: Churchill Livingstone.

Pracy,R., Siegler, J., Stell, P. M. (1974). *A Short Textbook. Ear, Nose and Throat*. London: English Universities Press.

Rains, A. J. H., Ritchie, H. D. (1981). *Bailey and Love's Short Practice of Surgery*. London: Lewis.

Reading, P. (1966). *Common Diseases of the Ear, Nose and Throat*. London: Churchill.

Robinson, J. O., Brown, A. (1980). *Surgery*. London: Heinemann.

Taylor, S., Cotton, L. (1982). *A Short Textbook of Surgery*. London: Hodder and Stoughton.

Wiles, P., Sweetman, R. (1965). *Essentials of Orthopaedics*. London: Churchill.

Terminology

Lennox, B. (1980). *Ffrangcon Roberts' Medical Terms*. London: Heinemann.

Journals

British Medical Journal. London: British Medical Association.
British Journal of Radiology. London: British Institute of Radiology.
Clinical Radiology. London: Royal College of Radiologists.
RAD. Harlow, Essex: Kingsmoor Publications.

Glossary

Some prefixes and suffixes, and other components of medical words

List of some important abbreviations which are used in medical notes

TABLE 1

Usage of some general prefixes, suffixes and other word components in medicine

This table shows some of the ways in which some prefixes and suffixes and other components of a general nature are used in medical words. The common usages given here may sometimes differ from the original literal meanings.

Components of words referring to the organs and tissues of the body are not included in Table 1 (pp 327–330), but the meanings of certain of these are indicated in Table 2 of this appendix.

Prefix, suffix or other component	Senses in which commonly used	Examples
a-	absence of	*aplasia*, absence of growth.
ab-	away from	*abduct*, move away from the median plane.
ad-	towards	*adduct*, move towards the median plane.
an-	absence of	*anaesthesia*, absence of sensation.
andr-	male	*androgens*, male hormones.
ante-	before, forward	*antenatal*, before birth.
anti-	opposed to	*antihistamine*, a drug acting in opposition to histamine.
auto-	self	*autograft*—a graft taken from one part of the body and implanted elsewhere in the body of the same individual.
baro-	pressure	*barotrauma*—injury due to pressure.
bi-	two	*bilateral*—on both sides.
bio-	life	*biopsy*—visual examination (usually microscopic) of tissue from a living subject.

Prefix, suffix or other component	Senses in which commonly used	Examples
calc-	calcium	*calcification*—deposition of calcium salts in the tissues.
circum-	around	*circumduct*, move in a circle.
con-	together with	*congenital*, together with (i.e. present at) birth.
cryo-	cold	*cryosurgery*, involving use of severe cold for tissue destruction.
crypto-	hidden, concealed	*cryptorchidism*, in which an undescended testis is concealed within the abdomen or inguinal canal.
dys-	difficult, disordered	*dysplasia*, disordered growth.
e-	out	*evert*, turn outwards.
-ectomy-	cutting out, removal	*splenectomy*, removal of the spleen.
end-	inside, inner	*endothelium*, the inner lining of various body structures.
epi-	upon	*epidermis*, on the skin, hence the outer layer of skin.
eu-	good, normal	*euthyroid*, normal function of the thyroid gland.
extra-	outside	*extrauterine*, outside the uterus.
gen-	referring to production, birth or reproduction	*genitalia*, reproductive organs.
-genic	producing	*pathogenic*, disease producing.
-graphy	recording	*radiography*, recording by use of ionising radiation.
gyn-	female	*gynaecology*—study of diseases of women.
haem-	blood	*haemorrhage*—bleeding.
hemi-	half	*hemiplegia*, paralysis of half of the body.
hetero-	other, differing	*heterogenous*—of differing type.
homo-	same	*homograft*—a tissue graft from one individual member of a species to another of the same species.
hydro-	fluid	*hydrothorax*—fluid in the thorax.
hyper-	above, in excess of normal	*hypertrophy*—growth in excess of normal.
hypo-	beneath, less than normal	*hypodermic*, beneath the skin. *hypoplasia*, growth of a degree less than normal.
in-	in	*inverted*, turned inwards (also, upside down).
infra-	below	*infraclavicular*, below the clavicle.

Prefix, suffix or other component	Senses in which commonly used	Examples
inter-	between	*interlobar*, between lobes.
intra-	within	*intracranial*, within the cranium.
iso-	same	*isotopes*, differing forms of the same element, possessing the same chemical properties and the same atomic number (but differing atomic weights).
-itis	inflammation	*osteitis*—inflammation of bone.
macro-	large	*macroradiography*, direct enlargement radiography.
mal-	bad	*malunited*, badly united.
mega-	big	*megacolon*, enlarged colon.
men-	month	*menopause*, cessation of the monthly periods.
micro-	small	*microcephalic*, having a small head.
multi-	many	*multicentric*, in many centres.
myco-, *myceto-*	fungus	*mycoses*, fungus diseases.
-myces	fungus	*Actinomyces*, a genus of fungi.
-natal	birth	*neonatal*, newly born.
-neo-	new	*neoplasm*, new growth.
normo-	normal	*normocyte*, a normal red blood cell particularly as regards size.
-oid	like	*osteoid*, like bone.
-ology	science	*radiology*—the science of radiation, esp. referring to medical use of ionising radiation.
-oma	tumour	*osteoma*, tumour of bone.
-ortho	straight, normal, upright	*orthopaedics*, a branch of surgery concerned with the correction of skeletal deformities.
-orrhoea	flow, discharge	*otorrhoea*, a discharge from the ear.
-osis	a condition of, or to indicate a degenerative disorder	*diverticulosis*—a condition or having diverticula. *spondylosis*—a degenerative spinal disorder.
-ostomy	making an opening into	*cholecystostomy*—making an opening into the gall bladder and inserting a tube for drainage.
-otomy	cutting into or through	*osteotomy*—cutting through a bone.
pan-	all	*pansinusitis*—inflammation of all the sinuses.
para-	beside, close to	*paramedian*, close to the midline.
-pathy	disease	*encephalopathy*, disease of the brain.

Prefix, suffix or other component	Senses in which commonly used	Examples
per-	through	*pertrochanteric*, through the femoral trochanters.
peri-	around	*periapical*, around the apex of a tooth root.
pneumo- } *pneumato-* }	air (or other gas)	*pneumoperitoneum*—air in the peritoneal cavity. *pneumaturia*—gas in the urine.
-pnoea	breath	*dyspnoea*, difficulty in breathing.
poly-	many	*polyarthritis,* simultaneous inflammation of many joints.
post-	after	*postnatal*, after birth.
pre-	before	*precancer*, a condition which is a forerunner of cancer.
pro-	before, in front	*prothrombin*, a precursor of thrombin, a substance concerned in the clotting of the blood.
pseudo-	false	*pseudoangina*, a condition simulating angina.
psych-	mind	*psychogenic*—produced in the mind.
py-	pus	*pyuria*, pus in the urine.
quadri-	four	*quadriplegia*—paralysis of all four limbs.
radio-	radiation	*radioactive*, emitting ionising radiation.
retro-	behind, backward	*retrosternal*—behind the sternum.
sub-	below	*subnormal*, below normal.
supra-	above	*supracondylar*, above the condyles.
syn-	with, union	*synthesis*, the artificial joining together of substances to form a new chemical compound.
tox-	poison	*toxin*, a poisonous substance.
tri-	three	*tri-iodide*, a compound with three iodine atoms in its molecule.
ultra-	beyond	*ultrasonics*, sound vibrations beyond the audible range.
uni-	one	*unilateral,* on one side.
-uria	urine	*albuminuria*, albumen in the urine.

TABLE 2

Some Components of Words Referring to Body Structures

Component	Pertaining to
aden-	gland(s).
angi-	vessel(s) (esp. blood vessel).
arthr-	joint(s).
aur-	ear(s).
cardi-	heart, or cardiac orifice of the stomach.
caud-	tail, hence the lower part of the human body.
cephal-	head.
cheilo-	lips.
cholangi-	bile ducts.
chole-	biliary system.
cholecyst-	gall bladder.
choledoch-	common bile duct.
chondr-	cartilage.
col-	colon.
cyst-	bladder (esp. urinary bladder).
dactyl-	digit(s), esp. finger(s).
derm-	skin.
encephal-	brain.
enter-	intestine.
epiphysi-	epiphysis(es).
fibro-	fibrous connective tissue.
gastr-	stomach.
gloss-	tongue.
hepat-	liver.
hyster-	uterus.
labio-	lips.
lien-	spleen.
lymphangi-	lymph vessels.
lymph-	lymphatic system.
mamm-, mast-	breast(s).
myel-	bone marrow or spinal cord.
myo-	muscle(s).
nephr-	kidney(s).
ocul-	eye(s).
onych-	nails.
ophthalm-	eye(s).
orchi-, orchid-	testis(es).
or-	mouth.
oste-	bone(s).
ot-	ear(s).
phleb-	vein(s).
pneumon-	lung(s).
port-	portal vein.

Component	Pertaining to
proct-	rectum.
pyel-	kidney pelvis(es).
pyle-	portal vein.
ren-	kidney(s).
rhin-	nose.
salping-	uterine tube(s).
sial-	salivary gland(s).
spondyl-	vertebra(ae).
stomato-	mouth.
vesic-	urinary bladder.

Some Important Abbreviations

AID	artificial insemination-donor.	*D & V*	diarrhoea and vomiting.
AIDS	Acquired immune deficiency syndrome.	*DVT*	deep vein thrombosis.
APH	antepartum haemorrhage.	*DXRT*	deep X-ray therapy.
APM	anterior poliomyelitis.	*ECG*	electrocardiography.
ASD	atrial septal defect.	*ECT*	electroconvulsive therapy.
bd	twice per day.	*EDD*	expected date of delivery (childbirth).
BI	bony injury.	*EEG*	electroencephalography.
BMR	basal metabolic rate.	*ENT*	ear, nose and throat.
BP	blood pressure, British Pharmacopoeia.	*ERCP*	endoscopic retrograde cholangiopancreato-graphy.
BSR	basal sedimentation rate.	*ESR*	erythrocyte sedimentation rate.
CIN	cervical intraepithelial neoplasia.	*EUA*	examination under anaesthesia.
CDH	congenital dislocation of the hip joint.	*FB*	foreign body.
CSF	cerebrosponal fluid.	*FDIU*	fetal death in-utero.
CNS	central nervous system.	*GI*	gastrointestinal.
CSOM	chronic suppurative otitis media.	*GU*	gastric ulcer, genitourinary.
CT	computerised tomography.	*Hb*	haemoglobin.
CVP	central venous pressure.	*HRT*	hormone replacement therapy.
CVS	cardiovascular system.	*HV*	hallux valgus.
D & C	uterine dilation and curettage.	*ICP*	intracranial pressure.
DLE	disseminated lupus erythematosus.	*IDK*	internal derangement of the knee joint.
DS	disseminated sclerosis.	*IM*	intramuscular.
DU	duodenal ulcer.	*Ig*	immunoglobulin.
		IOFB	intraocular foreign body.

ISQ	in status quo, i.e. unchanged.	PV	by (through) the vagina.
		RA	rheumatoid arthtiris.
IPPR	intermittent positive pressure respiration.	RBC	red blood cells.
		RDS	respiratory distress syndrome.
IPPV	intermittent positive pressure ventilation.	RE	rectal examination.
IUCD	intrauterine contraceptive device.	Rh	rhesus factor.
		RT	radiotherapy.
IUD	intrauterine death (or intrauterine contraceptive device).	Ski	skiagraph, i.e. a radiograph.
		SMR	submucous resection of nasal septum.
IV	intravenous.		
KUB	kidneys, ureter and bladder.	SOB	shortness of breath.
		SOL	space-occupying lesion.
LB	loose body.	SOS	if necessary.
MI	myocardial infarct, mitral incompetence.	TABC	vaccine against typhoid and paratyphoid A, B & C fevers.
MPV	metatarsus primus varus.		
MS	mitral stenosis, multiple sclerosis.	TB	tuberculosis or tubercle bacilli.
NAD	no abnormality demonstrated.	tds	three times per day.
		THR	total hip replacement.
NAI	non-accidental injury.	TPR	temperature, pulse and respiration.
NG	new growth.		
NYD	not yet diagnosed.	Ts and As	tonsils and adenoids.
OA	osteoarthritis.	TUR	transurethral resection of prostate.
OT	occupational therapy.		
PCM	protein-calorie malnutrition.	UG	urogenital.
		UTI	urinary tract infection.
PE	pulmonary embolism.	VD	venereal disease.
PID	prolapsed intevertebral disc.	VE	vaginal examination.
		VSD	ventricular septal defect.
PM	post mortem.	VVs	varicose veins.
POP	plaster of Paris.	WBC	white blood cells.
PPH	postpartum haemorrhage.	WR	Wassermann reaction.
PR	by (through) the rectum.	XR	X-ray.
PU	peptic ulcer.		
PUO	pyrexia of unknown origin.		

Index